A Comprehensive Overview of Telemedicine

Edited by Charles R. Doarn and Thomas F. Heston

Published in London, United Kingdom

A Comprehensive Overview of Telemedicine
http://dx.doi.org/10.5772/10.5772/intechopen.1002138
Edited by Charles R. Doarn and Thomas F. Heston

Contributors
Abhishek Jahagirdar, Alozie Emeonye, Amleset Kelati, Anik Debrot, Arimi Fitri Mat Ludin, Christine Goodchild, Daniela Sgroi, Digvijaysinh Parmar, Elizabeth Kagotho, Florence Nkwogu, Francesca Cioffi, Francesca Milito, Gregor Donaj, Hadassah Drukarch, Hannu Tenhunen, Jitesh V. Pimpale, Joseph Okeibunor, Joy Hanoun, Juan Vito-Antonio Held, Juha Plosila, Kamal El-Badawi, Katina Lang-Lindsey, Laurent Berthoud, Liliane Efinger, Mariana Orduz-Robledo, Marina Cerbo, Maya Kheyar, Michael John, Michael Wagner, Mirjam Sepesy Maučec, Muhuntha Sri-Ganeshan, Mónica P. Novoa-Candia, Nele Sassor, Peter Cameron, Rabih Hajj, Radhika Thakkar, Reabal Najjar, Robin Wicki, Serena Salvatore, Shivani Karre, Simon Onsongo, Suad J. Ghaben, Sunaina Swatantramath, Sunny Ibeneme, Thomas F. Heston, Tiziana Chiriaco, Valentino Pomini, Valeria Vela-Lopez, Vikranth Ravipati

First published in London, United Kingdom, 2024 by IntechOpen
IntechOpen is the global imprint of INTECHOPEN LIMITED, registered in England and Wales, registration number: 11086078, 167-169 Great Portland Street, London, W1W 5PF, United Kingdom

British Library Cataloguing-in-Publication Data
A catalogue record for this book is available from the British Library

Additional hard and PDF copies can be obtained from orders@intechopen.com

A Comprehensive Overview of Telemedicine
Edited by Charles R. Doarn and Thomas F. Heston
p. cm.

This title is part of the Biomedical Engineering Book Series, Volume 26
Topic: Bioinformatics and Medical Informatics
Series Editor: Robert Koprowski
Topic Editor: Slawomir Wilczynski

Print ISBN 978-0-85466-797-0
Online ISBN 978-0-85466-796-3
eBook (PDF) ISBN 978-0-85466-798-7
ISSN 2631-5343

For EU product safety concerns :
IN TECH d . o . o . , Prolaz Marije Krucifikse Kozulić 3 , 51000 Rijeka , Croatia ,
info@intechopen . com or visit our website at intechopen . com .

IntechOpen Book Series

Biomedical Engineering

Volume 26

Aims and Scope of the Series

Biomedical Engineering is one of the fastest-growing interdisciplinary branches of science and industry. The combination of electronics and computer science with biology and medicine has improved patient diagnosis, reduced rehabilitation time, and helped to facilitate a better quality of life. Nowadays, all medical imaging devices, medical instruments, or new laboratory techniques result from the cooperation of specialists in various fields. The series of Biomedical Engineering books covers such areas of knowledge as chemistry, physics, electronics, medicine, and biology. This series is intended for doctors, engineers, and scientists involved in biomedical engineering or those wanting to start working in this field.

Meet the Series Editor

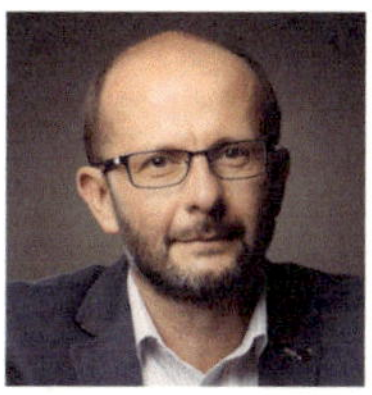

Robert Koprowski, MD (1997), Ph.D. (2003), Habilitation (2015), is an employee of the University of Silesia, Poland, Institute of Computer Science, Department of Biomedical Computer Systems. For 20 years, he has studied the analysis and processing of biomedical images, emphasizing the full automation of measurement for a large inter-individual variability of patients. Dr. Koprowski has authored more than a hundred research papers with dozens in impact factor (IF) journals and has authored or co-authored six books. Additionally, he is the author of several national and international patents in the field of biomedical devices and imaging. Since 2011, he has been a reviewer of grants and projects (including EU projects) in biomedical engineering.

Meet the Volume Editor

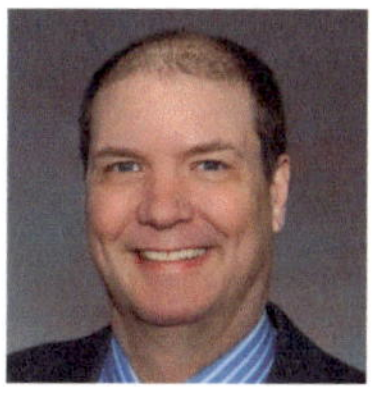

Thomas F. Heston, MD, is a board-certified physician with over 30 years of clinical experience, specializing in the integration of technology in healthcare. He holds faculty positions as clinical associate professor at Washington State University and clinical assistant professor at the University of Washington School of Medicine. A leader in telemedicine research, Dr. Heston's work spans artificial intelligence, blockchain technology, and digital health. He has published extensively on the adoption of telemedicine and innovations in digital healthcare. Board-certified in family medicine, nuclear medicine, and artificial intelligence in medicine, his multidisciplinary expertise uniquely positions him as a key voice in advancing telehealth. Dr. Heston's research continues to shape the future of digital health.

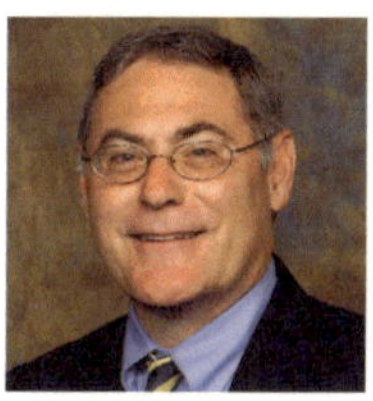

Charles Doarn is an emeritus professor in the College of Medicine, University of Cincinnati, and the director of the Armstrong Institute for Space, Technology and Research. For the past 33 years, he provided subject-matter expertise in aerospace medicine to NASA's chief health and medical officer and served as the co-chair of the Federal Telehealth Working Group for the U.S. government. He has worked with NATO, the Department of Defense, and the Department of State as a Fulbright specialist. Since 2005, he has served as the editor-in-chief of the Telemedicine and e-Health journal. He is a recognized leader in telemedicine and telehealth as a scholar and teacher, having published seven books; over 475 manuscripts, editorials, and federal reports; and more than 55 book chapters.

Contents

Preface

For more than a century, telemedicine has slowly emerged as a tool in the practice of medicine. The COVID-19 pandemic and the subsequent public health emergency accelerated its integration into everyday practice worldwide. While the pandemic was a catalyst, it was the development and evaluation of innovative technologies that have made it possible for a patient to be seen by their physician remotely. The breadth and scope of application are not limited to only a few clinical disciplines. It has been applied to literally all clinical needs. It also has been shown to be a significant tool in education. While the technology has continued its unabated march forward, the barriers to wider adoption are slowly being ameliorated. These include legislation, policy formulation, reimbursement, trust, and acceptance by providers and patients alike.

This book brings together a wide variety of authors from around the world. They present diverse thoughts on applications, research platforms, and clinical outcomes that can serve as another tool in our armamentarium for addressing patients' needs, increasing not only awareness but access as well. These 16 chapters provide unique perspectives on telemedicine at this point in time. This text will serve as a foundational instrument for all of those individuals interested in furthering their understanding of this field and how it can be beneficial to patients regardless of their location.

Telemedicine offers an approach that enables better access to healthcare and the needs of patients. The pages herein provide a ready reference for academics, clinical personnel, industrial innovators, and the lay public.

On behalf of all the authors, we hope you enjoy this text and find it useful in whatever stage you are in, whether a user or implementer.

Thomas F. Heston, MD, FAAFP
Washington State University School of Medicine,
Bellingham, Washington, USA

Charles R. Doarn, MBA, FATA, FAsMA
Armstrong Institute for Space, Technology, and Research,
Office of Research,
College of Medicine,
University of Cincinnati,
Cincinnati, Ohio, USA

Section 1

Telemedicine in Society

Chapter 1

Addressing True Health Disparities: The Imperative of Telehealth and Telemental Health Services for Rural Americans

Katina Lang-Lindsey

Abstract

This chapter explores the pressing issue of health disparities affecting rural Americans. It sheds light on the mortality rates associated with chronic conditions and behavioral health problems in these rural regions in the United States. The central focus revolves around identifying the underlying causes of these health disparities, encompassing limited knowledge about managing chronic diseases and behavioral health problems. These intertwined factors contribute significantly to the substantial health inequities experienced by rural residents. Furthermore, the chapter emphasizes the importance of introducing telehealth, telemental health services, and virtual visits as key options for closing the healthcare gap in rural areas. By embracing healthcare technology such as telemedicine, which includes virtual visits and telemental health treatments, rural areas can overcome distance barriers and ensure access to critical healthcare services and support. These tried-and-true strategies have the potential to close health disparities while also improving the overall health and quality of life for rural Americans living with chronic conditions. Additionally, the chapter explores the critical role of partnerships and paid apprenticeships in strengthening healthcare delivery and education in these underserved areas. This approach is instrumental in driving the broader objective of achieving health equity in rural regions across the United States.

Keywords: telemental health, disparities, chronic disease, rural, telehealth, mental health

1. Introduction

Rural residents in the United States face a wide range of health disparities compared to their urban counterparts, as highlighted in the CDC's report from 2023. According to the US Census Bureau, rural areas are home to over 46 million Americans, making up roughly 15% of the US population [1]. Particularly in southern rural areas, Americans are at a higher risk of premature death from the top five leading causes of death: heart disease, cancer, unintentional injury, chronic lower respiratory disease, and stroke [2]. These disparities in health outcomes can be attributed to various factors, including unhealthy lifestyle choices, limited access to healthcare services, and a lack of nutritious dietary options.

These challenges are further compounded by demographic factors such as advanced age, lower income levels, and reduced educational attainment, all associated with poorer health outcomes [3, 4]. In response to these healthcare disparities, the Centers for Disease Control and Prevention (CDC) have made it their mission to improve the well-being of rural populations.

Their approach involves accurate measurement and reporting of chronic diseases, comprehensive investigation of healthcare inequalities, and promoting programs like telehealth initiatives to reach and support these underserved communities [5]. The prevalence of chronic diseases in rural settings is exacerbated by distinct challenges, including geographical isolation, socioeconomic determinants, and a shortage of healthcare resources [6, 7]. These factors hinder timely diagnosis and effective management of chronic conditions, complicating the provision of long-term care for individuals with such health issues. This perpetuates the cycle of health disparities, leading to continued poor health outcomes and escalating healthcare costs [8].

This chapter's primary objective is to thoroughly examine the factors contributing to healthcare disparities in rural America. It will delve into the prevalence and consequences of chronic diseases, mental health needs, and the root causes of these disparities in the United States. Additionally, the chapter will examine the vital contributions of innovative solutions like telehealth and telemental health, alongside collaborative apprenticeship partnerships, in extending services to underserved rural communities. It will conclude with recommendations, highlighting these strategies as effective means for overcoming these areas' challenges.

2. Health disparities in rural America

Health disparities in the rural regions of the United States have been notably more pronounced than their urban counterparts. These areas grapple with significant challenges related to specific chronic diseases, including behavioral health issues such as alcohol and substance use disorders. The emergence of the COVID-19 pandemic has further exacerbated these disparities, emphasizing the crucial need for diverse, community-centered approaches in healthcare research [9]. Furthermore, it underscores the importance of allocating dedicated funding to support rural service agencies and populations, highlighting the pivotal need for innovations to meet these concerns.

Rural Americans, constituting 20% of the nation's population, equivalent to one in every five US residents, or approximately 60 million individuals, face more pronounced healthcare challenges than urban and suburban populations. Rural areas, encompassing more than 90% of the United States landmass and comprising any population, housing, or territory outside urban zones, present unique healthcare hurdles. According to a 2015 National Rural Health Association study, the mortality rate in rural areas stood at 830.5 deaths per 100,000 people in 2014, contrasting starkly with the 704.3 deaths per 100,000 people in non-rural regions [10].

These rural areas grapple with distinct healthcare barriers, contributing to higher mortality rates than urban areas [11]. Restricted availability of healthcare services often results in timely medical care, leading to favorable health outcomes. Over the two-decade period from 1999 to 2019, rural areas consistently reported the highest age-adjusted mortality rates in the US, underscoring their enduring vulnerability [12]. This disparity arises from a combination of factors, including restricted access to hospitals and healthcare providers, insufficient healthcare infrastructure, and elevated rates of chronic diseases [13].

Unequal access to healthcare services constitutes a significant component of health disparities in the United States [14]. However, many aspects of access still require a more profound understanding. Accessing healthcare entails recognizing healthcare needs, having available care providers and facilities, and successfully reaching, obtaining, and utilizing healthcare services. In comparison to urban areas, rural regions fall behind when it comes to healthcare access, resulting in higher mortality rates, premature morbidity, and limited access to preventive or mental healthcare services [15–22].

Health outcomes in rural areas consistently report higher rates of preventable deaths, mainly attributed to chronic diseases, accidents, and suicides. Health disparities manifest across multiple dimensions and impact populations differently. Addressing these disparities is complex and multifaceted, necessitating targeted interventions and policies. Finally, the urgency of addressing these disparities is underscored by stark statistics on death rates and health challenges, emphasizing that rural populations bear a disproportionately heavier burden of chronic diseases compared to their urban counterparts.

3. Chronic health issues in rural America

Rural Americans face a disproportionately high risk of chronic diseases, which appear to be the leading causes of death and disability in the United States [23]. These disparities in rural areas are driven by limited access to healthcare services and persistent socioeconomic challenges. In the deep rural regions, approximately 19% of the US population consists of rural residents, who confront significantly greater chances of premature death due to chronic illnesses when compared to their urban counterparts [23]. The prevalent chronic diseases contributing to this heightened risk include heart disease, chronic obstructive pulmonary disease (COPD), type 2 diabetes, obesity, hypertension, and strokes [24], along with chronic health conditions.

Chronic diseases pose significant concerns for both rural healthcare systems and residents, given their profound impact on quality of life, mortality rates, and healthcare expenditures [25]. Numerous studies underscore the prevalence of chronic conditions in rural areas of the southern United States. For instance, cardiovascular disease (CVD), the leading cause of death in the country, disproportionately affects residents in rural communities [26–30].

One study delved into the factors contributing to health disparities related to cardiovascular disease (CVD) and high blood pressure (HBP) among adults residing in three underserved rural communities in the South. The findings revealed that older men and male residents in rural Southern counties, regardless of their racial background, exhibited a significantly higher likelihood of being diagnosed with both high blood pressure and cardiovascular disease [31]. Conversely, women with a college education were notably less likely to have high blood pressure. Furthermore, the study found that married men had a significantly lower likelihood of having cardiovascular disease. Elevated and uncontrolled cholesterol levels were recognized as contributing factors to the onset of chronic high blood pressure and cardiovascular disease [31].

Another study focused on disparities in healthcare access, specifically examining variations in racial/ethnic and income disparities among individuals with chronic obstructive pulmonary disease (COPD) in urban and rural settings [32]. This research encompassed 34,439 participants and revealed that the prevalence of COPD was 8.6% in rural counties compared to 5.4% in urban counties. Rural residents with COPD faced challenges associated with lower socioeconomic status, limited education, compromised health, and elevated disability rates [32]. Additionally, a separate study aimed to explore differences in diabetes prevalence and adherence to guidelines between rural and urban areas, utilizing data from the Behavioral Risk Factor Surveillance System (BRFSS) [26]. The findings indicated a slightly higher diabetes prevalence in rural residents than in urban ones.

Lastly, another study delved into the rising obesity epidemic among adults residing in rural America, where obesity rates exceed those in urban regions. This research emphasized the significant health challenges faced by rural areas due to their heightened vulnerability to chronic conditions such as hypertension, obstructive sleep apnea (OSA), diabetes, and coronary artery disease, all of which are closely linked to obesity [33]. Furthermore, the study underscored the importance of addressing income inequalities as a critical aspect of mitigating the consequences of obesity and reducing mortality rates among rural Americans.

In conclusion, the body of research evidence highlights concerns about improving quality of life and healthcare access in hard-to-reach American communities. The residents of rural areas grapple with numerous diseases, only a few of which have been discussed here. However, comprehending the societal impact of chronic diseases requires innovative solutions and further evaluation.

4. Mental health problems in the rural United States

Approximately one-fifth of individuals in rural areas are affected by mental illness, as indicated by Refs. [34, 35]. While the prevalence of severe mental illness and most psychiatric disorders is similar among US adults residing in rural and urban settings [36, 37], adults in rural regions tend to receive mental health treatment less frequently, often from providers with less specialized training, in comparison to their counterparts in metropolitan areas. This mental health treatment disparity is well documented, and several factors contribute to it, including psychological well-being, opioids, and other substance use, suicide among adolescents, and the aging population in rural communities in America during COVID-19 [38, 39].

4.1 Psychological well-being

In the aftermath of the COVID-19 pandemic, the mental well-being of individuals residing in rural areas of the United States endured significant challenges. The pre-existing disparities in behavioral and mental health within these regions widened as COVID-19 took its toll on the country. Research suggests a substantial surge in mental health disorders during the pandemic, as evidenced by the works of Daly and Sutin [40] and Twenge and Joiner [41]. Notably, one study estimated a 28% increase in cases of major depressive disorder and a 26% rise in anxiety disorders in 2020 [42].

While extensive research has delved into understanding the prevalence of these mental health, less attention has been directed toward the utilization of mental health services, as indicated in Refs. [42, 43]. Moreover, studies that have explored the impact of the COVID-19 pandemic on mental health outcomes among rural and urban populations have predominantly focused on either rural or urban contexts independently, exemplified by the works of Riblet et al. [44] and Stack et al. [45]. To our knowledge, there have been no studies that have comprehensively examined shifts in depression or anxiety among rural and urban populations in the United States before and during the pandemic. Additionally, none have investigated how the utilization of mental health services may have influenced the severity of an individual's anxiety or depression during this challenging period [46].

In essence, several studies have endeavored to shed light on the changes in reported anxiety and depression levels in both rural and urban communities in the United States preceding and during the COVID-19 pandemic. The findings reveal that individuals living in urban areas were more prone to report heightened anxiety compared to their rural counterparts amid the COVID-19 pandemic. This discrepancy can be attributed to the fact that urban areas bore the brunt of the pandemic's impact earlier and more severely, serving as the initial epicenters of the COVID-19 outbreak in the United States, potentially contributing to increased anxiety among urban residents. Furthermore, our research suggests that these findings indicate differences in how urban and rural populations perceive and adhere to COVID-19 mitigation measures, such as lockdowns and social distancing policies.

4.2 Opioid and other substance

Since the advent of the COVID-19 pandemic, there has been a worrisome surge in fatalities linked to opioid overdoses in the United States, notably involving the illicit production of fentanyl [47]. This problem has extended its grip to rural regions, including the rural South [48] of the United States. In the year 2020 alone, the nation bore witness to a staggering count of over 100,000 deaths [49] attributed to drug overdoses, catapulting drug overdose to the position of the second most prevalent cause of mortality in the country. Unfortunately, the rural areas have experienced the most severe impact of this epidemic [49].

Furthermore, individuals grappling with substance use disorders (SUDs), encompassing opioid use disorder (OUD), frequently contend with concurrent health conditions, encompassing cardiovascular, pulmonary, and metabolic ailments and increased susceptibility to infections. These coexisting health issues served as risk factors for contracting COVID-19 [50]. A scrutiny of electronic health records within the United States, conducted by Wang and colleagues, brought to light that individuals afflicted by OUD faced a significantly elevated risk of contracting COVID-19, a risk even higher than that observed among individuals with other subtypes of SUD, despite sharing similar prevalence rates of established COVID-19 risk factors [51].

Even before the pandemic's onset, challenges revolving around organizational capacity and the availability of services had already been impeding the prompt treatment of OUD across various parts of the United States, particularly in predominantly low-income rural areas that had borne a disproportionate burden of opioid misuse, addiction, and fatal overdoses [52]. The advent of the COVID-19 pandemic merely exacerbated these obstacles and introduced novel challenges, including technological limitations, significantly affecting individuals in recovery and those providing services [53]. As a result, those responsible for offering OUD treatment and support services in rural areas were compelled to rapidly adjust their programming to ensure the continued accessibility of essential care and support for their clientele [54].

In a nutshell, the COVID-19 pandemic has further aggravated the opioid overdose crisis in the United States, with rural areas bearing the brunt of the impact. Individuals dealing with OUD face an elevated risk of contracting COVID-19, necessitating the development of innovative approaches to address their unique challenges. Rural OUD treatment and support service providers were forced to swiftly adapt to these evolving circumstances to guarantee that needy individuals could still obtain essential care and support.

4.3 Suicide among adolescents

The effects of COVID-19 on the mental well-being of teenagers remain uncertain, as there has been a lack of comprehensive research targeting this specific age group [55]. Adolescents are unequally influenced by concerns such as suicide and non-suicidal self-harm (NSSI) [56]. Suicide was already the second leading cause of death among youth before the pandemic [57], and a substantial percentage, ranging from 22 to 38% of adolescents, have reported experiencing thoughts of suicide at some point in their lives [58].

Furthermore, the pandemic introduced unique challenges for adolescents, including shifting to online classes, canceling extracurricular activities, and social isolation from peers. Peer connections are significant during the adolescent years [59]. Moreover, the loss of direct access to peers and friends due to school closures and social distancing may have significant consequences for their mental health. While some adults benefited from increased access to mental health support through telehealth services during the pandemic, adolescents may have experienced reduced access to support systems, such as teachers and counselors.

As a result, there is a possibility that rates of self-harm among adolescents have risen since the pandemic's onset. However, it is essential to consider potential protective factors unique to this age group, such as a decrease in school-related bullying and increased time spent with family members, both of which have been associated with reduced thoughts and behaviors related to self-harm [60].

In conclusion, the pandemic's impact on the mental health of adolescents remains uncertain, with potential risks and protective factors at play. Further research is needed to understand how this age group's rural disparity has been affected and develop appropriate interventions and support systems.

4.4 Aging population

Health disparities markedly impact the well-being of elderly residents in rural regions. Older adults in these areas face a 20% higher rate of mortality from all causes and have a life expectancy that lags over 3 years behind their urban peers. Additionally, there is an 11% higher incidence of hypertension, a 40% increase in diabetes, a 40% escalation in heart disease, a 30% rise in stroke occurrences, and a doubling in the prevalence of chronic obstructive pulmonary disease [61, 62].

The root causes of these health and longevity discrepancies are multifaceted. Rural inhabitants often grapple with challenges such as lower income levels, limited access to education, insufficient insurance coverage, subpar housing conditions, and a lack of supermarkets providing healthy food options. Moreover, the dearth of medical professionals, particularly in oncology, cardiology, and pulmonology, further aggravates these health disparities [62].

DOI: http://dx.doi.org/10.5772/intechopen.1004587

Addressing these health inequalities among the senior population is imperative to promote health parity between rural and urban regions. The National Institute of Minority Health and Health Disparities categorizes rural communities as a group experiencing health disparities, mainly due to higher instances of mental health concerns, chronic illnesses, and overall worse health outcomes than those in non-rural areas [63]. As a result, rural populations, especially the elderly, face increased morbidity rates, including conditions like obesity, diabetes, coronary artery disease, cancer, COVID-19, and higher mortality rates.

During the COVID-19 pandemic, elderly individuals in rural areas faced distinctive challenges. These regions, characterized by an aging demographic, a greater prevalence of underlying health conditions, and limited economic resources compared to urban areas, experienced unique vulnerabilities [63]. Restricted healthcare and technology access, along with connectivity issues, placed these older adults at a heightened risk, not only from the virus but also in fulfilling their healthcare, social, and fundamental needs.

Such disparities have led to increased instances of depression, suicide, and drug-related fatalities among this demographic. Research by Cohen and Greaney investigated differences in mental and social well-being between older adults in rural and urban settings during the early stages of the COVID-19 pandemic. Their study found similar mental health and social welfare outcomes among both groups, with rural participants exhibiting less anxiety about COVID-19 and a higher engagement with social media [64].

In conclusion, health disparities in rural elderly populations remain a critical issue, influenced by a variety of factors leading to poorer health outcomes. Addressing these disparities is vital for achieving health equity and enhancing the quality of life for the elderly in rural communities.

5. Root causes of health disparities

To gain insight into the underlying causes of health disparities and develop practical solutions, it is crucial to delve into the factors contributing to these disparities within rural communities. This discussion will comprise three key elements: the impact of social determinants of health, the constraints posed by limited healthcare and mental health providers, and the challenges arising from inadequate transportation infrastructure. Each of these factors plays a significant role in exacerbating health disparities among rural individuals. The subsequent sections will provide an evidence-based analysis to substantiate these claims, shedding light on the complex issues at the heart of health disparities in rural areas.

5.1 Social determinants of health

Around 3.6 million rural inhabitants, constituting 6.0% of the rural populace in the United States, self-identify as African Americans, making them the third-largest racial group in the nation. This demographic shows a notable concentration in the southern states, which can be attributed to historical patterns, where they make up 11.5% of the overall rural population. Interestingly, a substantial majority (90.4%) of African American individuals residing in non-metropolitan counties can be found in the South [1]. Social determinants, as delineated by the definitions provided by the World Health Organization (WHO) and the CDC [65, 66], encompass the conditions surrounding people's birth, growth, life, work, and aging.

These determinants encompass various factors, including income, education, access to healthcare, and community-related conditions like housing, safety, and employment prospects [67]. These determinants frequently pose considerable obstacles to accessing treatment, particularly in the context of substance use disorders, as they engender issues such as stigma, limited availability of treatment facilities, difficulties with transportation, and childcare necessities. These challenges disproportionately affect marginalized groups within rural regions [68, 69].

Collectively, these social determinants of health make a substantial contribution to the marked health disparities experienced by African American rural communities within the United States. The widespread presence of poverty and a dearth of educational attainment has led to a significant proportion of rural African Americans inhabiting suboptimal social and environmental circumstances, which exert a profound influence on their holistic health, social welfare, and economic outlook [70–72].

In the course of a comprehensive research investigation aimed at uncovering potential factors influencing the health of African American residents in a rural Deep South community, the findings revealed a range of determinants spanning multiple dimensions: individual, relational, environmental, structural, and superstructural. These determinants included a variety of challenges, including limited participation in personal health and health promotion endeavors, the notable scarcity of social capital due to generational disconnection, environmental issues related to access to physical activity and nutritious food, structural obstacles linked to disparities in employment opportunities, and superstructural elements involving heightened poverty rates and racial bias [73].

Each of these determinants directly impacts healthcare access and underscores health-related risks. To sum up, the multifaceted facets of social determinants of health occupy a central role in molding the health disparities experienced by African American rural populations. Acknowledging and targeting these determinants is pivotal for advancing health equity and overall well-being within these communities.

5.2 Limited health care and mental health providers

Access to primary care and mental health services in rural American regions has long been a persistent issue. These areas confront challenges such as a shortage of specialized healthcare and mental health professionals, obstacles to coordinating care within rural healthcare systems, and a tendency to underutilize available mental health services. Notably, reports reveal that up to 65% of non-metropolitan counties lack psychiatrists [39], and more than 60% of rural residents live in areas officially designated as lacking mental health service providers [74]. This dearth of specialized mental health services in rural locales unquestionably contributes to disparities in healthcare accessibility and delivery [75].

Rural mental health systems frequently function under a *de facto* status, diverging significantly from their urban counterparts [76]. These systems face limitations in service availability, shortages of resources, a significant deficit of specialized health and mental health professionals and providers, limited utilization of services, challenges in specialization, and the acknowledgment that clients require assistance beyond the boundaries of narrowly defined specialized mental health offerings [77]. Astoundingly, over 90% of psychiatrists, psychologists, and 80% of master's-level social workers exclusively practice in metropolitan areas—a workforce distribution that has endured for more than three decades, despite repeated efforts to address it and encourage mental health professionals to serve in rural areas. Mental health clinicians practicing in rural settings face formidable challenges, including treating patients outside their areas of expertise, making intricate decisions without the input of fellow professionals, adopting non-clinical roles in patient interactions, and contending with professional isolation and a heightened risk of burnout [78, 79].

Instead of aspiring to acquire potentially elusive resources, developing a comprehensive national rural mental health plan that rationalizes the existing system and harnesses available strengths and resources is imperative. This approach is pivotal in addressing the distinctive challenges faced by rural mental health systems and ensuring enhanced access to mental healthcare for rural communities.

5.3 Transportation access

Rural regions in the United States grapple with a complex issue regarding transportation limitations. This predicament emerges from a blend of geographical factors and personal situations. For instance, individuals residing in remote rural areas find themselves in a situation where access to private vehicles is restricted, impeding their ability to travel conveniently. In contrast to their urban counterparts, rural households and residents confront substantial challenges and hurdles concerning mobility due to the extensive distances to essential destinations and the scarcity of transportation alternatives. This situation becomes even more daunting when individuals lack access to a personal vehicle. Public transit services are scarcely available, on-demand mobility services can be expensive or simply unavailable, and the infrastructure for pedestrian and bicycle travel is often lacking [80].

This predicament may disproportionately affect people of color residing in rural areas, potentially leading to their exclusion from essential services compared to urban residents. Furthermore, rural areas typically have an aging population, with a decreasing number of working-age individuals, which may indicate an increasing demand for healthcare services among rural residents compared to their urban counterparts [81]. Recent research conducted in California sheds light on income disparities related to car ownership. The findings reveal that households without cars in rural areas earn 27% less than their non-rural counterparts. Additionally, rural Black individuals are 2.5 times more likely than their rural White counterparts lack access to a vehicle. Furthermore, unemployed and disabled rural residents are 1.7 times and 1.3 times more likely, respectively, to be without a car compared to their non-rural peers [82].

Access to affordable, high-quality transportation is a critical social determinant of health, profoundly influencing individuals' mental, physical, and emotional well-being. This is particularly vital for individuals with disabilities, those with low incomes, patients with chronic illnesses, families with children, older adults, and others who may not have reliable access to a vehicle or the ability to drive safely. Public and private transportation services are indispensable in facilitating access to healthcare, obtaining groceries and other essentials, and fostering community engagement [83].

A study conducted by Krasniuk and Crizzle [5] delved into the impact of health and transportation on rural adults who do not utilize healthcare services, family doctor services, or medical specialist services. The study compared individuals living in rural areas with those in small population centers. The research findings illuminated the significant influence of health status and transportation on the accessibility of medical specialist services among older adults residing in rural areas, as opposed to their counterparts in small communities. Factors such as perceiving one's health as poor, receiving assistance with transportation, and traveling to larger towns or cities emerged as predictors of older adults in rural communities utilizing medical specialist services [84].

In conclusion, the study's results support the idea that older individuals living in rural areas face more substantial difficulties concerning health, transportation, and healthcare accessibility in contrast to their counterparts in smaller population centers. Despite the possibility of having poorer health and a higher incidence of chronic ailments among older rural adults, they exhibit a greater tendency to utilize medical specialist services compared to individuals in smaller population centers.

6. Telemedicine and telemental health partnerships: a viable solution

Persistent healthcare disparities have long posed a challenge to the well-being and quality of life of residents in rural communities throughout the United States. To address these ongoing disparities, it is crucial to actively seek evidence-based solutions that can provide much-needed relief to individuals and families living in these underserved areas. This endeavor is in alignment with the principles of fairness and social justice, acknowledging the inherent value of every person's health, regardless of where they live.

This introductory statement establishes the foundation for a thorough examination of the use of telemedicine, also known as "telehealth," and telemental health services within rural US communities. It emphasizes the pressing need to identify evidence-based approaches to mitigate these challenges. Additionally, this section will explore potential community partnerships that could assist rural residents in meeting the growing demand for healthcare providers. By examining the available evidence and assessing effective interventions, the goal is to facilitate improved access to healthcare, enhance health outcomes, and ultimately elevate the overall quality of life for those residing in rural areas.

6.1 Understanding telehealth, and telemental health

Telemedicine encompasses a broad range of practices characterized by the American Telemedicine Association. It involves transferring medical data electronically across different locations to enhance patient health [85]. Telehealth and telemental health, on the other hand, extend the scope of telemedicine to include the provision of health and mental health evaluation and treatment from a distance [86], focusing on remote delivery of both primary care and mental health services.

The governance of telemedicine services varies significantly at the federal and state levels, influenced by each state's unique interpretation of what constitutes telemedicine. These interpretations are crucial in defining which services qualify for compensation through Medicaid and private insurers [87]. The Centers for Medicare and Medicaid Services (CMS) encourage states to use Medicaid's adaptable framework to develop new payment models that integrate telemedicine technologies [88]. Almost all states, except two, provide some level of Medicaid reimbursement for telemedicine-related services [89]. In addition, 39 states include coverage and reimbursement for telemental health services under Medicaid [90, 91].

In private insurance, 32 states have implemented specific telehealth policies, reflecting various covered services and varying compensation rates for healthcare providers [92]. Additionally, 23 states require reimbursement for telemental health services to align with traditional in-person consultations [93].

6.2 Evidence to support the utility and benefits telehealth and telemental health

An extensive collection of scholarly evidence firmly advocates for the implementation of telehealth in the rural sectors of the United States, significantly enhancing the availability of healthcare for susceptible demographics including seniors, persons with disabilities, and families with minors and teenagers who may face obstacles in accessing conventional in-person health services. Telehealth, propelled by advancements in digital technology, establishes an efficient platform for remote healthcare delivery, enabling instantaneous interaction between patients and medical practitioners [94]. This innovative healthcare paradigm extends the reach of medical treatments, diminishes hindrances to healthcare access in underserved rural localities, bolsters patient involvement and contentment, and plays a pivotal role in curbing the prevalence of chronic diseases. Numerous research endeavors have consistently affirmed the positive impact of telehealth in rural communities [1].

For instance, a study spearheaded by Huurne et al. [95] applied web-based technological solutions to amplify healthcare services for individuals grappling with chronic eating disorders, leading to marked enhancements in Body Mass Index, body satisfaction, overall life quality, and both physical and psychological health for over half of the participants [2].

Moreover, an exhaustive review of relevant literature conducted by Kruse and associates [96] revealed that telehealth effectively curtails travel requirements, enriches patient-healthcare provider communication, broadens healthcare accessibility, augments patient self-awareness, and empowers individuals in managing their chronic health conditions [3]. From the perspective of healthcare systems and providers, telehealth introduces a multitude of benefits, including a reduction in missed medical appointments, shortened waiting periods, lowered rates of patient readmission, heightened adherence to medication, and improved overall quality and timeliness in patient care, also serving as a robust educational resource. Particularly in rural areas grappling with shortages of medical professionals and provider burnout, telehealth has shown potential to alleviate these issues. Research by Ward et al. [96] indicated that three-quarters of family physicians in rural settings were required to provide coverage in local emergency departments, a mandate that often discourages practices in rural areas, yet telemedicine has been found to enhance the recruitment and retention of physicians in these regions [97].

Additionally, a comprehensive review by Butzner and Cuffee [5] on telehealth interventions in rural American communities, incorporating studies focusing on both patients and healthcare professionals, reported unanimously positive outcomes, high levels of acceptance, and increased satisfaction among participants, highlighting the efficiency and convenience of technological applications in delivering healthcare services in rural areas [98].

The evidence base suggests that telehealth, including its telemental health aspect, is instrumental in addressing mental health challenges like depression, anxiety, and suicidal tendencies in rural communities by improving access to mental health services and reducing care barriers.

The onset of the COVID-19 pandemic has particularly underscored the necessity for telemental health services in both urban and rural America, bringing to light issues such as social isolation, loneliness, depression, and anxiety, thereby spotlighting telemedicine and telemental health. Mental health specialties, including psychiatry and psychology, are at the forefront of employing telemedicine (*via* video conferencing platforms) for evaluations, therapeutic interventions, and distant patient education [99, 100]. Despite evidence indicating that delays in insurance reimbursements dampen providers' enthusiasm for telemedicine [101, 102], the uptake of telemental health has been gradual but consistent, increasing from 15% in 2010 to nearly 29% in 2017 [103]. This growth is particularly noteworthy in private clinics and facilities catering to medically underserved populations, including rural areas [104]. A study revealed a significant surge in the daily use of telemedicine by telemental health practitioners during the pandemic, with usage jumping from 17% before the pandemic to 40% during it. Additionally, the proportion of remotely served caseloads rose from 9.1% before the pandemic to 57.7% during it, and the comfort level of providers in telemedicine also saw substantial growth during this period [105].

In another investigation, researchers [106] assessed the initial phase of the COVID-19 pandemic, observing a swift transition to virtual and telephone consultations within the Veterans Health Administration (VA) to mitigate virus transmission. To address the evolving mental health requirements of elderly veterans, a novel 8-week virtual group treatment manual was developed and implemented. Despite technological hurdles encountered by older veterans, clinicians found this manual effective in addressing pandemic-related concerns and social isolation [18].

Telemedicine has been essential not only for mental and behavioral health issues but also in catering to telehealth and telemental health needs among vulnerable groups (e.g., people of color, those with compromised immune systems, the elderly, disabled, and families with children and adolescents) in rural counties. In a systematic review conducted by Appleton et al. [106], the adoption and impact of telemental health approaches during the COVID-19 pandemic were examined, along with facilitators and barriers to optimal implementation. The review, encompassing 77 papers, found that most contacts could be adapted to a remote format during the pandemic, with generally favorable acceptability reported by service users and clinicians, especially where the alternative was the interruption of care [19].

Furthermore, a national survey by the Bipartisan Policy Center (BPC) and Social Sciences Research Solutions (SSRS) involving 1776 adults sought to evaluate the effectiveness of telehealth services, investigate the motivations behind patients seeking remote care, and identify consumer barriers. The survey uncovered various motivations for using telehealth, such as annual physical or preventive services (24%), routine visits for chronic conditions like diabetes or high blood pressure (18%), consultations for surgical procedures (12%), immediate care for illnesses, injuries, or conditions (11%), prescription refills (10%), physical therapy (7%), and mental health or substance use treatment (5%). These findings offer valuable insights into the diverse applications of telehealth and the healthcare needs of the surveyed population [107, 108].

6.3 Advancing rural telehealth: Success stories, economic evaluation, and policy recommendations

While previous research studies have laid a strong foundation for understanding the impact and challenges of telehealth in rural America, there is a clear need for further refinement to maximize its applicability. In the following discussions, we will delve into successful instances of telehealth adoption in rural areas, scrutinize economic evaluations demonstrating cost savings and improved health outcomes, and emphasize the significance of recommending supportive policies and legislation to promote the expansion of telehealth services in rural regions.

In rural healthcare, a case study conducted at the White Earth Health Center (WEHC) shows the successful integration of telehealth. Situated in the northern rural regions of Minnesota, USA, WEHC operates under the umbrella of the Indian Health Service (IHS), serving approximately 10,000 American Indians and Alaska Natives annually. This specific case study aimed to explore the deployment and utilization of telehealth during the COVID-19 pandemic. Remarkably, prior to this crisis, WEHC did not possess a telehealth program, mainly due to Medicaid regulations restricting billing for outpatient encounters unless they were conducted in person. This posed a significant obstacle to continuous patient care. Initially, even the staff at WEHC had reservations about implementing on-site telehealth services, fearing potential inconvenience for patients and themselves. However, proactive measures taken by WEHC's administrators and leaders led to the swift adoption of a telehealth program, witnessing its peak utilization by the end of April 2020 [109]. This success story underscores the transformative potential of telehealth for vulnerable populations.

Furthermore, examining economic evaluations of telemedicine in numerous rural health facilities across the United States is paramount for its cost-saving attributes and capacity to enhance health outcomes. A study by Chen, Amaize, and Barath aimed to assess the cost-effectiveness of telemedicine interventions across various medical specialties in rural areas in the United States involved a comprehensive search of the Cochrane Library and the Center for Review and Dissemination for relevant studies up to February 2013.

The study encompassed 21 articles and revealed diverse outcomes across different medical domains. In cardiology, telemedicine has emerged as both practical and cost-effective. However, its impact on reducing fatalities through pre-hospital telemedicine diagnostics for acute myocardial infarction appeared limited. In pulmonary care, telemedicine was cost-effective, particularly in delivering outpatient services to rural populations with limited access to specialized care. In ophthalmology, specifically in diagnosing diabetic retinopathy, telemedicine was deemed a cost-effective tool [110].

The research extended its evaluation to various other medical fields, encompassing physical activity, diet, eating disorders, tele-ICU, psychotherapy for depression, and telemedicine on ships. Telemedicine was recognized as a cost-effective approach for delivering treatments and care in these areas.

Based on these significant findings, which underscore the growth of telehealth services in rural areas and their positive impact on health outcomes, there is a critical need to implement supportive policies and legislation to facilitate further telehealth expansion in rural America. As of 2023, the Biden and Harris Administration has taken proactive measures to enhance rural communities' well-being. These initiatives include:

1. We are expanding the Affordable Care Act and Inflation Reduction Act to enhance the availability of cost-effective health coverage and healthcare services for rural residents.

2. We are ensuring the sustained operation of rural hospitals to guarantee the continued provision of essential healthcare services to local communities.

3. We are strengthening the rural healthcare workforce, emphasizing addressing the needs of primary care and behavioral health professionals.

4. Facilitating access to essential healthcare, including behavioral health services, by promoting telehealth services to bridge geographical barriers and enhance healthcare accessibility.

These policy and legislative actions represent significant strides toward providing universal access to healthcare [111]. Healthcare services in rural communities need to catch up, but the importance of universal health coverage has now gained prominence. These measures are poised to improve the quality of life in rural communities across America by extending access to healthcare to more individuals.

6.4 Apprenticeships and academic university partnerships in rural America

One promising solution to address unmet disparities in underserved rural areas is the establishment of partnerships with apprenticeship programs affiliated with agricultural land-grant universities situated in rural America. Many of these universities boast departments specializing in social work, counseling, and psychology, offering students with bachelor's degrees an opportunity to pursue their master's degrees. These students are being prepared to work within apprenticeship settings, contributing to the efforts to bridge the provider gap prevalent in rural communities nationwide.

Apprenticeships represent a largely untapped resource that can leverage the behavioral workforce to enhance the well-being of rural residents. A notable example is the initiative of Alabama A&M University, a land-grant university in a rural and underserved area. In 2020, this institution secured funding from the Health Resources and Services Administration (HRSA) to establish a groundbreaking apprenticeship program—the first of its kind in the nation. This apprenticeship program focuses on training master's level social work students to serve in rural Alabama, partnering with community-based, primary, and behavioral health centers to support rural residents. These dedicated students receive certification in case management, telehealth, and telemental health, equipping them to work with families affected by opioid and other substance use challenges.

Such collaborations between land-grant universities and apprenticeship programs hold the potential to significantly expand telehealth and telemental health access while concurrently enhancing healthcare delivery and education in rural areas. These initiatives represent a crucial step toward addressing the unique healthcare needs of rural communities and reducing disparities in access to vital services.

7. Conclusion and implications for consideration

The comprehensive analysis of healthcare disparities in rural America, as discussed in this chapter, underscores the urgent need for targeted, evidence-based interventions to address the complex health challenges faced by this population. The data reveals that rural residents, particularly in the United States, face higher risks of chronic diseases, behavioral mental health issues, and overall poorer health outcomes compared to their urban counterparts. These disparities are further exacerbated by limited access to healthcare services, social determinants of health, and a lack of specialized healthcare providers.

Telemedicine, telehealth, and telemental health have emerged as practical solutions to bridge the gap in healthcare access. These technologies can significantly improve healthcare delivery by facilitating real-time communication between patients and providers, thereby overcoming geographical barriers. Substantial evidence suggests telemedicine can effectively manage chronic diseases, enhance patient satisfaction, and increase healthcare efficiency in rural settings. Implementing telehealth services, especially for primary care and mental health, can mitigate the impacts of physician shortages and provide much-needed care for vulnerable populations, including the elderly, disabled, and children.

The mental health challenges prevalent in rural communities, exacerbated by the COVID-19 pandemic, underscore the importance of telemental health. This approach can address issues like depression, anxiety, and substance use disorders by improving access to mental health services. Telemental health can reduce barriers to care, offer anonymity, and provide consistent support, which is crucial in areas with limited mental health resources.

Partnerships with agricultural land-grant universities in rural areas present a novel opportunity to address healthcare workforce shortages. Programs like the one initiated by Alabama A&M University demonstrate the potential of such collaborations. By training students in social work, counseling, and psychology through apprenticeships, these partnerships can prepare a new generation of healthcare providers equipped with skills in telehealth and telemental health. These providers can offer culturally competent care and are more likely to remain in rural communities, thereby sustainably addressing the shortage of healthcare professionals.

Supportive policies and adequate funding are crucial to realizing the full potential of telehealth and telemental health services. This includes reimbursement policies for telehealth services, incentives for healthcare providers to adopt telehealth, and grants for universities to establish and maintain apprenticeship programs. Such policies can create a conducive environment for the widespread adoption of telehealth services and training a new healthcare workforce.

7.1 Implications for future research and practice

Continued research into the effectiveness of telehealth and telemental health in rural settings is essential. This research should focus on identifying best practices, understanding patient and provider experiences, and exploring the long-term impacts of these services. Healthcare providers and educators should be encouraged to integrate telehealth training into their curricula and practice, ensuring that the future workforce is prepared to meet the unique needs of rural communities.

In summary, addressing the health disparities in rural America requires a comprehensive strategy that integrates telemedicine, telehealth, telemental health, and innovative educational partnerships. By leveraging technology and educational resources, we can enhance access to healthcare, improve health outcomes, and ultimately reduce the healthcare disparities that disproportionately affect rural populations.

Author details

Katina Lang-Lindsey
LMSW, Alabama A&M Universitys, Huntsville, Alabama, United States

*Address all correspondence to: katina.lindsey@aamu.edu

References

[1] Centers for Disease Control and Prevention. Rural public health. 2023. Available from: https://www.cdc.gov/ruralhealth/docs/ruralhealth-aag-508.pdf

[2] Warshaw R. Health Disparities Affect Millions in Rural US Communities. Washington DC, United States: The Association of American Medical Colleges (AAMC); 2017. Available from: https://www.aamc.org/news-insights/health-disparities-affect-millions-rural-us-communities [Accessed: June 22, 2020]

[3] U.S. Department of Agriculture, Economic Research Service. Rural poverty & well-being. Available from: https://www.ers.usda.gov/topics/rural-economy-population/rural-poverty-well-being/ [Accessed: December 13, 2021]

[4] USDA Economic Research Service (ERS). Nonmetro Population Change, 2010-17 [Chart]. Washington, DC; 2018. Available from: https://nca2018.globalchange.gov/chapter/10/

[5] Braveman P, Arkin E, Orleans T, Proctor D, Plough A. What is health equity? And what difference does a definition make? Princeton, New Jersey, United States: The Robert Wood Johnson Foundation; 2017. Available from: https://www.rwjf.org/en/library/research/2017/05/what-is-health-equity-.html

[6] Cockerham WC, Hamby BW, Oates GR. The social determinants of chronic disease. American Journal Preview Medice. 2017;**52**(1S1):S5-S12. DOI: 10.1016/j.amepre.2016.09.010

[7] Bhattacharya G. Self-management of type 2 diabetes among African Americans in the Arkansas Delta: A strengths perspective in social-cultural context. Journal of Health Care for the Poor and Underserved. 2012;**23**(1):161-178. DOI: 10.1353/hpu.2012.0035

[8] National Academies of Sciences, Engineering, and Medicine, Health and Medicine Division, Board on Population Health and Public Health Practice. Committee on community-based solutions to promote health equity in the United States. In: Baciu A, Negussie Y, Geller A, et al., editors. Communities in Action: Pathways to Health Equity. Washington (DC): National Academies Press (US); 2017. Chapter 3, The Root Causes of Health Inequity. Available from: https://www.ncbi.nlm.nih.gov/books/NBK425845/

[9] Cacari Stone L, Roary MC, Diana A, Grady PA. State health disparities research in rural America: Gaps and future directions in an era of COVID-19. The Journal of Rural Health. 2021;**37**(3):460-466. DOI: 10.1111/jrh.12562

[10] The United States Census Bureau. What is Rural America?. 2017. Available from: https://www.census.gov/library/stories/2017/08/rural-america.html [Accessed: January 15, 2020]

[11] Leider JP, Meit M, McCullough JM, et al. The state of rural public health: Enduring needs in a new decade. American Journal of Public Health. 2020;**110**(9):1283-1290. DOI: 10.2105/AJPH.2020.305728

[12] Cross SH, Califf RM, Warraich HJ. Rural-urban disparity in mortality in the US from 1999 to 2019. Journal of the American Medical Association. 2021;**325**(22):2312-2314. DOI: 10.1001/jama.2021.5334

[13] Rural Health Information Hub. Critical Access Hospitals. Available from: https://www.ruralhealthinfo.org/topics/critical-access-hospitals [Accessed: December 6, 2021]

[14] Riley WJ. Health disparities: Gaps in access, quality and affordability of medical care. Transactions of the American Clinical and Climatological Association. 2012;**123**:167-174

[15] Singh GK, Siahpush M. Widening rural-urban disparities in all-cause mortality and mortality from major causes of death in the USA, 1969-2009. Journal Urban Health. 2014;**91**(2):272-292

[16] Meit M, Knudson A, Gilbert T, et al. The 2014 Update of the Rural-Urban Chartbook. Bethesda, MD: Rural Health Reform Policy Research Center; 2014

[17] Blake KD, Moss JL, Gaysynsky A, Srinivasan S, Croyle RT. Making the case for investment in rural cancer control: An analysis of rural cancer incidence, mortality, and funding trends. Cancer Epidemiol Biomarkers Preview. 2017;**26**(7):992-997

[18] Singh GK, Daus GP, Allender M, et al. Social determinants of health in the United States: Addressing major health inequality trends for the nation, 1935-2016. International Journal of Maternal and Child Health and AIDS. 2017;**6**(2):139-164

[19] Zahnd WE, James AS, Jenkins WD, et al. Rural-urban differences in cancer incidence and trends in the United States. Cancer Epidemiology, Biomarkers & Prevention. 2017;**27**:1265-1274. DOI: 10.1158/1055-9965.EPI-17-0430

[20] Doescher MP, Jackson JE. Trends in cervical and breast cancer screening practices among women in rural and urban areas of the United States. Journal of Public Health Management Practices. 2009;**15**(3):200-209

[21] Cole AM, Jackson JE, Doescher M. Urban-rural disparities in colorectal cancer screening: Cross-sectional analysis of 1998-2005 data from the centers for disease control's behavioral risk factor surveillance study. Cancer Medicine. 2012;**1**(3):350-356

[22] Chen X, Cisse-Egbuonye N, Spears EC, Mkuu R, McKyer ELJ. Children's healthy eating habits and parents' socio-demographic characteristics in rural Texas, USA. Health Education Journal. 2018;**77**:444-457. DOI: 10.1177/0017896917752014

[23] Jean-Louis F. Overlooked Americans: The toll of chronic disease in rural America. RTI Health Solutions. 2023. Available from: https://healthcare.rti.org/insights/chronic-disease-and-rural-health-disparities

[24] Ward BW, Schiller JS, Goodman RA. Multiple chronic conditions among US adults: A 2012 update. Preventing Chronic Disease. 2014;**11**:E62

[25] Centers for Disease Control and Prevention (CDC). Potentially excess deaths from the five leading causes of death in metropolitan and nonmetropolitan counties — United States, 2010-2017. MMWR Supplements. 2019;**68**(10):1-11. Available from: https://www.cdc.gov/mmwr/volumes/68/ss/ss6810a1.htm

[26] Krishna S, Gillespie KN, McBride TM. Diabetes burden and access to preventive care in the rural United States. The Journal of Rural Health. 2010;**26**(1):102-109. DOI: 10.1111/j.1748-0361.2009.00259. x

[27] Ingram DD, Gillum RF. Regional and urbanization differentials in coronary

heart disease mortality in the United States, 1968-85. Journal of Clinical Epidemiology. 1989;**42**(9):857-868

[28] Brown JR, O'Connor GT. Coronary heart disease and prevention in the United States. New England Journal of Medicine. 2010;**362**(23):2150-2153

[29] Kochanek KD, Xu JQ, Murphy SL, Miniño AM, Kung HC. Deaths: Preliminary data for 2009. National Vital Statistics Reports. 2011;**59**(4):1-17

[30] Cosby AG, Neaves TT, Cossman RE, et al. Preliminary evidence for an emerging nonmetropolitan mortality penalty in the United States. American Journal of Public Health. 2008;**98**(8):1470-1147

[31] Amponsah WA, Tabi MM, Gibbison GA, et al. Health disparities in cardiovascular disease and high blood pressure among adults in rural underserved communities. Online Journal of Rural Nursing and Health Care. 2020;**15**(1):185-208. DOI: 10.14574/ojrnhc. v15i1.351

[32] Gaffney AW, Hawks L, White AC, Woolhandler S, Himmelstein DU, Christiani DC, et al. Health care disparities across the urban-rural divide: A national study of individuals with COPD. The Journal of Rural Health. 2022;**38**:207-216. DOI: 10.1111/jrh.12445

[33] Okobi OE, Ajayi OO, Okobi TJ, et al. The burden of obesity in the rural adult population of America. Census. 2021;**13**(6):e15770. DOI: 10.7759/cureus.15770

[34] Substance Abuse and Mental Health Services Administration. Results from the 2016 National Survey on Drug Use and Health: detailed tables. 2017. Available from: https://www.samhsa.gov/data/sites/default/files/NSDUH-DetTabs-2016/NSDUH-DetTabs-2016.htm

[35] United States Census Bureau. New Census Data Show Differences between Urban and Rural Populations. The U.S. Census Bureau; 2016. Available from: https://www.census.gov/newsroom/press-releases/2016/cb16-210.html

[36] McCall-Hosenfeld JS, Mukherjee S, Lehman EB. The prevalence and correlates of lifetime psychiatric disorders and trauma exposures in urban and rural settings: Results from the national comorbidity survey replication (NCS-R). PLoS One. 2014;**9**(11):e112416. DOI: 10.1371/journal.pone.0112416

[37] Stewart EG. Suicide in rural areas. In: Stewart EG, editor. Mental Health in Rural America: A Field Guide. New York: Routledge; 2018

[38] Kepley HO, Streeter RA. Closing behavioral health workforce gaps: A HRSA program expanding direct mental health service access in underserved areas. American Journal Preview Medicine. 2018;**54**(6S3):S190-S191. DOI: 10.1016/j.amepre.2018.03.006

[39] Andrilla CHA, Patterson DG, Garberson LA, Coulthard C, Larson EH. Geographic variation in the supply of selected behavioral health providers. American Journal Preview Medicine. 2018;**54**(6S3):S199-S207. DOI: 10.1016/j.amepre.2018.01.004

[40] Daly M, Sutin AR, Robinson E. Depression reported by US adults in 2017-2018 and March and April 2020. Journal Affective Disorders. 2021;**278**:131-135. DOI: 10.1016/j.jad.2020.09.065

[41] Twenge JM, Joiner TE. Mental distress among U.S. adults during the

COVID-19 pandemic. Journal of Clinical Psychology. 2020;**76**(12):2170-2182. DOI: 10.1002/jclp.23064

[42] Santomauro DF, Mantilla Herrera AM, Shadid J, Zheng P, Ashbaugh C, Pigott DM, et al. Global prevalence and burden of depressive and anxiety disorders in 204 countries and territories in 2020 due to the COVID-19 pandemic. Lancet. 2021;**398**(10312):1700-1712. DOI: 10.1016/S0140-6736(21)02143-7

[43] Vindegaard N, Benros ME. COVID-19 pandemic and mental health consequences: Systematic review of the current evidence. Brain Behavior Immunity. 2020;**89**:531-542. DOI: 10.1016/j.bbi.2020.05.048

[44] Riblet NBV, Stevens SP, Shiner B, Cornelius SL, Forehand J, Scott RC, et al. A longitudinal examination of COVID-19 public health measures on mental health for rural patients with serious mental illness. Military Medicine. 2021;**186**(9-10):e956-e961. DOI: 10.1093/milmed/usab099

[45] Stack E, Leichtling G, Larsen JE, Gray M, Pope J, Leahy JM, et al. The impacts of COVID-19 on mental health, substance use, and overdose concerns of people who use drugs in rural communities. Journal of Addiction Medicine. 2021;**15**(5):383-389. DOI: 10.1097/ADM.0000000000000814

[46] Danek R, Taylor H, Hilts KE. Changes in reported levels of depression and anxiety among rural and urban populations during the COVID-19 pandemic. Mental Health Science. 2023;**1**:128-135. DOI: 10.1002/mhs2.24

[47] O'Donnell J, Tanz LJ, Gladden RM, Davis NL, Bitting J. Trends in and characteristics of drug overdose deaths involving illicitly manufactured fentanyls—United States, 2019-2020. MMWR Morbidity and Mortality Weekly Report. 2021;**70**:1740-1746. DOI: 10.15585/mmwr.mm7048a1

[48] Centers for Disease Control and Prevention. Drug Overdose Deaths in the U.S. Top 100,000 Annually. 2021. Available from: https://www.cdc.gov/nchs/pressroom/nchs_press_releases/2021/20211117.htm [Accessed: August 20, 2022]

[49] Commonwealth of Kentucky Justice & Public Safety Cabinet. Overdose Fatality Report. 2020. Available from: https://odcp.ky.gov/Documents/2020%20KY%20ODCP%20Fatality%20Report%20(final).pdf [Accessed: August 20, 2022]

[50] Bahorik AL, Satre DD, Kline-Simon AH, Weisner CM, Campbell CI. Alcohol, cannabis, and opioid use disorders, and disease burden in an integrated healthcare system. Journal of Addiction Medicine. 2017;**11**:3. DOI: 10.1097/ADM.0000000000000278

[51] Centers for Disease Control and Prevention. People with Certain Medical Conditions. 2022. Available from: https://www.cdc.gov/coronavirus/2019-ncov/need-extra-precautions/people-with-medical-conditions.html [Accessed: August 20, 2022]

[52] Friedman H, Pross S, Klein TW. Addictive drugs and their relationship with infectious diseases. FEMS Immunology and Medical Microbiology. 2006;**47**(3):330-342. DOI: 10.1111/j.1574-695X.2006.00097. x

[53] National Institute on Drug Abuse. Health consequences of drug misuse. Available from: https://www.drugabuse.gov/drug-topics/health-consequences-drug-misuse/hiv-hepatitis-other-infectious-diseases [Accessed: August 20, 2022]

[54] Richardson S, Hirsch JS, Narasimhan M, Crawford JM, McGinn T, Davidson KW, et al. Presenting characteristics, comorbidities, and outcomes among 5700 patients hospitalized with COVID-19 in New York city. Journal of the American Medical Association. 2020;**323**(20):2052-2059. DOI: 10.1001/jama.2020.6775

[55] Octavius GS, Silviani FR, Lesmandjaja A, Angelina JA. Impact of COVID-19 on adolescents' mental health: A systematic review. Middle East Current Psychiatry. 2020;**27**(1):72. DOI: 10.1186/s43045-020-00075-4

[56] Nock MK, Green JG, Hwang I, McLaughlin KA, Sampson NA, Zaslavsky AM, et al. Prevalence, correlates, and treatment of lifetime suicidal behavior among adolescents: Results from the national comorbidity survey replication adolescent supplement. JAMA Psychiatry. 2013;**70**(3):300-310. DOI: 10.1001/2013.jamapsychiatry.55

[57] Hedegaard H, Warner M. Suicide Mortality in the United States, 1999-2019. NCHS Data Brief, no 398. Hyattsville, MD: National Center for Health Statistics; 2021. DOI: 10.15620/cdc:101761

[58] Nock MK, Borges G, Bromet EJ, Cha CB, Kessler RC, Lee S. Suicide, and suicidal behavior. Epidemiologic Reviews. 2008;**30**(1):133-154. DOI: 10.1093/epirev/mxn002

[59] Victor SE, Hipwell AE, Stepp SD, Scott LN. Parent and peer relationships as longitudinal predictors of adolescent non-suicidal self-injury onset. Child Adolescent Psychiatry Mental Health. 2019;**13**(1):1-13. DOI: 10.1186/s13034-018-0259-3

[60] Esposito C, Bacchini D, Affuso G. Adolescent non-suicidal self-injury and its relationships with school bullying and peer rejection. Psychiatry Research. 2019;**274**:1-6. DOI: 10.1016/j.psychres.2019.01.068

[61] Harrington RA, Califf RM, Balamurugan A, Brown N, Benjamin RM, Braund WE, et al. Call to action: Rural health: A presidential advisory from the American Heart Association and American Stroke Association. Circulation. 2020;**141**(10):e615-e644. DOI: 10.1161/CIR.0000000000000755

[62] Croft JB, Wheaton AG, Liu Y, Xu F, Lu H, Matthews KA, et al. Urban-rural county and state differences in chronic obstructive pulmonary disease — United States, 2015. MMWR Morbidity and Mortality Weekly Report. 2018;**67**(7):205-211. DOI: 10.15585/mmwr.mm6707a1

[63] Henning-Smith C, Meltzer G, Kobayashi LC, Finlay JM. Rural/urban differences in mental health and social well-being among older US adults in the early months of the COVID-19 pandemic. Aging Mental Health. 2022;**27**:505-511. DOI: 10.1080/13607863.2022.2060184

[64] Cohen SA, Greaney ML. Aging in rural communities. Current Epidemiology Reports. 2023;**10**(1):1-16. DOI: 10.1007/s40471-022-00313-9

[65] World Health Organization. Social Determinants of Health. 2018. Available from: http://www.who.int/social_determinants/sdh_definition/en/

[66] Centers for Disease Control and Prevention. Social Determinants of Health: Know What Affects Health. 2018. Available from: https://www.cdc.gov/socialdeterminants/

[67] Madras BK, Ahmad NJ, Wen J, Sharfstein J. Improving access to evidence-based medical treatment

for opioid use disorder: Strategies to address key barriers within the treatment system. NAM Perspective. 2020:1-37. DOI: 10.31478/202007b

[68] Schalkoff CA, Lancaster KE, Gaynes BN, Wang V, Pence BW, Miller WC, et al. The opioid and related drug epidemics in rural Appalachia: A systematic review of populations affected, risk factors, and infectious diseases. Substance Abuse. 2020;**41**(1):35-69. DOI: 10.1080/08897077.2019.1580239

[69] Lagisetty PA, Ross R, Bohnert A, Clay M, Maust DT. Buprenorphine treatment divide by race/ethnicity and payment. JAMA Psychiatry. 2019;**76**(9):979-981. DOI: 10.1001/jamapsychiatry.2019.0876

[70] Woolf SH, Braveman P. Where health disparities begin: The role of social and economic determinants—And why current policies may make matters worse. Health Affairs (Millwood). 2011;**30**(10):1852-1859. DOI: 10.1377/hlthaff.2011.0685

[71] Joint Economic Committee. Economic challenges in the black community. 2015. Available from: https://www.jec.senate.gov/public/index.cfm/minorities?page=32

[72] Braveman P, Gottlieb L. The social determinants of health: It's time to consider the causes of the causes. Public Health Reports. 2014;**129**(Suppl. 2):19-31. DOI: 10.1177/00333549141291S206

[73] Scott AJ, Wilson RF. Social determinants of health among African Americans in a rural community in the deep south: An ecological exploration. Rural and Remote Health. 2011;**11**:1634. DOI: 10.3316/informit.338952398784368

[74] Health Resources and Services Administration. Designated Health Professional Shortage Areas Statistics. Department of Health and Human Services: Bureau of Health Workforce. U.S; 2019. Available from: https://ersrs.hrsa.gov/ReportServer?/HGDW_Reports/

[75] Cheesmond NE, Davies K, Inder KJ. Exploring the role of rurality and rural identity in mental health help-seeking behavior: A systematic qualitative review. Journal of Rural Mental Health. 2019;**43**:45-59. DOI: 10.1037/rmh0000121

[76] Lambert D, Hartley D. Linking primary care and rural psychiatry: Where have we been? Where are we going? Psychiatry Service. 1998;**49**(7):965-967. DOI: 10.1176/ps.49.7.965

[77] Beeson P, Britain C, Howell M, Kirwan A, Sawyer D. Rural mental health at the millennium. In: Manderscheid R, Henderson M, editors. Mental Health, United States. Rockville, MD: Center for Mental Health Services; 1998. pp. 82-97

[78] Roberts L, Battaglia J, Epstein R. Frontier ethics: Mental health care needs and ethical dilemmas in rural communities. Psychiatry Service. 1999;**50**(4):497-503. DOI: 10.1176/ps.50.4.497

[79] Beeson P. The successful rural mental health practitioner: Dimensions of success, challenges, and opportunities. Rural Community Mental Health. 1991;**18**(4):4-7

[80] Centers for Disease Control and Prevention. Older Adult Drivers. 2015. Available from: http://bit.ly/224S0O9

[81] Davis JC, Rupasingha A, Cromartie J, Sanders A. Rural America at a Glance. 2022nd ed. USDA: Economic Research

Service; 2022. Available from: https://www.ers.usda.gov/webdocs/publications/102076/eib-230.pdf?v=5000.7

[82] Barajas JM, Wang W. Mobility justice in rural California: examining transportation barriers and adaptations in carless households. 2022. DOI: 10.7922/G2X928NC. Available from: https://escholarship.org/uc/item/8pk0h9zr

[83] Wang W, Espeland S, Barajas JM, et al. Rural–nonrural divide in car access and unmet travel need in the United States. Transportation. 2023. DOI: 10.1007/s11116-023-10429-6

[84] Krasniuk S, Crizzle AM. Impact of health and transportation on accessing healthcare in older adults living in rural regions. Transportation Research Interdisciplinary Perspectives. 2023;**21**:100882. DOI: 10.1016/j.trip.2023.100882

[85] American Telemedicine Association. Telemedicine glossary. Available from: http://thesource.americantelemed.org/resources/telemedicine-glossary

[86] Hilty DM, Ferrer DC, Parish MB, Johnston B, Callahan EJ, Yellowlees PM. The effectiveness of telehealth: A 2013 review. Telemedicine e-Health. 2013;**19**(6):444-454. DOI: 10.1089/tmj.2013.0075

[87] Blackman K. Covering and Reimbursing Telehealth Services. The National Institutes of Health (NIH); 2016. Available from: http://www.ncsl.org/documents/health/lb_2404.pdf

[88] Center for Medicare and Medicaid Services. Telemedicine. Available from: https://www.medicaid.gov/medicaid/benefits/telemed/index.html

[89] Center for Connected Health Policy. Telehealth Medicaid and state policy. Available from: http://www.cchpca.org/telehealth-medicaidstate-policy

[90] American Telemedicine Association. State Medicaid Best Practices: Telemental and Behavioral Health. Available from: https://www.americantelemed.org/resources/state-medicaid-best-practices-telemental-and-behavioral-health/

[91] U.S. Health Resources and Services Administration. Increasing access to behavioral health care through technology. Available from: https://www.hrsa.gov/publichealth/guidelines/behavioral-health

[92] National Conference of State Legislatures. State coverage for telehealth services. 2016. Available from: https://www.ncsl.org/research/health/state-coverage-for-telehealth-services.aspx

[93] Pew Charitable Trusts. How teletherapy addresses mental health needs. 2016. Available from: https://www.pewtrusts.org/en/research-and-analysis/blogs/stateline/2016/10/26/how-teletherapy-addresses-mental-health-needs

[94] Orlando JF, Beard M, Kumar S. Systematic review of patient and caregivers' satisfaction with telehealth videoconferencing as a mode of service delivery in managing patients' health. PLoS One. 2019;**14**(8):e0221848. DOI: 10.1371/journal.pone.0221848

[95] ter Huurne ED, Postel MG, de Haan HA, Drossaert CHC, DeJong CAJ. Web-based treatment program using intensive therapeutic contact for patients with eating disorders: Before-after study. Journal of Medical Internet Research. 2013;**15**(2):e12. DOI: 10.2196/jmir.2211. Available from: https://www.jmir.org/2013/2/e12/

[96] Kruse CS, Krowski N, Rodriguez B, Tran L, Vela J, Brooks M. Telehealth, and patient satisfaction: A systematic review and narrative analysis. BMJ Open. 2017;7(8):e016242. DOI: 10.1136/bmjopen-2017-016242. Available from: https://bmjopen.bmj.com/content/7/8/e016242

[97] Ward MM, Merchant KAS, Carter KD, Zhu X, Ullrich F, Wittrock A, et al. Use of telemedicine for ED physician coverage in critical access hospitals increased after CMS policy clarification. Health Affairs (Millwood). 2018;**37**(12):2037-2044. DOI: 10.1377/hlthaff.2018.05103

[98] Butzner M, Cuffee Y. Telehealth interventions and outcomes across rural communities in the United States: Narrative review. Journal of Medical Internet Research. 2021;**23**(8):e29575. DOI: 10.2196/29575. Available from: https://www.jmir.org/2021/8/e29575/

[99] Robeznieks A. Which Medical Specialties Use Telemedicine the Most. Chicago, Illinois, United States: The American Medical Association; 2019. Available from: https://www.ama-assn.org/practice-management/digital/which-medical-specialties-use-telemedicine-most

[100] Gershkovich M, Herbert JD, Glassman LH, et al. Clinicians' attitudes and experiences regarding telemental health services. Behavior Therapy. 2016;**39**:14-20. Available from: https://www.sciencedirect.com/science/article/abs/pii/S0005789416301161

[101] Wilson FA, Rampa S, Trout KE, et al. Telehealth delivery of mental health services: An analysis of private insurance claims data in the United States. Psychiatry Service. 2017;**68**(12):1303-1306. DOI: 10.1176/appi.ps.201700017

[102] Bunnell BE, Barrera JF, Paige SR, et al. Acceptability of telemedicine features to promote its uptake in practice: A survey of community telemental health providers. International Journal of Environmental Research and Public Health. 2020;**17**(22):8525. DOI: 10.3390/ijerph17228525. Available from: https://www.mdpi.com/1660-4601/17/22/8525

[103] Spivak S, Spivak A, Cullen B, et al. Telepsychiatry use in US mental health facilities, 2010-2017. Psychiatry Service. 2020;**71**(2):121-127. DOI: 10.1176/appi.ps.201900249

[104] Patel SY, Huskamp HA, Busch AB, et al. Telemental health and US rural-urban differences in specialty mental health use, 2010-2017. American Journal of Public Health. 2020;**110**(S2):S130-S136. DOI: 10.2105/AJPH.2020.305784

[105] Weiskittle R, Tsang W, Schwabenbauer A, Andrew N, Mlinac M. Feasibility of a COVID-19 rapid response telehealth group addressing older adult worry and social isolation. Clinical Gerontologist. 2022;**45**(1):129-143. DOI: 10.1080/07317115.2021.1906812

[106] Appleton R, Williams J, Vera San Juan N, et al. Implementation, adoption, and perceptions of telemental health during the COVID-19 pandemic: A systematic review. Journal of Medical Internet Research. 2021;**23**(12):e31746. DOI: 10.2196/31746. Available from: https://www.jmir.org/2021/12/e31746

[107] Panzirer W. Survey confirms effectiveness of telehealth in rural America and beyond. In: Health Affairs Blog. Washington, DC, United States: Project Hope; 2021. DOI: 10.1377/hblog20211019.985495

[108] Prina LL. Foundation funding in telehealth. Health Affairs. 2021. DOI: 10.1377/hlthaff.2021.00746

[109] Indian Health Service (IHS). About IHS – Indian health service (IHS). Available from: https://www.ihs.gov/ [Accessed: March 10, 2021]

[110] Chen J, Amaize A, Barath D. Evaluating telehealth adoption and related barriers among hospitals located in rural and urban areas. The Journal of Rural Health. 2020. DOI: 10.1111/jrh.12534

[111] HHS.gov. The Biden-Harris Administration is taking actions to improve the health of rural communities and help rural health care providers stay open. Available from: https://www.hhs.gov/about/news/2023/11/03/department-health-human-services-actions-support-rural-america-rural-health-care-providers.html [Accessed: November 3, 2023]

Chapter 2

Perspective Chapter: Recognition of Activities of Daily Living for Elderly People in the Era of Digital Health

Mirjam Sepesy Maučec and Gregor Donaj

Abstract

People around the world are living longer. The question arises of how to help elderly people to live longer independently and feel safe in their homes. Activity of Daily Living (ADL) recognition systems automatically recognize the daily activities of residents in smart homes. Automated monitoring of the daily routine of older individuals, detecting behavior patterns, and identifying deviations can help to identify the need for assistance. Such systems must ensure the confidentiality, privacy, and autonomy of residents. In this chapter, we review research and development in the field of ADL recognition. Breakthrough advancements have been evident in recent years with advances in sensor technology, the Internet of Things (IoT), machine learning, and artificial intelligence. We examine the main steps in the development of an ADL recognition system, introduce metrics for system evaluation, and present the latest trends in knowledge transfer and detection of behavior changes. The literature overview shows that deep learning approaches currently provide promising results. Such systems will soon mature for more diverse practical uses as transfer learning enables their fast deployment in new environments.

Keywords: digital health, elderly, activities of daily living, recognition of activities, sensors, machine learning

1. Introduction

Today, most people can expect to live over 60 years. Projections by the World Health Organization indicate that by 2050, the global population of people aged 60 and older will double. The number of persons aged 80 or older is expected to triple between 2020 and 2050 to reach 426 million. The shift in the distribution of a country's population toward older ages is known as population aging. Initially, it took place in high-income countries. However, nowadays, the most significant shifts are observed in low- and middle-income countries. Population aging has many consequences, such as increased household costs, strains on public finances and healthcare providers, and decreasing economic growth. It requires transforming healthcare services and demanding new approaches to optimize costs.

Aging is a physiological process that cannot be prevented, but efforts can be made to improve its quality. The World Health Organization defines digital health as the field of knowledge and practice associated with developing and using digital technologies to improve health. It expands the concept of eHealth to include artificial intelligence, machine learning, big data, the Internet of Things (IoT), etc. If incorporated into the broader care system, it could help elderly people and their caregivers.

As life expectancy increases, the number of requests for nursing homes increases as well, and applicants often face long waiting times because the demand exceeds available capacities. Also, many elderly people cannot afford to stay there.

It is often the case that people do not want to leave their home environment where they have spent the majority of their lives and go to a nursing home. The question is, can technology help them to stay independent and safe at home longer? Today, there is a wide range of aids that can help the elderly feel safer: emergency call necklaces, mobile phones with fall sensors, and applications to automatically notify emergency services, etc. However, these aids are mostly closed, standalone systems that the elderly often struggle to use, either because they do not know how to use them, forget to use them in critical situations, or simply forget to change or charge the batteries. When the elderly person might need help could be assessed by monitoring Activities of Daily Living (ADL) [1], which is the topic of this chapter.

The chapter is organized as follows. In Section 2, the basics of ADL recognition are described. Sensors and networks that are commonly used for ADL recognition are given in Section 3. Once the network is set up, the next step is data collection. Because this is a time-consuming and expensive task, some publicly available datasets are referenced in Section 4. Sections from 5 to 7 describe major steps in ADL recognition system construction, from data preprocessing to evaluating the final system. ADL recognition environments differ in user types, sensor technologies, and environmental conditions. Section 8 is about transfer learning approaches in which previously learned knowledge in one ADL recognition environment is utilized to model a new but related ADL recognition environment. One of the goals of ADL is early anomaly detection in user behavior. Section 9 is devoted to this topic. The chapter concludes with some problems that are still open and some ideas for future work.

2. Recognition of activities of daily living

2.1 Activities of daily living

Activities of daily living were defined in the 1950s by geriatrician Sidney Katz [2]. He determined six basic ADLs: bathing, dressing, toileting, transferring (i.e., getting in and out of a chair or bed without assistance), continence, and feeding. In the late 1960s, Instrumental ADLs were additionally defined to measure a greater range of activities needed for independence and indicate disabilities that might not show up using the ADL alone (e.g., managing finances and taking medications). Instrumental ADLs are more complex and challenging to recognize. Although both types of activities are important, basic ADLs are usually recognized by ADL recognition systems. The set of daily activities varies from study to study. Some studies, especially those based on wearable sensors, instead of basic activities, recognize movement-related activities like walking, walking upstairs, walking downstairs, sitting, standing, etc.

2.2 ADL recognition system

ADL recognition and monitoring systems in Ambient Assisted Living (AAL) environments automatically recognize the daily activities of residents in smart homes. In contrast to using elderly aids, in most cases, residents do not interact directly with such systems as they are part of their environment or installed in their homes. These systems aim to enable elderly people to live longer in their home environment, be independent, have a high quality of life, and ultimately reduce the costs of society and healthcare systems. Automated monitoring of the daily routines of older individuals could recognize early indicators of needing assistance. It is important to mention that such systems must ensure residents' confidentiality, privacy, and autonomy.

ADL recognition systems can be broadly classified into vision-based and sensor-based systems. Historically, vision-based systems appeared first. They use cameras to capture information and computer vision techniques to recognize activities. There are many issues related to these approaches. Privacy is the primary concern. Today, sensor-based approaches are much more popular due to low costs and advancements in sensor technology. These are technologies that intrude significantly less into the user's privacy. Sensor-based approaches are further divided into solutions based on wearable sensors, solutions based on sensors attached to objects, solutions based on environmental sensors, and solutions based on a combination of different types of sensors. In approaches based on wearable sensors, users must carry the sensors with them as they perform activities. As mentioned in the introduction, this could be problematic for elderly people. They do not want to use them or forget to use them. In approaches based on sensors attached to objects, users must use these objects when performing daily activities. This can also be problematic, as we force them to change their habits. The advantage of approaches based on environmental sensors is that they do not alter how a person performs any activity. These approaches bring new problems that need to be addressed, such as noise and interference in sensor data caused by the environment.

In this chapter, we focus on sensor-based approaches. The setup of the ADL recognition system for research purposes is depicted in **Figure 1**. The central part of

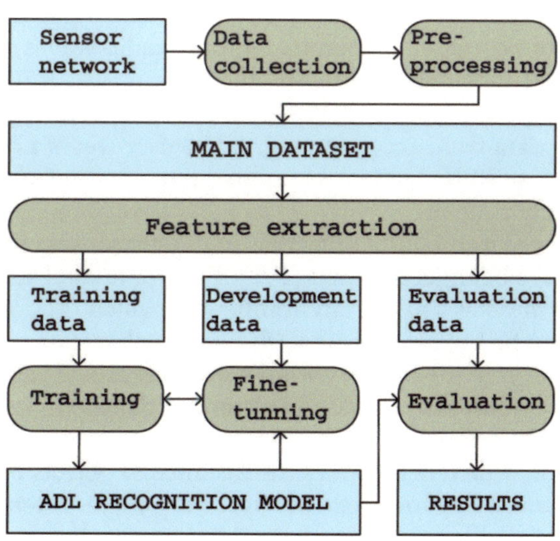

Figure 1.
General data flow for training and evaluating ADL systems.

the system is the ADL recognition model. Each step in the system's development is described in a separate section. In the continuation of the chapter, instead of ADL recognition system, we will use the term ADL system.

3. Sensors and networks

The first step in building an ADL system is selecting and deploying sensors and setting up the network for data transmission.

Wearable sensors are attached to the person's body to measure parameters of interest. Accelerometers are the most broadly used wearable sensors [3]. In some cases, they are combined with other sensors, such as a gyroscope, magnetometer, GPS, and pressure sensor. To measure physiological signals, additional biometric sensors would be required, such as those for body temperature, ECG, blood pressure, oxygen, etc. However, many of them are not useful in the context of ADL recognition. For example, after performing physically demanding activities (e.g., running), the heart rate remains high for a while, even if the individual is lying or sitting. ADL system can utilize the sensor data from a smartphone [4]. In the case of using one smartphone, we have a single point of contact. To have more of them, smartphones are combined with other wearable sensors on different body parts to capture the subject's movements fully. The popularity of wearable sensors has given rise to a new technology called Body Sensor Network (BSN). BSNs collect data from wearable sensors, process them, and extract useful information. As pointed out in the previous section, wearing sensors is not often feasible. Wearable sensors are well-suited for applications in physical therapy, enabling accurate recognition of movements. They are probably not the best choice for ADL recognition for elderly people.

Objects of daily use could be tagged with RFID tags [5]. Tags are small chips that can be easily attached to any object. These tags could be active or passive. Active tags have their own power supply, while passive tags are battery-less and harvest their energy from the radio waves of the RFID readers. Active tags have a longer range as compared to passive tags. A reader is a device employed for gathering information from RFID tags. Equipped with an antenna emitting radio waves, the reader interacts with RFID tags by receiving and modulating the radio waves. RFID tags transmit information, including their unique identifier. Data from RFID tags is commonly used in combination with data from accelerometers. The user wears a device consisting of an accelerometer and an RFID reader. As pointed out, wearing an RFID reader is problematic for elderly people.

The idea of using environmental sensors is to deploy sensors in the environment where the activities are being performed [6–8]. Environmental sensors are static devices that capture measures in the environment in which they are deployed. Environmental sensors can be binary sensors with two possible states (e.g., ON/OFF) or numerical sensors that provide values within a predetermined range. In most studies, passive infrared (PIR) sensors are utilized to monitor daily activities. With the help of this sensor, general movement or presence in a room can be detected. The next sensor is an ultrasonic sensor, which determines the distance to objects or presence in a precisely defined location due to its narrow operating angle. A temperature sensor detects changes in the ambient temperature. They can also be used near heat sources such as a stove to detect meal preparation. Magnetic sensors can be used to determine whether doors of rooms or apartments are open or closed. This can help determine which rooms the observed person has entered. The power consumption sensor indicates the use of electrical devices. A water flow sensor can show water use in a sink or shower, indicating the resident's personal care. Pressure sensors can be used on different surfaces such as the floor, chair, toilet, or under the bed mattress. Information from these sensors can reveal how much time a person has spent sitting on a chair while eating a meal or using the toilet. A carbon dioxide (CO_2) sensor can also be used to detect the presence of a person by measuring the amount of CO_2 in the room.

Careful placement of sensors at crucial locations in an apartment enables accurate recognition of activities, given that most activities are significantly dependent on their location. **Figure 2** shows the recommended sensor locations.

Communication is often the most expensive operation. Sensors in the network can be connected by wires or by wireless connections. With a wired connection, communication between sensors and the base station is very fast and reliable. However, this type of connection is only suitable for a smaller number of sensors, as wiring becomes challenging and cost-intensive for a larger number of sensors. It is much easier to use wireless connections. In most cases, short range wireless networks are preferred over long-range networks as the former require lower power, and wireless communication usually constitutes the largest part of the power consumption. Radiofrequency (RF) and WiFi technologies are the most frequently used. For RF, the frequency bands are 433 MHz and 868 MHz (in some regions, 915 MHz). In the case of WiFi, data could be exchanged on two frequency bands, at 2.4 GHz and 5 GHz. The idea is to minimize the amount of transmitted data. If feature extraction and ADL recognition are performed

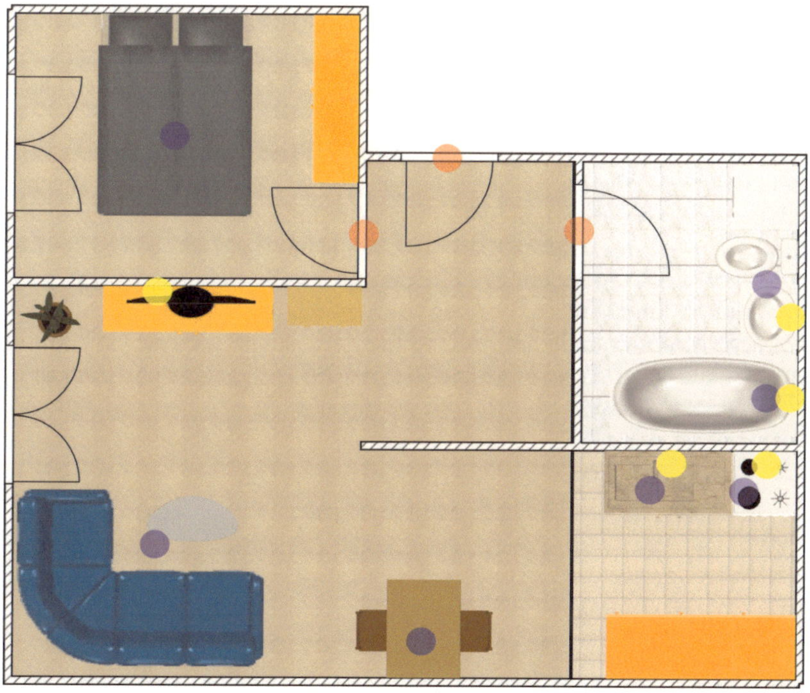

Figure 2.
Locations of environmental sensors in a hypothetical apartment. Motion sensors are marked in blue, door sensors are marked in red, and power/waterflow sensors are marked in yellow.

on integrated devices, raw signals do not have to be continuously sent to the server, and network traffic is minimized.

4. Data collections

For training ADL systems, large collections of data are needed. Collecting proprietary data is a very time-consuming and costly process. It could be avoided by using a publicly available dataset. Another advantage of using public datasets is the performance evaluation and comparison to published research. The research community has developed many datasets. We review the ones that have provided the most significant impact on the development of research related to ADL recognition.

Table 1 lists datasets where data was captured by the use of wearable sensors. The Opportunity dataset [9] allows multi-patient experimentation. Residents were monitored in the kitchen performing daily morning activities: waking up, grooming, making breakfast, and cleaning. Sensors were located on the participant's body, attached to objects, and fixed in the environment. The mHealth dataset [10] contains body motion and vital sign recordings for persons performing several physical actions, like standing still, cycling, jogging, running, jumping front and back, etc. Sensors were located on each person's chest, right wrist, and left ankle. Similar activities were performed by participants in the SBA dataset [11]. Each participant performed each activity for 3–4 minutes. Participants were equipped with five smartphones in five body positions. In the USC-HAD dataset [12], persons perform 12 different activities of the same type as in the previous two datasets. The sensing hardware was attached to the person's front right hip. All referenced datasets are labeled with activities. In recent years, datasets containing no prior labeling of the activities have been studied [13]. Interpreting and using such data imposes significant challenges in developing appropriate ADL recognition techniques.

Especially for elderly people, wearing sensors all the time is problematic. **Table 2** lists datasets where data is captured exclusively by using environmental sensors. Van Kasteren dataset [7] contains data of 14 environmental sensors that changed the state when a resident acted, for example, opened, or closed the door. The stored sensor values are binary. CASAS repository [6] contains a wide variety of datasets. Datasets differ in the number and types of sensors from which data is collected and the number and type of activities manually assigned to the data. ARAS dataset [14] contains binary sensor readings of 2 residents for 30 days. MIT [15] is a small dataset of 17 days collected with approximately 80 PIR sensors installed in everyday objects such as

Dataset	Occupancy	Size	Sensors
Opportunity [9]	12	25 hours	W + O + E
mHealth [10]	10	196,608 samples	W
SBA [11]	10	630,000 samples	W
USC-HAD [12]	14	84 hours	W

Table 1.
Datasets collected by wearable sensors. The sensors used are as follows: wearable (W), object-tagged (O), environmental (E).

Dataset	Occupancy	Size	Sensors
Van Kasteren [7]	1 (in 2 houses)	19/25 days	M, D, I
CASAS Cairo [6]	2 + dog	57 days	M, T
CASAS Milan [6]	1 + pet	72 days	M, D, T
CASAS Kyoto 7 [6]	2	46	M, D, I, B, HW, CW
CASAS Kyoto 8 [6]	2	62	M, D, I, T, Pwr
CASAS Kyoto 11 [6]	2	232	M, D, I, T, Pwr
ARAS [14]	2	30 days	F, D, M, P, L, T, IR
MIT [15]	1	17 days	I, B, D, A, HW, CW, LS

Table 2.
Datasets collected by environmental sensors. The sensors used are as follows: Motion (M, on/off), temperature (T, numeric), door, drawer, cabinet, etc. (D, open/close), item (I, present/absent), power consumption (Pwr, numeric), burner (B, on/off), hot and cold water sensors (HW and CW, numeric), light switch (LS, on/off), force/pressure (F, on/off), IR receiver (IR active/not active), appliances (a, on/off), proximity (P, on/off), light detection (L, on/off).

drawers, refrigerators, containers, etc. All datasets reported in **Table 2** contain prior labeling of user activities. Some datasets lack labels for activities, while others are only partially labeled [6].

5. Data preprocessing, feature extraction, and feature selection

Data from sensors is stored in the form of time series. Datasets collected by wearable sensors consist of raw accelerometer and gyroscope data, possibly augmented with data from other sensors. Every sensor data point is recalculated into a data point representing the relative change of the position and orientation of the sensing device.

Datasets collected by environmental sensors have different structures. **Figure 3** shows an excerpt of the CASAS Kyoto7 dataset, where each line has a time stamp, the ID of the sensor, the sensor state, and in certain cases, the start or end of the activity tag. Other datasets with environmental sensors have similar structures.

It often happens that some data is missing or disturbed by environmental noise. Some preprocessing is usually required to complete the missing data. The typical approaches to dealing with missing values include: manually adding missing values that can be trivially determined; removing the examples with missing values from the dataset (that can be done if the dataset is big enough to sacrifice some training examples); keeping data with missing values if using a machine learning algorithm for ADL recognition that can deal with missing values; using a data imputation technique to replace the missing values with average values or values in the middle of the range. In some cases, raw data is passed through a segmentation process in which the continuous sequence of sensor data is divided into individual segments. Each segment represents a specific activity.

Data preprocessing is followed by feature extraction and feature selection. A set of features with good discrimination can yield better recognition results. Various features can be extracted from the preprocessed sensor data. The same features are used in the training and evaluation of ADL systems. There are two main types of data

```
2009-02-03 06:15:36.11346    M48 OFF
2009-02-03 06:18:18.364049   M47 ON
2009-02-03 06:18:23.87538    M47 OFF    R2_bed_to_toilet end
2009-02-03 06:32:54.238749   M48 ON     R2_groom begin
2009-02-03 06:32:58.748349   M49 ON
2009-02-03 06:33:02.762109   M46 OFF
            • • • •
2009-02-03 07:07:53.272209   M48 ON
2009-02-03 07:07:53.59907    M49 ON
2009-02-03 07:07:53.764689   M44 OFF    R2_groom end
2009-02-03 08:06:10.968039   M19 ON     R1_breakfast begin
2009-02-03 08:06:12.582469   M18 ON
2009-02-03 08:06:16.502799   M19 OFF
            • • • •
2009-02-03 08:09:30.278039   D10 CLOSE
2009-02-03 08:09:35.469739   M19 ON
22009-02-03 08:09:35.93771   M18 ON
2009-02-03 08:09:44.219059   M17 OFF
2009-02-03 08:09:44.384449   M19 OFF
```

Figure 3.
Excerpt from raw sensor data in CASAS Kyoto7 dataset. Colored parts represent different activities; the dark-shaded part is an example of an error in the dataset.

features: time- and frequency-domain features. However, time-domain features are more commonly used [16]. Frequency-domain features are used in the case of wearable sensors. They have higher computation costs because of the extra Fourier transform calculation. In [17], time-domain statistical features (i.e., mean, variance, standard deviation) were combined with frequency-domain features (mel-frequency cepstral coefficients extracted from mobile phone microphone data).

When using environmental sensors, the number of features is usually the same as the number of sensors installed in a smart home. Since all the sensors are part of a feature set, the features representing inactive sensors are assigned zeros.

Not all features are helpful in recognizing the activities effectively. In the process called feature selection, the most informative features are chosen. In [18], information gain was used to identify the important sensors in multienvironment sensor data. Principal Component Analysis (PCA) was used in [19] to reduce the dimensionality of the features extracted from the accelerometer sensor embedded in a smartphone.

Feature extraction and feature selection pack data into feature vectors, which are then used as input data to train ADL recognition algorithms. If neural network models are used for ADL recognition, feature extraction and feature selection are embedded into a model, as neural networks can automatically extract the relevant features [20].

6. ADL recognition algorithms

ADL recognition can be formulated as a classification problem. The task of the ADL algorithm is to classify feature vectors into a predefined number of classes, where each class represents one activity. Different classification techniques can be applied.

The Naïve Bayes classifier was one of the first classifiers used for ADL recognition [21]. It is based on the Bayes theorem for conditional probability and assumes conditional independence of the feature vectors. It classifies feature vectors into classes by maximizing the posterior probability.

The early work on ADL also used the hidden Markov model (HMM) to recognize activities from sensor data. The basic model was advanced in different ways to model long-range dependencies. In [7], a hidden semi-Markov model (HSMM) was used, which models the duration of the hidden state. It outperformed basic HMM. Conditional random fields (CRFs) also show good performance in modeling duration. In [22], HMM was extended with a Markov chain model suitable for activity sequences, which can model longer dependencies between activities. A large number of transitions between activities were avoided by introducing the cost of activity transition.

Support vector machines (SVM) are better adapted to problems with small datasets. SVM is a binary classifier but can be transformed to solve multiclass problems. In [23], a "one-vs-rest" approach with a majority vote was used.

In [16], variants of the K-nearest neighbor (KNN) classifier were used with datasets from CASAS. One modification of KNN was based on belief assignment. The first belief represented the overall probability of an activity instance belonging to a particular activity class, and the second belief, also known as plausibility, was the conditional probability of an activity instance belonging to a particular class, given that the class of its neighbors is known. Another modification called Fuzzy KNN assigned a degree of class membership to an activity instance rather than associate the instance to a particular activity class.

In recent years, neural networks and deep learning-based methods have gained popularity. Neural networks inherently learn features from raw data, eliminate noise from data, and solve the problems of intraclass differences and interclass similarities. Convolutional neural networks (CNN) can capture the local dependency and scale invariance of a signal. In [20], CNN was used for ADL recognition using mobile sensors. Good results were obtained with the Opportunity dataset. CNNs were used with environmental sensors as well. In [24], activity data was segmented using a sliding window and then converted into binary activity images. 2D CNNs were used for classification. The architecture of the CNN classifier consisted of three convolutional layers followed by pooling layers as a feature extraction part and neural networks with three fully connected layers as a classification part. In [25], colored pixels were proposed to encode sensor information that is not binary. CNNs were also used in [18], where the spatial distance matrix was constructed, in which distances between sensors were stored. A wide time-domain CNN was applied with a larger convolution kernel size, two fully connected layers, and a softmax activation function. Increasing the convolution kernel size can capture more time-related relationships in the time-series data.

Recurrent neural networks (RNN) are suitable for processing time-series data of environmental sensors because they can remember early information in the sequence. When the time-series span is large, the phenomenon of gradient disappearance can occur. LSTM has difficulty finding a suitable time scale to balance long-term and short-term temporal dependencies. Long short-term memory (LSTM) with a stacked structure was a powerful approach in [26]. The drawback of RNN is its slow speed.

ADL system can employ different base classifiers with complementary characteristics to enhance the recognition performance [27, 28].

7. Evaluation of results

For evaluation, the data is split into three subsets: training, development, and evaluation. The ratios of the sets can be, for example, 80–10–10%. Classification models are trained using a training set, parameters are fine-tuned using a development set, and the performance of the final system is evaluated using the evaluation set. There should be no intersection between these three sets. In cases of small datasets, 3-fold cross-validation solves the problem.

Different measures assess the performance of an ADL system. The confusion matrix summarizes how successful the system is at predicting examples belonging to various activities. Rows in the confusion matrix represent the activities that the model predicted, and the columns represent the actual activities. The confusion matrix for the case of three activities is given in **Table 3**.

For a long time, accuracy was the only metric in use:

$$accuracy = \sum_{i=1}^{N} \frac{TP_i}{Total}. \tag{1}$$

Accuracy computes how many times an ADL system made a correct prediction across the entire dataset, which remains valid if the dataset is activity-balanced. In real-world scenarios, this is not the case. *Precision, recall,* and *F*1 score are better choices.

$$precision = \sum_{i=1}^{N} \frac{TP_i}{TI_i} \tag{2}$$

$$recall = \sum_{i=1}^{N} \frac{TP_i}{TT_i} \tag{3}$$

N denotes the number of activities. The accuracy, precision, and recall are calculated for each activity separately, and then the average over all activities is taken.

The F1 score combines precision and recall using their harmonic mean.

$$F1 = \frac{2 \cdot precision \cdot recall}{precision + recall} \tag{4}$$

		Predicted		
Actual	**1**	**2**	**3**	
1	TP_1	ϵ_{12}	ϵ_{13}	TT_1
2	ϵ_{21}	TP_2	ϵ_{23}	TT_2
3	ϵ_{31}	ϵ_{32}	TP_3	TT_3
	TI_1	TI_2	TI_3	Total

Table 3.
Confusion matrix. TP_i denotes true positive for class i. TT_i denotes the number of occurrences of activity i. TI_i denotes the number of times activity i was infered. ϵ_{ij} denotes the number of times activity i was predicted as activity j.

Because, in most cases, datasets are unbalanced, *weighted* $F1$ score is used.

$$weighted\,F1 = \sum_{i=1}^{N} w_i \cdot F1_i \tag{5}$$

$$w_i = \frac{TT_i}{Total} \tag{6}$$

$F1_i$ is $F1$ score of activity i.

Evaluation is closely connected to the size and characteristics of the dataset. ADL systems also differ in activity sets, approaches, and experimental setups.

Tables 4 and **5** report cited ADL systems from the literature. The effectiveness of learning techniques is not directly comparable because they use different datasets and consequently different splits into training, development, and evaluation subsets. The systems also recognize various sets of activities. There is no standard setup or benchmark (i.e., benchmark dataset) for comparable evaluation of an ADL system performance. However, the general observation is that the obtained results show promise for practical use. It is also evident that they have improved over time.

In some real-world scenarios, correct recognition of activity sequences is more important than individual activities. Therefore, it is even more difficult to compare ADL systems for evaluation.

	Sensors	Activities	Ref.
1.	Wearable	Walking, running, typing, etc.	[13]
2.	Wearable	Walking, running, typing, etc.	[13]
3.	Environmental	Brush teeth, showering, toileting etc.	[7]
4.	Environmental	Breakfast, dinner, snack, etc.	[7]
5.	Environmental	Breakfast, dinner, snack, etc.	[22]
6.	Wear. + envir. + mic.	Toilet use, eating, communication, etc.	[23]
7.	Environmental	Toilet, leave home, dinner, etc.	[16]
8.	Wearable	Jogging, walking, descending stairs, etc.	[20]
9.	Environmental	Leave home, meal preparation, relax	[24]
10.	Environmental	Leave home, dinner, laundry, etc.	[25]
11.	Environmental	Leave home, dinner, laundry, etc.	[25]
12.	Environmental	Leave home, dinner, laundry, etc.	[18]
13.	Environmental	Leave home, dinner, laundry, etc.	[18]
14.	Environmental	Leave home, sleeping, dinner, etc.	[28]
15.	Environmental	Leave home, sleeping, dinner, etc.	[28]
16.	Wearable	Walking, running, sitting, standing, etc.	[27]

Table 4.
ADL recognition systems based either on wearable or environmental sensors, except for system number 6, which utilizes both and includes speech recognition. Only a few activities are listed. For the complete list of activities, the reader is referred to the associated reference.

	Learning algorithm	Accuracy	F1
1.	KNN	—	75.73%
2.	Random forest	—	88.75%
3.	HSMM	—	76.4%
4.	CRF	—	67.0%
5.	Extended HMM	94.52%	—
6.	SVM	86%	—
7.	Fuzzy kNN	97.44%	—
8.	CNN	96.88%	—
9.	CNN	—	79%
10.	CNN	95.2%	—
11.	CNN	97.8%	—
12.	LSTM	96.46%	—
13.	CNN	97.08%	—
14.	Hybrid HMM + SVM	—	76%
15.	Hybrid HMM + NN	—	71%
16.	Ensemble	95%	—

Table 5.
*Learning algorithms used for recognizing activities in ADL systems, reported in **Table 4** along with the obtained ADL recognition results expressed as average accuracy or F1 score. Results are not directly comparable.*

8. Transfer learning

ADL systems and datasets reported in the literature are very diverse. They differ in the type of residents, sensor types and layout, environmental conditions, and activities recognized. Transfer learning is an approach in which previously learned knowledge is utilized to model a new but related setting. For example, the setting of environmental sensors in new apartments is different, or the residents in the apartment change. Transfer knowledge from one setting to the other can reduce the need to collect and label new data and to train a new recognition model from scratch.

Transfer knowledge was most frequently used with data from mobile and other wearable devices with sensors such as accelerometers and gyroscopes. Instance transfer and feature-representation transfer are the two most common techniques utilized in transfer learning.

Instance transfer was used in [29]. In their experiment, accelerometer data was collected from the user, who was asked to perform a specific task such as walking, running, and bicycle riding. Two new users did not want to label their accelerometer data. The data of the first user was reweighted by the covariate shift adaptation technique and combined with a probabilistic classification algorithm to recognize the activities of the new users. The idea of covariate shift is that even though the distributions of input points change from one user to another, the conditional distribution of class labels given input points remains unchanged.

Feature-representation transfer was applied in [8] in an experiment with two apartments. One apartment had labeled data available, while another had only unlabeled data. The arrangement and installation of sensors in both apartments were different, along with the profiles of the residents. Sensor mapping and a semi-supervised learning approach, in which labeled and unlabeled training data were combined to find the parameters for the HMM, improved the ADL recognition results.

Deep neural networks are particularly suited to transfer learning, as learning is achieved layerwise, enabling the transfer of selected layers from one network to the other. In [30], layers of the target network were progressively added, and weights of only the most recently added hidden layer and the classification layer were trained by gradient descent. All previous layers were frozen. A new hidden layer and classification layer were trained with features transferred from the source network.

9. Anomaly detection in user behavior

The existing solutions are mainly dealing with recognizing individual activities. The idea of behavior recognition is to infer a person's behavior by studying the activity sequences. Any abnormality in a person's behavior can be detected by knowing how to characterize normal behavior. This is particularly important in cases of elderly people. If abnormal behavior of an elderly person is detected, the concerned people can be informed of the situation.

There is no uniform definition of abnormal activity or abnormal behavior. In general, this is the activity or behavior that occurs rarely or is not expected to occur [31]. In literature, abnormal activities were mainly recognized through visual data [32], which is beyond the scope of the chapter.

In [5], an RFID-based system for monitoring the activities of Alzheimer's patients was set. The basic idea was to track a user's movement from one room to another and report any abnormal situation (e.g., staying in the washroom for a longer time).

With the help of medical models provided by cognitive neuroscience researchers, techniques to identify short-term and long-term abnormal activity routines were developed [33]. The focus was on instrumental ADLs. Short-term behavioral anomalies that were recognized were categorized as omissions, commissions, and additions. The omission occurs when an action or a sequence of actions that constitute an instrumental ADL is not carried out (e.g., "the elderly person forgets to consume a meal after having prepared it"). The commission occurs when instrumental activity is performed inaccurately (e.g., "putting butter in a nonrefrigerated storage"). The addition takes place when unnecessary actions are carried out to complete the current activity. (e.g., "the elderly retrieves a food item not needed for lunch preparation"). Long-term abnormal behaviors refer to groups of activities and anomalies observed over relatively extended periods (ranging from one week to several months). These behaviors exhibit significant deviations from the typical trends observed in the past and may signal the onset of cognitive impairment. Long-term abnormal behaviors were personalized and tailored to trends observed as "normal" for a specific person or person's profile. In their ADL system, different sensing devices like environmental sensors and RFID-tagged objects were used.

In [31], a causal association rule mining algorithm was proposed to detect abnormal behavior. The sensor data was annotated with anomalies by experts. Anomaly causes were afterward automatically extracted from the dataset using causal association rules. To also consider data uncertainty, a Markov logic network was used to predict anomalies. Their system also recommends suitable actions to avoid the occurrence of an actual anomaly.

Identifying the habits of a resident is crucial to distinguish between common and uncommon behavior. In [34], usual behavior patterns were defined as partitions in a clustering algorithm used with ADL data. Changes in those patterns could be declared as unusual and may be indicators of declining health.

In [35], sensor data of multiple smart home residents were investigated to detect differences between groups of people. Group-level discrepancies may help isolate behaviors that manifest in a routine of daily activities due to health problems. A framework called Behavior Change Detection for Groups was developed based on change point detection methods for analyzing changes in time series data. Experiments included two groups of people. One group contained individuals with the same health/behavioral trait, and the second group contained age-matched individuals who did not exhibit the same health/behavioral trait as the first group. Statistically significant changes were detected, including changes in duration, complexity, and pattern of ADL.

Smart home technologies provide a new paradigm to deliver remote health monitoring. In [36], a clinician-in-the-loop visual interface was designed that provides clinicians with patient behavior patterns derived from smart home data. Clinicians can observe behavior fluctuations, which allows for early detection of health events and decline. Making recommendations in the healthcare domain is not an easy task due to its complexity. In [37], a framework is presented that includes a fuzzy logic-based decision support system that provides information about the suspected disease of an elderly person and its severity. The system is based on the similarity score computed for each activity during a day concerning the same activity in the normal behavior pattern. Consequently, these scores serve as a marker for changes in the typical behavior of the elderly person during a specific activity. A significant decline in these scores over an extended period, ranging from a few days to a few weeks, could serve as an early indicator of deterioration, prompting a notification to the caregivers or family members.

10. Challenges for further work

Recognition of activities of daily living for elderly people has seen tremendous improvements. Challenges seem to be well tackled by deep learning algorithms. State-of-the-art developments are mostly based on either LSTM or CNN. However, current ADL recognition systems still have some problems that need to be addressed in the future. Multi-resident scenarios pose problems as the activities of two or more residents intertwine. Concurrent activities (i.e., multiple activities simultaneously) are also challenging for future work. Current systems can also not cope with the variability between different residents in performing the same activity. If a different person performs the same activity or the same person performs the activity at a different pace, the performance of a system degrades.

Recent advances in machine learning from other fields offer opportunities for significant advances in smart homes. For example, advances in natural language processing could be adopted to infer semantic knowledge between activities [38].

Fusing data from heterogeneous sources is also a challenge, as it has been shown that a model developed using one data type does not perform well with other data types. There is still a lack of real data collected with residents who have developed signs of dementia or cognitive ability loss in general.

Many challenges still have to be faced for ADL recognition and monitoring systems to be deployed in real-use cases. The research community needs to define benchmarks and standardize the evaluation metrics to reflect the requirements for a real-use deployment and enable fair algorithm comparison.

11. Conclusion

In this chapter, we reviewed the core literature on methods and systems for ADL recognition. After a thorough literature review, we can conclude that the field has developed rapidly in the last two decades. If enough data is available, deep learning and neural network architectures provide very good results. In cases where we do not have enough data, transfer learning could mitigate the problem.

ADL systems based on environmental sensors are better accepted among final users as they do not unveil too much private information. Their advantage is also that they do not require a change in the way the residents perform daily activities. However, social barriers still impede the adoption of smart homes and must be addressed in the future. Overcoming these barriers necessitates trustworthy privacy-preserving data management and reliable cyber-secure ADL systems.

Acknowledgements

This work was supported by the Slovenian Research and Innovation Agency ARIS (research core funding No.P2-0069-Advanced Methods of Interaction in Telecommunications).

Author details

Mirjam Sepesy Maučec* and Gregor Donaj
University of Maribor, Slovenia

*Address all correspondence to: mirjam.sepesy@um.si

References

[1] Mlinac ME, Feng MC. Assessment of activities of daily living, self-care, and independence. Archives of Clinical Neuropsychology. 2016;**31**(6):506-516

[2] Wallace M, Shelkey M, et al. Katz index of independence in activities of daily living (ADL). Urologic Nursing. 2007;**27**(1):93-94

[3] Lara OD, Labrador MA. A survey on human activity recognition using wearable sensors. IEEE Communications Surveys & Tutorials. 2012;**15**(3): 1192-1209

[4] Shoaib M, Bosch S, Incel OD, Scholten H, Havinga PJ. A survey of online activity recognition using mobile phones. Sensors. 2015;**15**(1):2059-2085

[5] Raad MW, Sheltami T, Soliman MA, Alrashed M. An RFID based activity of daily living for elderly with Alzheimer's. In: Internet of Things (IoT) Technologies for HealthCare: 4th International Conference, HealthyIoT 2017; October 24-25, 2017; Angers, France, Proceedings 4. Angers, France: Springer; 2018. pp. 54-61

[6] Cook DJ, Crandall AS, Thomas BL, Krishnan NC. CASAS: A smart home in a box. Computer. 2012;**46**(7):62-69

[7] Van Kasteren T, Englebienne G, Kröse BJ. Activity recognition using semi-Markov models on real world smart home datasets. Journal of Ambient Intelligence and Smart Environments. 2010;**2**(3):311-325

[8] van Kasteren T, Englebienne G, Kröse BJ, et al. Recognizing activities in multiple contexts using transfer learning. In: AAAI Fall Symposium: AI in Eldercare: New Solutions to Old Problems. Washington, DC, USA: Association for the Advancement of Artificial Intelligence; 2008. pp. 142-149

[9] Roggen D, Calatroni A, Rossi M, Holleczek T, Förster K, Tröster G, et al. Collecting complex activity datasets in highly rich networked sensor environments. In: 2010 Seventh International Conference on Networked Sensing Systems (INSS). Kassel, Germany: IEEE; 2010. pp. 233-240

[10] Banos O, Garcia R, Holgado-Terriza JA, Damas M, Pomares H, Rojas I, et al. mHealthDroid: A novel framework for agile development of mobile health applications. In: Ambient Assisted Living and Daily Activities: 6th International Work-Conference, IWAAL 2014; December 2-5, 2014; Belfast, UK Proceedings 6. Belfast, United Kingdom: Springer; 2014. pp. 91-98

[11] Shoaib M, Bosch S, Incel OD, Scholten H, Havinga PJ. Fusion of smartphone motion sensors for physical activity recognition. Sensors. 2014; **14**(6):10146-10176

[12] Zhang M, Sawchuk AA. USC-HAD: A daily activity dataset for ubiquitous activity recognition using wearable sensors. In: Proceedings of the 2012 ACM Conference on Ubiquitous Computing. Pittsburgh, PA, United States: Association for Computing Machinery; pp. 1036, 2012-1043

[13] Bai L, Yeung C, Efstratiou C, Chikomo M. Motion2Vector: Unsupervised learning in human activity recognition using wrist-sensing data. In: Adjunct Proceedings of the 2019 ACM International Joint Conference on Pervasive and Ubiquitous Computing and Proceedings of the 2019 ACM International Symposium on Wearable Computers. London, United Kingdom:

Association for Computing Machinery; 2019. pp. 537-542

[14] Alemdar H, Ertan H, Incel OD, Ersoy C. ARAS human activity datasets in multiple homes with multiple residents. In: 2013 7th International Conference on Pervasive Computing Technologies for Healthcare and Workshops. Venice, Italy: IEEE; 2013. pp. 232-235

[15] Tapia EM, Intille SS, Larson K. Activity recognition in the home using simple and ubiquitous sensors. In: International Conference on Pervasive Computing. Vienna, Austria: Springer; 2004. pp. 158-175

[16] Fahad LG, Tahir SF. Activity recognition in a smart home using local feature weighting and variants of nearest-neighbors classifiers. Journal of Ambient Intelligence and Humanized Computing. 2021;**12**:2355-2364

[17] Ferreira JM, Pires IM, Marques G, Garcia NM, Zdravevski E, Lameski P, et al. Activities of daily living and environment recognition using mobile devices: A comparative study. Electronics. 2020;**9**(1):180

[18] Li Y, Yang G, Su Z, Li S, Wang Y. Human activity recognition based on multienvironment sensor data. Information Fusion. 2023;**91**:47-63

[19] Sukor AA, Zakaria A, Rahim NA. Activity recognition using accelerometer sensor and machine learning classifiers. In: 2018 IEEE 14th International Colloquium on Signal Processing & its Applications (CSPA). Penang, Malaysia: IEEE; 2018. pp. 233-238

[20] Zeng M, Nguyen LT, Yu B, Mengshoel OJ, Zhu J, Wu P, et al. Convolutional neural networks for human activity recognition using mobile sensors. In: In 6th International Conference on Mobile Computing, Applications and Services. Austin, TX, United States: IEEE; 2014. pp. 197-205

[21] Chen L, Hoey J, Nugent CD, Cook DJ, Yu Z. Sensor-based activity recognition. IEEE Transactions on Systems, Man, and Cybernetics, Part C (Applications and Reviews). 2012;**42**(6): 790-808

[22] Donaj G, Maučec MS. Extension of HMM-based ADL recognition with Markov chains of activities and activity transition cost. IEEE Access. 2019;**7**: 130650-130662

[23] Fleury A, Vacher M, Noury N. SVM-based multimodal classification of activities of daily living in health smart homes: Sensors, algorithms, and first experimental results. IEEE Transactions on Information Technology in Biomedicine. 2009;**14**(2):274-283

[24] Gochoo M, Tan T-H, Liu S-H, Jean F-R, Alnajjar FS, Huang S-C. Unobtrusive activity recognition of elderly people living alone using anonymous binary sensors and DCNN. IEEE Journal of Biomedical and Health Informatics. 2018;**23**(2):693-702

[25] Tan T-H, Gochoo M, Huang S-C, Liu Y-H, Liu S-H, Huang Y-F. Multi-resident activity recognition in a smart home using RGB activity image and DCNN. IEEE Sensors Journal. 2018;**18**(23): 9718-9727

[26] Liciotti D, Bernardini M, Romeo L, Frontoni E. A sequential deep learning application for recognising human activities in smart homes. Neurocomputing. 2020;**396**:501-513

[27] Khowaja SA, Yahya BN, Lee S-L. Hierarchical classification method based on selective learning of slacked hierarchy

for activity recognition systems. Expert Systems with Applications. 2017;**88**: 165-177

[28] Ordónez FJ, De Toledo P, Sanchis A. Activity recognition using hybrid generative/discriminative models on home environments using binary sensors. Sensors. 2013;**13**(5):5460-5477

[29] Hachiya H, Sugiyama M, Ueda N. Importance-weighted least-squares probabilistic classifier for covariate shift adaptation with application to human activity recognition. Neurocomputing. 2012;**80**:93-101

[30] Du X, Farrahi K, Niranjan M. Transfer learning across human activities using a cascade neural network architecture. In: Proceedings of the 2019 ACM International Symposium on Wearable Computers. London, United Kingdom: Association for Computing Machinery; 2019. pp. 35-44

[31] Hela S, Amel B, Badran R. Early anomaly detection in smart home: A causal association rule-based approach. Artificial Intelligence in Medicine. 2018; **91**:57-71

[32] Dhiman C, Vishwakarma DK. A review of state-of-the-art techniques for abnormal human activity recognition. Engineering Applications of Artificial Intelligence. 2019;**77**:21-45

[33] Riboni D, Civitarese G, Bettini C. Analysis of long-term abnormal behaviors for early detection of cognitive decline. In: 2016 IEEE International Conference on Pervasive Computing and Communication Workshops (PerCom Workshops). Sydney, Australia: IEEE; 2016. pp. 1-6

[34] Sepesy Maučec M, Donaj G. Discovering daily activity patterns from sensor data sequences and activity sequences. Sensors. 2021;**21**(20):6920

[35] Sprint G, Cook DJ, Fritz R. Behavioral differences between subject groups identified using smart homes and change point detection. IEEE Journal of Biomedical and Health Informatics. 2020;**25**(2):559-567

[36] Ghods A, Caffrey K, Lin B, Fraga K, Fritz R, Schmitter-Edgecombe M, et al. Iterative design of visual analytics for a clinician-in-the-loop smart home. IEEE Journal of Biomedical and Health Informatics. 2018;**23**(4):1742-1748

[37] Zekri D, Delot T, Thilliez M, Lecomte S, Desertot M. A framework for detecting and analyzing behavior changes of elderly people over time using learning techniques. Sensors. 2020; **20**(24):7112

[38] Bouchabou D, Nguyen SM, Lohr C, LeDuc B, Kanellos I. A survey of human activity recognition in smart homes based on IoT activity recognition using semi-Markov models on real world smart home datasets. Sensors algorithms: Taxonomies, challenges, and opportunities with deep learning. Sensors. 2021;**21**(18):6037

Chapter 3

Exploring Telemedicine: The Perceptions and Utilization among Patients

Rabih Hajj and Joy Hanoun

Abstract

This chapter explores into the dynamic terrain of telemedicine, focusing on the nuanced perceptions and usage trends across a diverse patient population. Through a careful examination of cultural influences, technological intricacies and regulatory framework, it seeks to provide a holistic understanding of how patients interact with telemedicine. By exploring how cultural nuances can shape attitudes, assessing the impact of technology on accessibility, and navigating the regulatory landscape, the chapter provides key insights. Ultimately, it aims to contribute to a comprehensive understanding of patient engagement with telemedicine, highlighting potential implications for healthcare practice and policy considerations in this evolving landscape of telehealth.

Keywords: telemedicine, perceptions, utilization, telehealth, cultural factors, regulations, patient engagement

1. Introduction

Telemedicine adoption has skyrocketed in recent years experiencing an unprecedented surge that has been catalyzed in particular by the global COVID-19 pandemic. As reported by a study of Ray et al. in the Journal of Medical Internet Research, a 154 per cent increase in the number of telemedicine visits during the last week of March 2020, compared to the same period in 2019 [1].

One of the key benefits of telemedicine is its ability to bridge the gap in access to healthcare by bringing vital healthcare services to remote and underserved areas, reducing travel time and associated costs for patients. It has dramatically improved access to care for patients in rural areas where healthcare facilities are often scarce [2].

The acceptance and perception of telemedicine by both patients and providers are vital for its adoption. A McKinsey & Company study in 2020 highlighted a dramatic increase in its use among both consumers and providers compared to the previous year [3]. However, despite these positive trends, privacy and security concerns continue to pose significant challenges, underscoring the necessity for stringent cybersecurity measures and adherence to regulations like HIPAA in the United States to maintain patient trust [4].

Telemedicine is not just a temporary response to a global crisis, but a fundamental component of future healthcare. Its growing importance, driven by technological advances, regulatory support, and the changing nature of the, and changing perceptions, marks a transformative stage in healthcare delivery.

2. The cultural influences on perception of telemedicine

Cultural factors significantly shape patient attitudes towards telemedicine. Deeply embedded in societal norms and values, these influences can facilitate or hinder the acceptance and use of telemedicine services.

Cultural attitudes and perceptions significantly influence telemedicine acceptance, shaped by how different cultures view health and healthcare. For instance, in Middle Eastern cultures, where there's a strong emphasis on physical presence in healthcare, the inclination towards telemedicine is lower, as found in a study by Al Ghamdi et al. [5]. For instance, this study reported that only 20% of surveyed patients in a Middle Eastern country were willing to use telemedicine services compared to 80% in South Korea, vividly highlighting the cultural disparity. In contrast, technologically advanced societies like South Korea show a greater tendency to embrace telemedicine, indicating cultural variability. Moreover, trust and privacy concerns vary across cultures, affecting the adoption of telemedicine. A German study by Zimmermann revealed higher skepticism towards digital healthcare due to privacy concerns compared to Scandinavian countries where there's more trust in digital services [6]. In this paper, 70% of German respondents expressed concerns about data privacy in telehealth, compared to only 30% in Scandinavian countries, thus quantifying the cultural impact on trust and privacy perceptions. This disparity significantly impacts telemedicine's uptake in different regions. Language barriers also play a crucial role, as non-native English speakers in the U.S. often struggle with telehealth services, leading to miscommunication, as highlighted by Torres et al. [7]. Offering multilingual services and culturally competent providers can mitigate these issues. Health literacy and technology familiarity, influenced by cultural and educational backgrounds, also affect telemedicine usage, as patients with lower health literacy have difficulties understanding the technology. Finally, the socio-economic and digital divide, linked to cultural contexts, plays a role. A World Bank report [8] notes that in cultures with a significant digital divide, 40% of individuals in lower socio-economic groups have access to the necessary technology for telehealth compared to 90% in higher brackets, thus underlining the intersection of cultural and economic factors [8].

The intersection of cultural factors with telehealth highlights the need for culturally sensitive telehealth services. Understanding these nuances is critical for healthcare providers and policy makers to design and implement telehealth solutions that are effective and equitable across diverse.

3. The impact of technology on patient utilization of telemedicine

The impact of technology on patient utilization of telemedicine can indeed be expanded upon, especially by diving deeper into specific aspects such as accessibility, patient engagement, data management, and the overall shift towards a patient-centered healthcare model.

Telemedicine technologies, especially in remote or underserved areas, have reduced barriers to healthcare access. For instance, mobile health applications enable patients to consult healthcare professionals without the need for physical travel. A study by Totten et al. highlighted that telemedicine had a significant positive impact on rural healthcare delivery, offering services previously unavailable in these areas [9].

Technologies like interactive patient portals and video conferencing tools have enhanced patient engagement. These platforms offer personalized healthcare experiences, enabling patients to be active participants in their health management. A report in the " Journal of Health Policy and Management" found that interactive telemedicine tools lead to higher patient satisfaction and engagement, fostering a more collaborative patient-provider relationship [10].

Wearable devices and health monitoring apps have revolutionized the way health data is managed and monitored. These technologies provide real-time health data, facilitating proactive disease management. A study by Mattison et al. demonstrated that continuous data monitoring via wearable technology significantly improves chronic disease management by providing patients and healthcare providers with timely and accurate health information [11].

The integration of technology in healthcare has been pivotal in transitioning towards a more patient-centered model. Telemedicine offers tailored healthcare solutions, respecting patients' preferences and needs. A research by Rubeis et al. suggests that telemedicine has been instrumental in making healthcare more patient-centric, leading to better health outcomes and increased patient autonomy [12].

Telemedicine effectively addresses issues like geographical distance and time constraints. This is particularly crucial for patients with mobility issues or those living in areas with limited healthcare facilities. A publication in the "Journal of Medical Internet Research" emphasized how telemedicine has made healthcare more accessible and convenient, especially for patients with chronic conditions requiring regular consultations [13].

In summary, the technological advancements in telemedicine have significantly enhanced patient accessibility, engagement, and the overall quality of healthcare delivery. These changes mark a substantial shift towards a more efficient, effective, and patient-centered healthcare system.

4. The impact of regulations on perception and utilization of telemedicine

The regulatory environment surrounding telemedicine has a significant impact on its adoption and use, affecting patient confidence and access to healthcare services. A study published in Nutrition in Clinical Practice reviewed legislative and regulatory changes and discussed issues such as disparities in access to telehealth, payment for telehealth versus in-person care, and concerns about fraud, quality and safety. This study illustrated how regulatory frameworks affect the delivery and effectiveness of telehealth services [14].

In discussing the regulatory barriers to telehealth before and after COVID-19, the importance of data collection on telehealth administrators and programmers and the need for regulatory flexibility to accommodate a range of use cases was highlighted. The recommendations were to use telehealth services for primary care to avoid redundant services. The impact of regulation on the role of telehealth in healthcare delivery was also discussed [15].

These sources suggest that the regulatory landscape is a critical factor in shaping the future of telehealth. Regulations play an important role in determining how telemedicine is implemented and perceived, and influence patient confidence and healthcare utilization. The ongoing evolution of these regulations, particularly in response to the COVID-19 pandemic, continues to shape the telehealth landscape, presenting both challenges and opportunities for healthcare providers and patients.

Another critical aspect of healthcare delivery is the influence of regulatory frameworks on patient confidence and, thus, use of telehealth services. Regulations affect various facets of telemedicine, including patient privacy, data security, service quality and accessibility.

1. *Patient privacy and data security*: Patient confidence can be enhanced by strong regulatory standards that ensure patient privacy and data security. For example, compliance with regulations such as HIPAA in the United States reassures patients that their sensitive health information is protected. When patients feel confident about the security of their data, they are more likely to use telehealth services [16].

2. *Quality of service and professional standards*: Patients' confidence in telemedicine services can be enhanced by regulations requiring certain quality and professional standards for telemedicine services. For example, requiring providers to be licensed and to adhere to specific standards of practice for telemedicine can increase patient confidence, leading to higher utilization rates [17].

3. *Accessibility and reimbursement policies*: Patient uptake can be significantly influenced by policies that expand insurance coverage and reimbursement for telehealth services. For example, changes in Medicare policy in the US during the COVID-19 pandemic, which allowed broader coverage of telehealth services, led to a significant increase in the use of these services [18].

4. *International licensure*: Regulations that facilitate or restrict the ability of health care providers to offer telemedicine services across state lines and countries borders can also have an impact on the use of telemedicine. Facilitating cross-state licensure can expand access to telehealth services, particularly for people in remote or underserved areas, potentially increasing utilization [19].

Overall, a regulatory environment that prioritizes patient safety, data security and accessibility of telehealth services is likely to foster greater patient confidence and higher utilization rates. Ongoing adjustments and updates to these regulations are essential to keep pace with technological advances and evolving healthcare needs [20].

5. Patient engagement and experience

Patients have increasingly embraced telemedicine for its convenience, accessibility and time-saving benefits, particularly those in remote areas or with mobility issues. Research suggests that patient satisfaction is higher due to the ease of accessing healthcare services from home and the efficiency of consultations. A study in the Journal of Telemedicine and Telecare highlights the positive impact of telemedicine in the management of chronic conditions, highlighting the benefits of convenience and reduced travel [21].

Despite these benefits, telemedicine also presents challenges, including technical issues, reduced face-to-face interaction with healthcare providers, and concerns about quality of care and privacy. Some patients, particularly the elderly or those less familiar with technology, may feel uncomfortable with virtual consultations. This issue is highlighted in a Health Affairs study, which emphasizes the need for user-friendly technology and better patient education to improve the usability of telemedicine [22].

Telemedicine has significantly improved access to and engagement in health care, particularly for chronic disease management and for remote or underserved populations. High levels of satisfaction have been reported due to the convenience and comfort of receiving care at home. For example, telemedicine has been shown to be effective in rural mental health services and in the management of chronic conditions such as diabetes that require continuous monitoring [23].

However, improvements are needed, including overcoming the digital divide, ensuring the quality of care is equivalent to face-to-face visits, and better integrating telehealth into health systems. Overcoming technical barriers, privacy issues, and improving patient and provider education in the use of telemedicine are critical to its optimization [24].

In conclusion, although telemedicine has significantly improved healthcare, concerted efforts are needed to address its current limitations and fully realize its potential in healthcare.

6. Challenges and solutions

The challenges to the use of telehealth are many and varied and include technology barriers, socio-demographic barriers and language barriers. The RAND Corporation report highlights a preference for audio-only telehealth in behavioral health services, particularly among non-white and older people, due to technology access issues. Digital literacy is a key challenge. It particularly affects vulnerable populations and those without stable housing. Broadband access remains a significant barrier, affecting millions in the U.S.

Language barriers further complicate the use of telehealth, with limited English proficiency leading to reduced use of video-based services. Addressing these challenges requires a comprehensive approach, including the provision of bilingual staff and video interpretation services, to ensure telehealth is accessible and effective for diverse patient populations. This approach is a step towards creating more inclusive and equitable telehealth solutions [25].

Practical solutions and strategies to overcome the challenges of using telemedicine include increasing digital literacy through patient education programs, expanding broadband access, especially in underserved areas, and providing technological support such as medical assistants to help with videoconferencing. Implementing bilingual staff and video interpretation services can overcome language barriers and ensure inclusivity. In addition, adapting telehealth platforms to be user-friendly for diverse populations, including the elderly, and raising awareness of the benefits of telehealth can also encourage wider use. For broader solutions to telehealth challenges, consider initiatives such as community-based digital training to improve technological literacy, partnerships with technology companies to provide affordable devices and internet services, and policy advocacy for telehealth-friendly legislation. Working with patient advocacy groups can help tailor services to specific needs, while feedback mechanisms allow for continuous improvement. It's also vital to integrate telehealth into mainstream healthcare services to ensure seamless continuity of care and collaboration between providers.

A multi-faceted approach is needed to develop solutions to overcome the challenges of telemedicine. This includes:

1. *Partnerships with educational institutions*: Work with schools and community colleges to offer digital literacy courses specifically tailored to telehealth.

2. *Telehealth training for healthcare providers*: Equip healthcare professionals with the skills to effectively conduct telehealth visits, addressing both technical and patient communication aspects.

3. *Public awareness campaigns*: Widespread campaigns to educate the public about the benefits and use of telemedicine, dispelling myths and addressing privacy concerns.

4. *Investment in telemedicine infrastructure*: Advocate for increased funding and investment in telehealth infrastructure, especially in rural and underserved communities.

7. Telemedicine perception future implications

The future impact of evolving telemedicine trends on patient care covers several key areas. With advances in technology, better perception and wider acceptance, telemedicine is poised to significantly improve access to healthcare, particularly in remote or underserved regions. It offers the potential for more personalized and convenient care, greater patient engagement and improved chronic disease management. However, it also brings challenges such as ensuring quality of care, addressing privacy concerns and maintaining the human touch in patient interactions. As telehealth trends continue to evolve, they are likely to reshape the healthcare landscape, making it more accessible, efficient and patient-centered.

The evolving trends in telehealth have significant implications for various stakeholders. Healthcare providers have the opportunity to expand their reach and streamline care delivery, but they must adapt to new technologies and maintain patient trust. Policymakers play a critical role in shaping regulations and infrastructure investments to support the growth of telemedicine. Technology developers must innovate and create user-friendly, secure solutions to meet the evolving needs of healthcare providers and patients in the changing healthcare landscape. These collaborative efforts are essential to ensure the continued advancement of telemedicine and its positive impact on patient care.

8. Conclusion

Telemedicine has developed rapidly, driven by technology and regulatory changes. It offers improved access to healthcare, particularly in remote areas. The various forms of telemedicine, including live video conferencing and remote patient monitoring, improve patient-centered care. However, cultural influences, digital literacy and language barriers affect its uptake. Patients appreciate the convenience, but face challenges such as technical issues. Overcoming these challenges requires digital literacy programs, increased broadband access, bilingual support, user-friendly platforms and public awareness campaigns. The future impact of telemedicine includes more accessible and personalized care, but will require continued efforts to address the challenges. Healthcare providers, policy makers and technology developers must work together to shape its future positively.

Acknowledgements

The authors wish to acknowledge the general support and resources provided which facilitated the completion of this project. While this work did not receive any specific grant from funding agencies in the public, commercial, or not-for-profit sectors, the contributions of our peers and colleagues in providing an intellectually stimulating environment are greatly appreciated.

Conflict of interest

The authors declare no conflict of interest.

Author details

Rabih Hajj[1*] and Joy Hanoun[2,3]

1 Bellevue Medical Center, Mansourieh, Lebanon

2 Antonine University, Baabda, Lebanon

3 Faculty of Medicine, EpiMaCT, Institute of Epidemiology and Tropical Neurology, Limoges University, France

*Address all correspondence to: rabihhajj@gmail.com

References

[1] Ray KN, Wittman SR, Burns S, Doan TT, Schweiberger KA, Yabes JG, et al. Parent-reported use of pediatric primary care telemedicine: Survey study. Journal of Medical Internet Research. 2023;**25**:e42892. DOI: 10.2196/42892

[2] Haleem A, Javaid M, Singh RP, Suman R. Telemedicine for healthcare: Capabilities, features, barriers, and applications. Sensors International. 2021;**2**:100117. DOI: 10.1016/j.sintl.2021.100117

[3] McKinsey & Company. Telehealth: A quarter-trillion-dollar post-COVID-19 reality? [Rapport]. 2020. Available from: https://www.mckinsey.com/industries/healthcare/our-insights/telehealth-a-quarter-trillion-dollar-post-covid-19-reality#/

[4] Privacy and security risk factors related to telehealth services – A systematic Review. Perspectives in Health Information Management. Available from: https://perspectives.ahima.org/privacy-and-security-risk-factors-related-to-telehealth-services-a-systematic-review/

[5] Alghamdi K, Aljohani A, Taha J, Qari L, Demyati M, Alzahrani S. Public awareness and utilization of the primary health care services in Al-Madinah, Saudi Arabia. Middle East Journal of Family Medicine. 2020;**18**(2):33-41

[6] Zimmermann BM, Fiske A, Prainsack B, Hangel N, McLennan S, Buyx A. Early perceptions of COVID-19 contact tracing apps in German-speaking countries: Comparative mixed methods study. Journal of Medical Internet Research. 2021;**23**(2):e25525

[7] Pinedo-Torres I, Garcia-Villasante EJ, Gutierrez-Ortiz CC et al. The doctor-patient relationship and barriers in non-verbal communication during teleconsultation in the era of COVID-19: A scoping review [version 1; peer review: 2 approved with reservations]. F1000Research. 2023;**12**:676. DOI: 10.12688/f1000research.129970.1

[8] World Bank. Socioeconomic impact on digital health adoption. 2020

[9] Totten AM, Womack DM, Griffin JC, McDonagh MS, Davis-O'Reilly C, Blazina I, et al. Telehealth-guided provider-to-provider communication to improve rural health: A systematic review. Journal of Telemedicine and Telecare, 1357633X221139892. 2022. DOI: 10.1177/1357633X221139892

[10] Atmojo JT, Sudaryanto WT, Widiyanto A, Ernawati E, Arradini D. Telemedicine, cost effectiveness, and patient's satisfaction: A systematic review. Journal of Health Policy and Management. 2020;**5**(2):103-107. Available from: https://thejhpm.com/index.php/thejhpm/article/view/172

[11] Mattison G, Canfell O, Forrester D, Dobbins C, Smith D, Töyräs J, et al. The influence of wearables on health care outcomes in chronic disease: Systematic review. Journal of Medical Internet Research. 2022;**24**(7):e36690. DOI: 10.2196/36690

[12] Rubeis G, Schochow M, Steger F. Patient autonomy and quality of care in telehealthcare. Science and Engineering Ethics. 2018;**24**(1):93-107. DOI: 10.1007/s11948-017-9885-3

[13] Lewinski AA, Walsh C, Rushton S, Soliman D, Carlson SM, Luedke MW, et al. Telehealth for the longitudinal

management of chronic conditions: Systematic review. Journal of Medical Internet Research. 2022;**24**(8):e37100. DOI: 10.2196/37100

[14] Shah ND, Krupinski EA, Bernard J, Moyer MF. Regulatory and legislative issues on telehealth. Nutrition in Clinical Practice. 2021;**36**(4):739-749. DOI: 10.1002/ncp.10740

[15] Milne R, Costa A. Disruption and dislocation in post-COVID futures for digital health. Big data & society. 2020;**7**(2):2053951720949567. DOI: 10.1177/2053951720949567

[16] Wright JH, Caudill R. Remote treatment delivery in response to the COVID-19 pandemic. Psychotherapy and Psychosomatics. 2020;**89**(3):130-132. DOI: 10.1159/000507376

[17] Snoswell CL, Caffery LJ. The role of telehealth in reducing the mental health burden from COVID-19. Telemedicine and e-Health. 2020;**26**(4):377-379. DOI: 10.1089/tmj.2020.0068

[18] Dorsey ER, Topol EJ. Telemedicine 2020 and the next decade. The Lancet. 2020;**395**(10227):859. DOI: 10.1016/S0140-6736(20)30424-4

[19] Yellowlees P, Shore JH. Telepsychiatry and Health Technologies: A guide for mental health professionals. Washington, D.C.: American Psychiatric Publishing; 2018

[20] Keesara S, Jonas A, Schulman K. Covid-19 and health care's digital revolution. New England Journal of Medicine. 2020;**382**(23):e82. DOI: 10.1056/NEJMp2005835

[21] Smith AC, Caffery LJ. Patient perceptions of telehealth services for the management of chronic conditions: A review of reviews. Journal of Telemedicine and Telecare. 2020;**26**(5):311-321. DOI: 10.1177/1357633X20930495

[22] Anderson M, Perrin A. Tech adoption climbs among older adults. Health Affairs. 2020;**39**(5):850-857. DOI: 10.1377/hlthaff.2020.01245

[23] Sands DZ. Beyond the EHR: How digital health tools foster participatory health and self-care for patients with diabetes. American Journal of Medicine Open. 2023;**10**:100043. ISSN: 2667-0364. DOI: 10.1016/j.ajmo.2023.100043

[24] Bashshur RL, Howell JD, Krupinski EA, Harms KM, Bashshur N, Doarn CR. The empirical foundations of telemedicine interventions in primary care. Telemedicine and e-Health. 2020;**26**(5):579-599. DOI: 10.1089/tmj.2019.0187

[25] mHealth Intelligence. Understanding key telehealth disparities & patient-facing barriers. mHealth Intelligence. 6 May 2022. Available from: https://www.ncbi.nlm.nih.gov/pmc/articles/PMC7857524/

Section 2

Technologies

Chapter 4

Analysis and Development of Telemonitoring Applications: A Model-Based Approach

Michael John, Juan Vito-Antonio Held, Nele Sassor and Michael Wagner

Abstract

In our article, we introduce a method for the model-based analysis and development of telemonitoring applications for the German healthcare system. Based on data from two exemplary telemonitoring applications in the fields of Parkinson's disease and heart failure, we show which barriers exist to the widespread introduction of digital health applications (DHA) and what positive effects a consistent digitization of the interacting IT components and process steps would have. The method presented combines approaches from process modeling using business process model and notation (BPMN) and the consistent application of quality metrics to the modeled processes, the actors involved, and the IT components used or to be developed. By modeling different evolutionary stages of digitalization of medical care processes, the positive effects and possible barriers in terms of resource consumption, effectiveness, security, and efficiency can be identified on the basis of the metrics used. The aim of the article is to use the developed methods to identify critical process steps at an early stage of product development or transition from a research project to standard care and to identify potential for improvement in the interaction between organizations, service providers, patients, and technology providers.

Keywords: telemonitoring-applications, business process modeling, model-based metrics and software development, telemedicine, telematics infrastructure, Parkinson's disease, cardiology

1. Introduction

The digitalization of the German healthcare system is still at a low level compared to other European countries [1, 2]. Examples of this are the physician's letter, medical prescriptions, doctor's appointments, or the storage of treatment and personal health data [3]. While it was possible to provide unlimited treatment services with the help of video consultations during the coronavirus pandemic, this exceptional arrangement has been limited again to 30 percent of the number of cases and service volumes [4]. According to recent surveys, a majority of German citizen welcome the use of digital medical solutions [5, 6], digital or telemedical health applications

(DHA) that enable patients to manage themselves. Nevertheless, DHAs primarily focusing on therapy-supporting processes so far have not been widely used to date [7].

The reasons for this are mainly the skepticism of the healthcare providers towards new, digital applications, the lack of evidence due to heterogeneous or inconsistent data from clinical studies, the complexity of DHAs, and the sometimes-missing therapeutic adherence of the patients themselves. As of today there exist a large number of telehealth applications that are used in projects or operated on the basis of selective contracts. So far they have not yet been integrated into standard care, at least not into the German healthcare system. In addition, the current Telematics Infrastructure 1.0 of the German healthcare system prevents the integration of mobile and telemedical solutions from third-party providers due to the restrictive, hardware-based access of the eHC to the secured network [8].

Only a comprehensive, end-to-end digitalized healthcare system offers the advantage of reducing frequent media disruptions and thus accelerating process chains between doctors, patients, health insurance companies, and manufacturers. In order to intensify the use of digital health applications, the necessary awareness and user skills also must be improved on both, doctor's and patient's side. In a broader context, this also requires the digitalization of administrative processes in health care so that both doctors and patients experience positive user experiences.

The German government recognized this challenge and took up several political initiatives in order to accelerate the end-to-end digitalization of the German healthcare system. With the corresponding legislative procedures, the Federal Ministry of Health has recently shown how a common platform for digital applications can be established in Germany's federal and self-governing healthcare system [9–11]. At a technical level, the first underlying conditions for this have already been defined by the integration of DHAs into the German telematics infrastructure (TI) [8]. For example, approved DHAs will in future have to write their recorded health data into the electronic patient record (ePA) via a backend interface according to Section 374a SGB V [12]. The establishment of standardized data structures (so-called DiGA MIOs [13]), e.g., for the integration of measurement data from medical devices or wearables into the ePA, is also central to this.

One of the central tasks in the German healthcare system is therefore to successively integrate the stand-alone DHAs into the future IT healthcare infrastructure TI 2.0 and to define the necessary technical and organizational steps towards this. With digitalization of healthcare processes, doctors and patients could access the same treatment data in order to keep themselves closely informed about the course of disease. The data collected via telemedicine could be used by physicians to make data-driven therapeutic decisions and motivate patients in their everyday lives. Prescription or ordering processes for apps and medical devices could also be faster, and digital services could be accessed more quickly. As with conventional therapies, the acceptance of digital applications and adherence are crucial factors for the positive, sustainable effect of a DHA.

2. DiGA.Pro project goals and impact on telemonitoring applications

For this reason, an analysis of exemplary DHAs is to be carried out as part of the DiGAPro project in order to identify the optimization potential for even more patient-centered digitalized care services [14]. Current "Digitale Gesundheitsanwendungen" (dt. DiGA/engl. DHA) listed in the BfArM directory are predominantly focusing on patient self-management [15]. The existing reimbursement model of the "App on prescription" does not yet cover data access by doctors or remote interventions in the therapy process based on digitally assessed data. Therefore, based on an analysis of the current state of DHAs one project objective is to demonstrate the possibilities of a more comprehensive and consistent interaction of IT-based care processes and their associated potential. Digital health applications should therefore be an integral part of digitally supported care and not only cover the narrowly defined subprocess of self-management.

How can such comprehensive care processes be created around DHA in the future? The DiGA.Pro project aims to investigate how linking DHA with other digital applications or analog healthcare services leads to overarching care processes in such a way that good and needs-based processes are created not only for patients, but also to the same extent for healthcare service providers, which effectively support everyday treatment. The project aims to develop solutions how DHA's, in conjunction with the eHR and other digital applications and services, can support data-driven, patient-centered, and hybrid care processes. The project takes up gematik's considerations on the further development of the Telematics Infrastructure (TI 2.0) and fits in with the BMG's activities to implement its digital strategy.

By analyzing innovative approaches on the market, from German Innovation Fund projects [16], from special care contracts, and from good practices in the healthcare systems of other countries, the DiGA.Pro project designs how user-centered digitalization can create added value for patients and other stakeholders in specific care scenarios. The considered scenarios range from technology-driven topics such as connecting aids to DHA to integrated forms of care across sectors and professions, such as digitalized Disease Management Programs (DMP). All scenarios considered in the DiGA.Pro project are hybrid, i.e., they aim to integrate medical, nursing, and digitally provided services. Patient-centricity, personalization, and performance measurement form cross-sections across all scenarios considered. In order to develop and analyze these care scenarios, a model-based approach was chosen.

3. The DiGA.Pro approach

The fact that the end-to-end digitalization of care and administrative processes can have many positive effects is to be verified in this article using the model-based approach and proven on the basis of the quality metrics applied. For this purpose, individual care processes such as the prescription of a DHA, the ordering of a medical device, or access to treatment data by the doctor are broken down into their atomic process steps and modeled. In this way, the basic interactions can be assessed, typified, and stored with value sets so that a more in-depth analysis of the enabling and hindering parameters is possible. In contrast to the large number of telemedical test projects carried out, a model-based approach has the advantage that, based on prior knowledge and empirically collected values, more generalized considerations can lead to comparability, harmonization, and standardization of care processes and environmental parameters. The model-based approach also has the advantage that the graphical notation can be used to visualize the complex relationships between care processes, IT infrastructures, and digital health or sensor applications in order to understand their workflows. An initial analysis of these relationships can be carried out during the requirements analysis and design phase to identify necessary features and interactions even before the actual implementation of the functionality starts. A model-based approach can also be used to visualize and analyze the processes and relationships for already existing IT applications.

Based on the case studies, this article will show how DHAs are used in their status quo and what the migration path toward end-to-end digitalized processes chains would look like. In particular, the detailed concept for TI 2.0 will be used to compare the status quo and the target picture [8]. The model-based approach can be used to identify the underlying process and software architecture patterns of DHAs that are similar to the components and services of the TI of the German healthcare system. This allows us to identify the potential for adapting these components to the concepts of the TI and, vice versa, the potential for aligning the components and services of the TI with the DHAs. Finally, by modeling different evolutionary phases of development, the migration path for a gradual integration of DHAs into the TI 2.0 can be shown.

4. The German telematic infrastructure 2.0

The Telematic Infrastructure (TI) 2.0 aims to increase acceptance through a user-centric approach. To reach this goal a technology leap is deemed necessary to establish an architecture enabling developments in new areas besides outpatient and inpatient care like digital health apps (DHA). To reach this goal the TI must become more technology independent and dissolve data silos to enable mobile patient-centric solutions. Hence, key properties of the TI 2.0 are:

- A flexible and user-friendly identity management
- Universal availability of TI services
- Robustness and adaptive modern security concepts (zero-trust)
- Intersectoral and international interoperability (FHIR and more)
- Data sovereignty in distributed services
- Services and application over spanning integration of data.

In the TI 1.0 service availability is limited through the necessary use of the so-called TI Konnektors functioning as secure hardware or cloud gateways. This necessity will be obsoleted through the introduction of the zero-trust concept in the TI 2.0, where services and users are constantly monitored and evaluated against a security model. This environment will be part of the basic services provided by the gematik upon which enhanced services can be provided by trusted and certified third-party vendors. Together with the new federated identity management, this will enable a more open participation of new user groups interacting with a broader range of services.

Through the TI 2.0, the gematik will still provide core infrastructure services such as OSCP and VSDM used for key functionality like key and certificate management and encryption. On top of these services, the gematik will provide additional services in cooperation with partners like:

- Basic services of the health insurance like:
  - ePA ("elektronische Patientenakte") which is the electronic health record containing all the recorded relevant data about the patient.
  - eID ("GesundheitsID" /identity) represents the digital identification mechanism for the patient within the TI.
  - eMP ("elektronischer Medikationsplan") represents the electronic medication plan stored in the ePA to be accessed by physicians.
  - NFDM ("Notfalldatenmanagement") contains the important data about a patient in case of an emergency.
- Services provided by billing centers of pharmacies like:
  - eRezept allowing pharmacies to hand out prescriptions and to bill them accordingly.
- Mostly independent third party will provide additional services like:
  - KIM ("Kommunikation im Medizinwesen") is secure email-like asynchronous communication.
  - TIM (TI Messenger) provides messaging capabilities to the TI 2.0.

Every service and service provider will need to be certified by the gematik to participate in the TI 2.0. This is also valid for typical TI 2.0 client systems like:

- DHA ("Digitale Gesundheitsanwendung") is a personal digital health app for patients.
- PVS ("Praxisverwaltungssystem") is a practice management system for general practitioners.
- KIS ("Krankenhausinformationssystem") is a hospital information system.

Based on these new concepts, the TI 2.0 is likely to become an innovative ecosystem for user-centric applications, medical research, and industry [17].

5. A model-based approach for analysis and adaptation of telemonitoring applications in healthcare processes

Model-based approaches encompass a set of methodologies that revolve around the utilization of models for comprehending, designing, and developing complex systems. Models can serve as abstract representations of real-world characteristics, system's structures, behavior, and requirements, capturing its essence and facilitating communication among stakeholders and system developers. By employing models as central elements, model-based approaches aim to enhance the consistency, accuracy, and efficiency of system development.

The core principle of model-based approaches lies in creating a common language and shared understanding of the system through the use of models. Models serve as blueprints, enabling stakeholders across various disciplines to collaborate effectively and ensure that the system aligns with their expectations. By establishing a common language for communication, models break down knowledge silos and foster a cohesive approach to system development [18]. Model-based approaches also promote the reusability of design elements and specifications, streamlining the development process and minimizing redundancies. By capturing the essence of the system in models, developers can easily reuse and adapt existing models, reducing the need for repetitive work and accelerating the development cycle [18]. Furthermore, through models, systems also can be simulated and analyzed, providing valuable insights into their functionalities and potential areas of improvement. Hence, model-based approaches facilitate early detection of errors and inconsistencies within the system. As models become integral to the development process, they serve as testing grounds for identifying and addressing potential issues before implementing them. This proactive approach to error detection saves time and resources in the long run [19].

A primary challenge in applying the model-based approach is finding the right level of abstraction. Too much simplification can lead to the loss of crucial details, while insufficient abstraction can result in overly complex models that are difficult to interpret and use. To be able to compare alternatives in processes and models it must be ensured that the models are modeled at the same abstraction to gain meaningful insight. In our project, the chosen modeling language must also be able to capture healthcare processes and reflect the dynamic nature of health care.

To analyze and improve telemonitoring applications and their surrounding processes in the DiGA.Pro project, a model-based approach has been chosen. Modeling of conventional and digitalized care processes can help to define patterns for needed harmonization and standardization of care processes and IT infrastructures. Up to the present day, BPMN has been recognized for its graphical notation, which is intended to be comprehensible by all business users. The model-based simulation of potential process outputs can result in cost-effectiveness before implementing and evaluating these processes in real life.

By providing a reliable description of the care process underlying information exchange and data management, the application of standard-based solutions becomes more straightforward. This is particularly crucial in healthcare settings, where multiple systems need to interact seamlessly to provide efficient and effective patient care [20–22]. Despite its potential to facilitate common understanding and promote automation, BPMN has witnessed some usage in health care, attributed to the complexity inherent in healthcare processes and the domain's highly regulated environments [23].

The utilization of a model-based approach in health care is illustrated by studies like those of Bowles et al. [24] and De Ramón Fernández et al. [25]. These studies demonstrate the effectiveness of business process management (BPM) in optimizing healthcare resource planning and improving process efficiency in clinical settings. Such evidence underscores the usefulness of model-based approaches in enhancing healthcare process efficiency and quality. Bowles et al. annotated BPMN models for optimized healthcare resource planning. Through the utilization of precise metrics on BPMN diagrams, a quantitative examination of healthcare processes was made feasible, facilitating a more focused and significant analysis that ultimately produced valuable insights into the annotated BPMN models [24].

In their 2020 study, De Ramón Fernández et al. delve into the application of BPM in the healthcare sector, focusing specifically on clinical processes. The research aims to assess the effectiveness and quality improvements gained through BPM methodology in clinical settings. A systematic literature review was conducted, analyzing 18 articles that met predefined criteria. The findings indicate that BPM is an effective tool for designing, optimizing, and automating clinical processes. The study also highlights the need for comprehensive follow-up, better technological support, and greater clinical staff involvement to fully realize BPM's potential in health care. This research supports the use of BPM as a methodology to enhance process efficiency and quality in healthcare environments [25].

By mapping out the sequence of activities, decision points, and interactions between healthcare professionals, BPMN diagrams provide a comprehensive view of how patient care unfolds. This visualization aids in identifying bottlenecks, redundancies, and opportunities for improvement [26]. BPMN models can be used for what-if analysis. By altering process parameters or introducing hypothetical scenarios, healthcare organizations can anticipate the impact of changes before implementing them. This proactive approach minimizes risks and ensures that process modifications are evidence-based [27]. BPMN models can be enriched with additional information, highlighting touchpoints and interactions from the patient's perspective. This perspective ensures that healthcare processes are designed with the patient's well-being and experience in mind [24].

Nevertheless, evaluating DHA and care processes has several challenges when using the model-based BPM approach: The lack of harmonized evaluation methods across various domains creates a significant barrier to comparing and assessing the effectiveness of solutions, impeding informed decision making and adoption of optimal practices [25]. Generic BPMN models, while useful, often fail to fully represent the intricacies of health care, overlooking factors like patient outcomes and healthcare provider satisfaction [28]. Data integration difficulties with existing healthcare systems further are leading to data silos and hampering effective data utilization [29]. Additionally, data quality and reliability concerns significantly impact decision making, necessitating robust data management strategies [30]. Finally, the fragmented ownership and decision making in digital health initiatives hinder collaboration and effective implementation in care processes, calling for a more coordinated approach to ensure alignment and shared responsibility [31].

Addressing these challenges is crucial for modeling and analyzing digital health solutions in the healthcare sector. Furthermore, to apply models effectively in health care, the definition and application of appropriate metrics are crucial. Therefore, these metrics should accurately reflect the analysis goals, aiding in the measurement and evaluation of process efficiency and effectiveness. Only by this the model-based approach allows for identification of improvement areas, leading to optimized healthcare processes.

5.1 The DiGA.Pro metamodel

In the DiGA.Pro-project a metamodel and an analysis matrix were defined to analyze the underlying technical and application processes. The metamodel (**Figure 1**) describes all actors, the processes, and process steps, the communication paths used, and the processed data as classes in object-oriented modeling using UML class

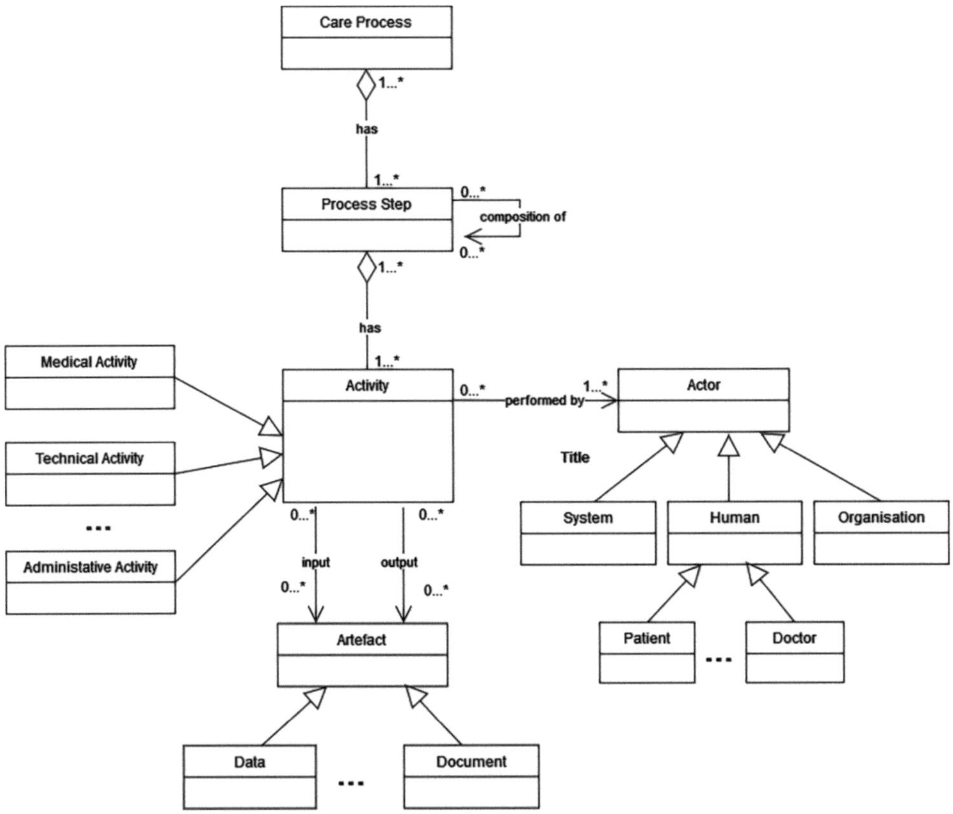

Figure 1.
DiGA.Pro metamodel.

notation. Based on the DHAs considered, the overarching system relationships were reflected in a metamodel, which serves as the basis for analyzing the processes and applying the metrics. It allows the assignment of individual activities for composite care and treatment processes. Each class of the analysis matrix contains individual value sets. The value sets make it possible to assign attributes to the classes of the metamodel. In the DiGA.Pro metamodel, the following classes are represented:

A care or treatment process consists of one or more process steps. The process step is defined as a semantic unit in order to group inherent or successive activities. In a process step, one or more activities can be carried out by one or more actors. Activities are divided into medical, technical, or organizational activities. They can be carried out by a technical system (a technical component), a physical person (doctor, patient, administrator, etc.), or an organization (practice, health insurance company, etc.) and can have various artifacts (data, documents, etc.) as input or output.

For concretization of the metamodel, the business process model and notation framework (BPMN) was used. The BPMN standard is maintained by the Object Management Group and is supported by several tool manufacturers [32]. Providing a set of standardized graphical elements and an underlying XML-based syntax, BPMN allows to represent activities, messages, or data flows carried out by the participating actors within complex and parallel processes. This allows to create and to visualize complex process maps. In the DiGA.Pro project the concepts of flow object (activity, gateway, and event), connecting object, pool, and swimlane, were primarily used to record and subsequently to analyze the different implemented telemonitoring applications at the process-level theses. The open-source desktop modeler Camunda 8, which supports all standardized BPMN 2.0 elements, was used to model the care and application processes [33]. For each subprocess, we created different process models. In total, we modeled 36 subprocesses (see therefore also chapter 5).

The exemplary model in **Figure 2** shows which optimization potentials arise with end-to-end digitized process chains on the future Telematics Infrastructure 2.0 of the German healthcare system.

After developing the metamodel, the appropriate metrics were chosen. The selection and application of metrics were important for evaluating and comparing different DHAs and their corresponding processes. Each metric chosen has its relevance and potential to provide insights into the evaluation of the DHA underlying a certain care process. Therefore, the selected metrics should:

- enable the evaluation of the number of interactions between people and system
- provide the ability to quantify the amount of manually entered data
- assess the number of duplicate manual data entries in order to quantify the degree of duplication in manual data entry
- quantify the time for data entry by doctors, patients, and practice staff in order to evaluate the efficiency of documentation and system usage.
- enable the evaluation of the number of media disruptions to identify inefficient communication or lack of integration
- assess the number of analog (paper) and digital data transmissions to quantify the degree of digital transmission methods and identify potential bottlenecks or inefficient use
- assess the number of different digital services used in a system or organization.

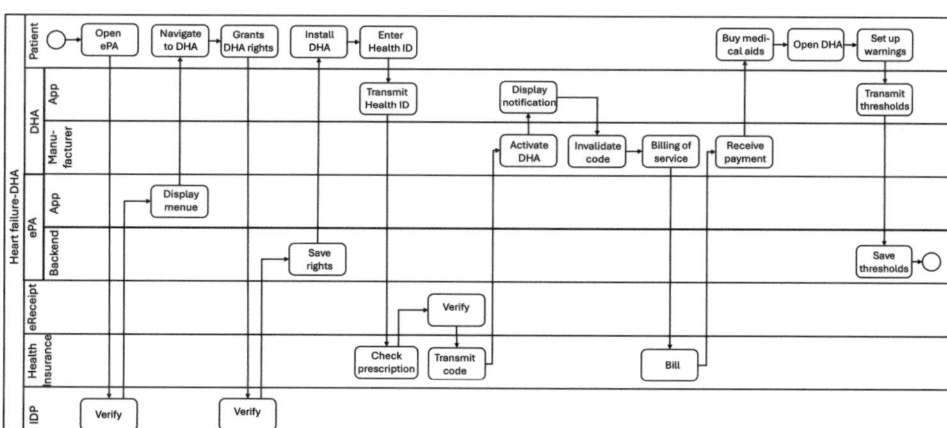

Figure 2.
BPMN notation of ePrescription process.

Goal	Question	Metric
Reduce manual data entry	How often is data put in manually?	• Number of manually entered data • Number of twice manually entered data
Make communication more efficient	How frequently does switching between digital and analog and analog and digital occur?	• Number of media disruptions
Make interaction more efficient	How time consuming is the usage of the applications?	• Time for data input • New, additional time expenses • Time to reach a process or subprocess goal
Understand the IT-landscape	How many different digital services are used?	• Number of different digital services and applications
Improve communication efficiency	How frequent are data transmissions?	• Number of digital data transmissions • Number of analog data transmissions
Improve security	How frequent are verification steps taken and how many steps are there?	• Number of verification steps

Table 1.
Selected metrics for DHA process evaluation.

- evaluate the quality of information based on various criteria such as completeness, timeliness, accuracy, consistency, and comprehensibility.
- enable the recording and evaluation of the technical quality of a medical device or a medical service, including security, availability, reliability, accuracy, performance, and safety.

Each metric was derived using the GQM approach [34]. This involves setting a specific goal, formulating a relevant question, and then determining the appropriate metric. For example, in analyzing "Interactions Between People and Systems," the goal might be to enhance communication efficiency in healthcare processes. The corresponding question could examine the frequency and effectiveness of these interactions, while the metric would involve counting occurrences of actor and communication keywords in BPMN diagrams. This systematic approach allows for a detailed and objective evaluation of each aspect of healthcare processes. In detail in the DiGA.Pro project, the following GQM metrics were applied (**Table 1**).

The metrics were then applied to the BPMN models in order to quantify individual results of the analysis (for results see Chapter 9).

6. Modeling of telemonitoring applications and healthcare processes

Once the metamodel had been developed, the object of the study was narrowed down. For this purpose, the care scenario to be examined was defined as "telemonitoring with reduced monitoring requirements." In this type of therapy-accompanying telemonitoring, vital and health data are recorded on an ad hoc or less continuous basis, because the diseases to be observed require a lower density of measurement points. The patients in question are not high-risk patients, but primarily patients with chronic or long-term diseases. Telemonitoring is carried out by general practitioners as part of their everyday practice and must therefore be as easy as possible to integrate into the outpatient treatment process.

Use cases for telemonitoring with reduced monitoring requirements are therapies that require frequent individual adjustment of the therapy or medication plan, based on symptoms or certain parameters that are collected *via* health assessments or measurements of vital and movement data. Examples include treatment of cancer, neurological diseases (multiple sclerosis and Parkinson's disease), chronic respiratory diseases (asthma and COPD) as well as cardiovascular diseases such as heart failure or chronic heart failure. The different types of telemonitoring applications were defined as follows:

Telemonitoring is generally defined as remote monitoring and analysis of health-related data [35]. This also includes the collection of health data on patient's site in everyday life and the transmission of this data to medical staff [36]. Areas of application for telemonitoring differ in particular with regard to the density of data collection from the patient. Depending on the clinical picture, a distinction can be made between continuous 24/7 monitoring and punctual monitoring. Continuous forms of 24/7 telemonitoring are often used in high-risk patients to monitor vital parameters (especially in cardiology) [37]. Punctual types of telemonitoring are used for indications with a reduced need for monitoring (e.g., high blood pressure) [38].

The building blocks of telemonitoring applications for patients and practitioners are shown in **Figure 3**. They include functionalities for planning and visualization of therapy measures and medication (e.g., medication plan), assessment of health condition and therapy progress (e.g., diaries or questionnaires), vital data acquisition

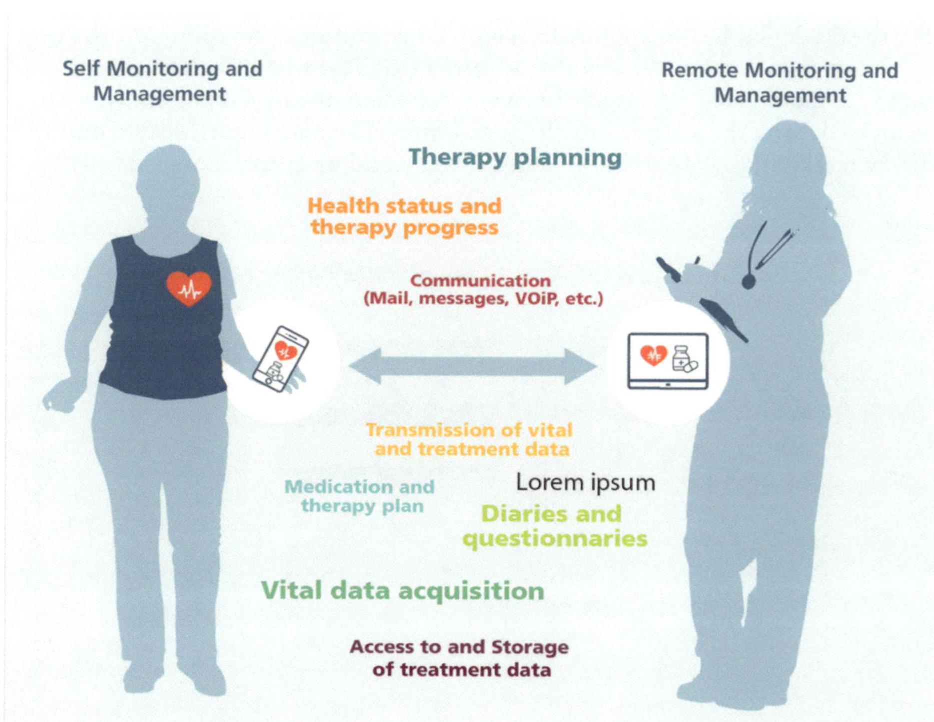

Figure 3.
Building blocks of telemonitoring applications.

by sensors or medical devices, integrated communication features (e.g., mail, messages, or videoconferencing), secure transmission of vital and treatment data, and storage of health data.

7. Data acquisition and analysis

After defining the scope of the study, a systematic review of the current DHA directory [39] and the German Innovation Fund projects [40] of the last 3 years was carried out. Therefore, publicly available sources of the projects (including project and application descriptions, publications, operating instructions, etc.) were considered.

A total of 48 DHAs and 118 innovation fund projects (focus on new concepts of care services—status ongoing) were documented. Of the 48 DHAs, a majority of 28 applications contained telemonitoring components. Especially DHAs have a high number of monitoring components overall (28 out of 48), particularly due to the automatic recording of therapy or program progress in self-study courses for improving health competence.

In innovation fund projects, telemonitoring has so far been used to a lesser extent. Of the 118 projects, only 32 integrated telemonitoring components in their application. In the analyzed projects predominated digital forms of medical documentation (e.g. case records) for cross-sectoral treatment, the usage of telemedical consultation services and questionnaire-based digital data collection to answer scientific questions. For five innovation fund projects, no final classification could be made due to insufficient information.

For the 60 digital health applications with telemonitoring components, the way in which way data is collected was also acquired (see **Figure 4**). To date, the data required for monitoring has largely been entered manually by the patient (n = 40). This can be data on the state of health (questionnaires, assessments, scales, and medication taken), diary entries, or notes. The second most common method

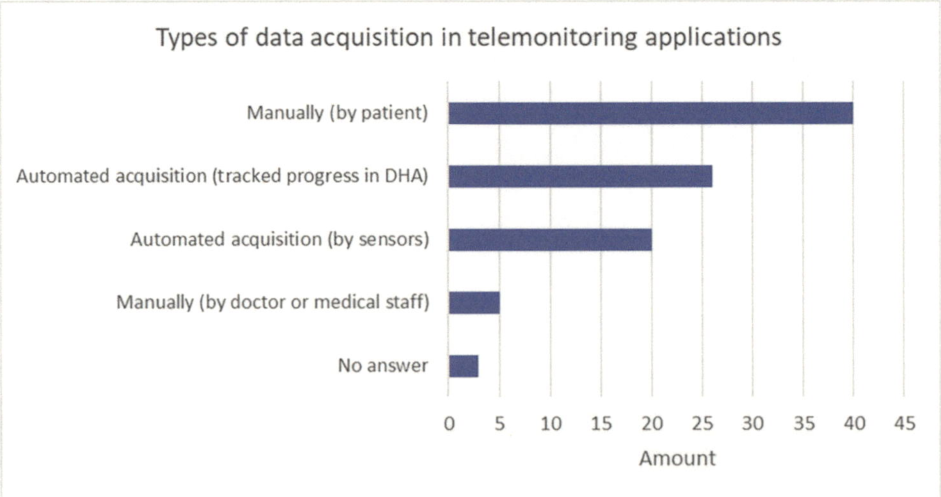

Figure 4.
Types of data acquisition in telemonitoring applications (multiple answers possible).

identified was the automatic recording of progress (e.g., for a completed learning unit or therapeutic exercise) in the therapy program (n = 26). Recording of vital data by sensors is also quite common (n = 20). Manual input by medical staff on site (n = 5) is predominantly used in geriatric applications.

The analysis showed that a good third of the DHA (60 out of a total of 166) include monitoring components. So far, however, simple forms of monitoring have predominated, such as manual data entry and occasion-related transmission by patients or periodic retrieval of health data by practitioners. This indicates that the data is not time critical for treatment and is therefore loosely related to the actual treatment process. The majority of the projects examined are still at the testing stage or in a scientific evaluation process. None of the projects or digital applications have standardized interfaces to services of the Telematics Infrastructure (TI) of the German healthcare system.

After the systematic review, expert interviews were conducted for seven selected digital applications to identify all central and secondary processes of the actors involved in the care scenarios. In detail, it was determined which processes and treatment steps are supported by the digital application and which actor or which technical component collects and processes the data in which situation and for what purpose. This step served as preparation for modeling the technical processes and the interactions between doctor, patient, digital application, and other actors within the care scenario. After the detailed modeling of user interactions and analysis of the technical components, it was worked out which of the components contain their own application-specific logic and which components are generic and therefore could be implemented using standard components of the TI.

8. Analysis and modeling of the DiGA.Pro care scenarios

For analysis and modeling of the whole processes, two care scenarios were examined in more detail using the elements of the metamodel. Resulting from the real-life scenarios, the process patterns and architectural software patterns should be identified. These process and architecture patterns can help future providers of telemonitoring applications to adapt their software components to the requirements for integration into the TI. The two care scenarios are described in detail below.

8.1 Care scenario1: motion monitoring for patients with Parkinson's disease

The analyzed telemonitoring system for Parkinson's patients is primarily used in the outpatient care sector. The system consists of a mobile app for patients, a motion sensor, and a web application for healthcare professionals. Using the app, patients can view exercise videos and receive advice on how to deal with Parkinson's disease. It is also possible to answer questionnaires and keep a symptom diary in the app. *Via* a secure web portal, practitioners receive aggregated reports on the gait quality and symptom patterns of their patients as well as their well-being and difficulties in everyday life. The telemonitoring component primarily serves to provide better data for medication therapy, in particular for planning medication therapy and measuring its effects.

The sensor and app-based system accompanies Parkinson's patients in their everyday lives. Movement sensors are attached to the shoes and continuously record the patient's gait patterns throughout the day. In addition, a standardized movement test is carried out three times a day. After the local data analysis from the movement tests, questions about the current state of health have to be answered. The gait quality, symptom patterns, and difficulties in everyday life are analyzed using algorithmic and pattern recognition methods from the long-term measurement data and the movement tests. Individualized coaching measures such as training exercises and tips are also derived from this.

Through situation-specific movement exercises, patients learn to better manage their symptoms themselves and make their everyday lives more active. In case of a change in the dosage of medication, the movement sensor system can record the changes in gait parameters and display them for both patients and remote doctors or specialized telenurses. However, medication is still prescribed in direct contact between the doctor and patient.

8.2 Care scenario 2: monitoring of vital data for patients suffering from heart failure

The system for monitoring vital data was designed for patients and users with heart failure to support self-management and as an early warning system for detecting changes in the disease. The mobile app aims to improve patients' state of health, quality of life, and disease-specific knowledge.

Similar to the telemonitoring system for Parkinson's patients, the system consists of a mobile app, various measuring devices, and a web application for healthcare professionals. The patients can use the measuring devices to measure their blood pressure, oxygen saturation, pulse, temperature, and weight on a daily basis. The recorded data is transferred to the server *via* the mobile app and displayed in the app as progress curves. After each measurement, patients receive a classification of their vital signs according to a traffic light system. Questionnaires on quality of life and individual symptoms are used to record the patient's general state of health. This approach can help to identify warning signs and deviations from the state of health at an early stage.

As a result of the analysis of the vital signs and the questionnaire-based assessments, the patient is automatically sent short educational content or recommendations for specific health measures *via* the app. This includes information on the current state of health, the correlation of specific symptoms, and the course of treatment. This is supplemented by information on nutrition, exercise, and other everyday topics, which are communicated through in-app messages.

Particular emphasis is placed on the implementation of guideline-based therapy and the recognition and interpretation of early warning signs so that emergency situations can be prevented. The app also offers a document repository for doctor's letters, imaging documents, ECG findings, laboratory reports, hospital letters, powers of attorney, and directives. All information can be exported by the user and sent to the doctor, creating transparency about the state of health and treatment over the selected period.

In addition to the basic model, personalized health coaching and further remote risk prevention measures can be implemented in a self-payer or intensive care model based on the data collected and the individual health profile. This includes patients being able to create a medication plan in the app that reminds them to take their medication every day. In addition, medical staff can send individualized messages to patients depending on their state of health after viewing the recorded patient data.

8.3 Identified processes

From the modeling and analysis of the two care scenarios, it became apparent that the process steps for prescribing, obtaining, and using a DHA are largely similar despite some slight differences in detail. For this reason, only the generalizable process steps for both applications are shown in **Figure 5**. To simplify the readability, only the process steps and activities from user's and from system's perspective are described in accordance with the DiGA.Pro metamodel. To improve the overall clarity of the diagram, the temporal relationships between input and output and the assignment of actors to the activities have been not considered. At the level of the analysis model, however, this information was considered with its corresponding level of detail.

The user's process steps can be taken to reconstruct the usage and functional scope of DHAs. This ranges from the prescription of the app by the doctor (1), the

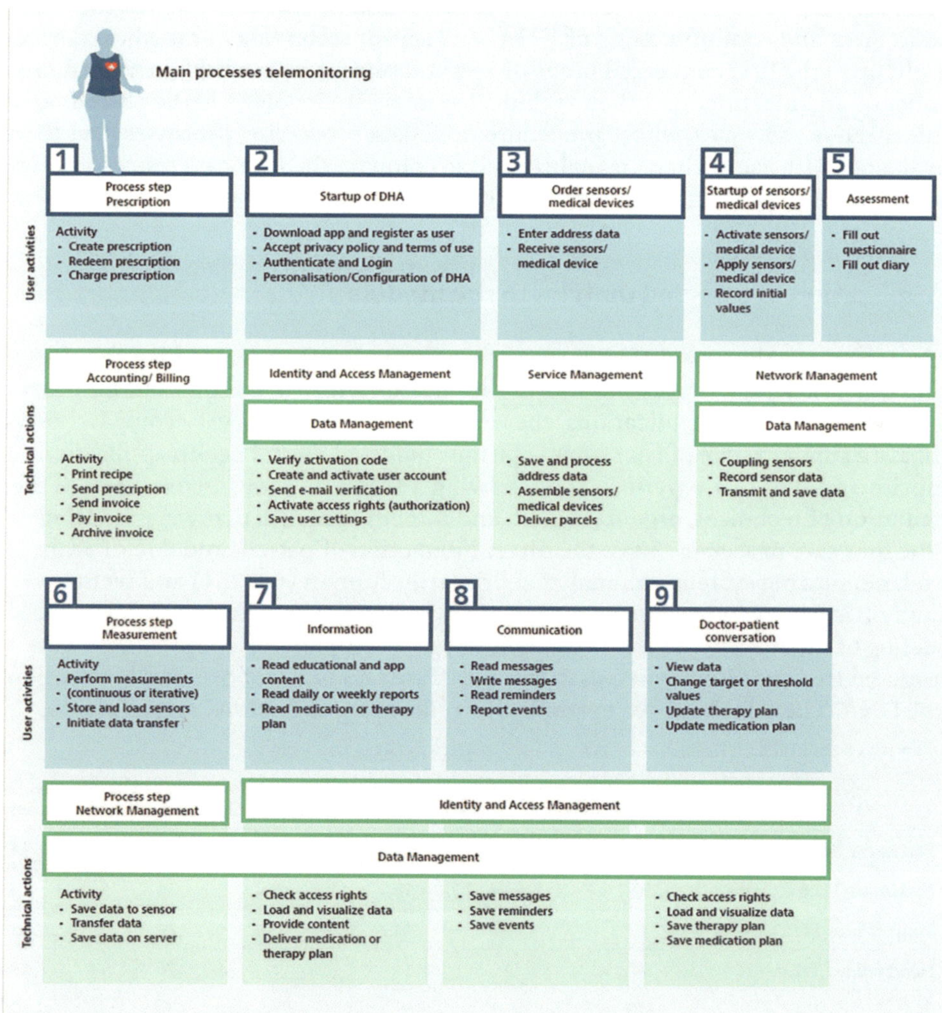

Figure 5.
Tableau of process steps and activities (human and technical).

commissioning of app (2) and sensors or medical devices (3–4) to its use (5–8), and remote care or follow-up visits to the doctor (9). Depending on the design of the DHA, process steps for information, communication, measurement, and assessment are also integrated. However, the process steps and corresponding activities can vary in their chronological sequence depending on the application logic and the built-in treatment process of the DHA. Information (7) and communication (8) are mostly accompanying process steps alongside the lifecycle of the DHA. They are separated here only for better readability of the illustration.

In the next step, user activities were assigned to technical actions and responses from a system perspective, thereby identifying the technical process steps and activities. For the use of a DHA, the central technical process steps for rollout and operation of an IT application are carried out. These range from accounting functions (1), the installation (2, 4) and secure operation of IT applications (5–9), customer relationship systems (3, 9) as well as user and problem management right up to dedicated technical processes such as network and database management.

The correlation of user and technical processes illustrates how complex the procurement and commissioning of DHAs and sensor technology or medical devices is, right up to the first connected usage of app and sensors or medical devices. A large number of organizations and their technical systems are involved in the preceding administrative processes, whose procedures and data processing processes have to be coordinated with each other. To analyze and to compare the four care processes more in detail, we applied selected metrics to the BPMN models.

9. Application of selected metrics to the models

By comparing the four different care processes in detail, we gained the following insights: Although the telemonitoring applications for Parkinson's and for heart failure address different indications, they are currently used in a very comparable way and have a similar range of functions. The four modeled digital health applications comprise a total of 623 activities. The following **Table 2** provides an overview of the distribution of technical, organizational, and human activities that were modeled for the four care processes. Since the direct interaction of patient and doctor with the telemonitoring system was analyzed primarily, human (n = 254) and technical activities (n = 310) predominate over organizational activities (n = 59). For the modeling of organizational activities, only those accompanying subprocesses were considered that are directly necessary for purchase and usage of a digital application of the DHA. These include, for example, the redeeming of doctors' prescriptions,

	Technical actions	Organizational activities	Human activities	*Sum:*
Parkinson_SOTA	69	17	56	**142**
Parkinson_TI2.0	92	15	36	**143**
Heart failure_SOTA	55	13	86	**154**
Heart failure_TI2.0	94	14	76	**184**
Sum:	**310**	**59**	**254**	**623**

Table 2.
Total number of technical, organizational, and human activities.

the dispensing of medication in the pharmacy, the ordering and shipping of medical aids, or the billing of services by the health insurance companies. To this extent, it is plausible that there are no major differences in the number of organizational activities between the current status of implementation and the porting of care processes to TI 2.0 (SOTA = 30/TI = 29).

When analyzing the aggregated activities, it is also noticeable that porting the current telemonitoring applications to the TI 2.0 can reduce the number of necessary human activities for both care processes (SOTA = 142/ TI = 112). This indicates a moderately optimized interaction between users (patient/doctor) and technical systems, as the migration of individual user's process steps to technical actions of the TI 2.0 allows them to run more automatically in the background. Again, this includes redeem of prescriptions, registration processes, ordering processes, and doctor-patient appointments. As a result, the number of technical actions increases significantly when porting the current DHAs to the TI 2.0 (SOTA = 124/TI = 186). The significant increase in technical activities is plausible insofar as the services available *via* TI 2.0 are more modularized and must be addressed individually due to its zero-trust architecture.

In the following sections, the analysis results based on the aggregated data will now be examined in more detail. The following observations for the entire care process were made using the metrics (**Table 3**).

From interpretation of the metrics, we derived the following results: Porting the telemonitoring applications onto the TI 2.0 is accompanied by a significant reduction in "manual data entry" (SOTA = 27/TI = 5). This is due to the central authorization and identity management of the TI 2.0. In contrast to the stand-alone telemonitoring applications, the use of the TI infrastructure eliminates inconvenient registration and authorization processes, as they can be configured either centrally by the user in the ePA or by the identity providers of the health insurance companies. Due to the centrally implemented set of access rules, the TI 2.0 services exchange authentication and authorization information during the subprocesses "installation of the DHA" and "doctor-patient conversation" in the background.

Surprisingly, we found little or no evidence of "duplicate manual data entry" in the processes (SOTA = 2/TI = 0). This is obviously due to the fact that DHAs with telemonitoring are only involved in a specific part of the care process, namely digital therapy support. As the treatment is largely based on digital technologies, the amount of duplicate data entered manually is low or negligible overall. Nevertheless, a large

Applied metrics for the entire process	Parkinson _SOTA	Parkinson _TI2.0	Heart failure _SOTA	Heart failure _TI2.0
Number of manually entered data	11	3	16	2
Number of twice manually entered data	2	0	0	0
Number of media disruptions	19	8	23	11
Number of paper-based interactions	10	0	9	0
Number of digital data transmissions	18	21	18	22
Used number of different digital services and applications	27	31	29	32
Number of verification steps	10	16	10	18

Table 3.
Metrics applied in DiGA.Pro to the entire process.

number of manual data entries must be made, especially for the use of the proprietary DHA, as was determined with Metric 1.

As can be seen from the "Media disruptions" metric, porting the stand-alone telemonitoring applications to TI 2.0 would reduce the number of media disruptions by half (SOTA = 42/TI = 19). The large number of media disruptions in the stand-alone applications results on the one hand from the conventional prescription and billing processes for medicines and medical aids and on the other hand from the fact that patients still have to make appointments by telephone. The introduction of the ePrescription service and electronic appointment allocation *via* TIM or other appointment allocation services could minimize these media disruptions.

We arrive at an even better result by the metric "paper-based interactions" (SOTA = 19/TI = 0). This includes printing out prescriptions, submitting prescriptions to the health insurance company, or sending activation codes for a DHA by letter. All of these paper-based interactions can be eliminated with end-to-end digitization of these processes on the TI 2.0.

However, the "number of digital data transmissions" is slightly increasing due to the fact that more data must be transferred between the DHAs and the corresponding distributed TI 2.0 applications, in particular ePA or health insurance app (SOTA = 36/ TI = 43).

As can be seen from the metric "Used number of different digital services and applications," the complexity of the overall systems is approximately the same. All DHAs must support the processes "installation and startup," "access and identity management," and "data transfer" between sensor, smartphone, and backend in the same way. In addition, they are integrated into the same healthcare system environment (e.g., for billing or ordering). The metrics differ only slightly, as the TI 2.0 architecture names the individual components in a more differentiated way and provides them as separate services (SOTA = 56/TI = 63).

Using the "Number of verification steps" metric, we were able to show that there are more verification steps on the TI 2.0 than in the stand-alone applications (SOTA = 20/TI = 34). However, this does not mean more effort for users, as the verification steps usually run in the background. The TI 2.0 was designed as a zero-trust architecture in which the services and devices encapsulated must temporarily verify themselves for each interaction and data transfer. It also can be assumed that the stand-alone telemonitoring applications have integrated sufficient security-relevant verification steps into their overall systems in order to meet the high data protection requirements when processing health data.

When analyzing the subprocesses in more detail, we made the following findings based on the metrics:

9.1 Prescription and payment

Porting the DHA to TI 2.0 eliminates media disruptions (SOTA = 8/ TI = 0) and paper-based interactions (SOTA = 16/ TI = 0). As a result of end-to-end digitization in central TI components, previous hardware-based interactions (e.g., printing and scanning prescriptions, inserting the eHC) can be virtualized in the future (SOTA = 4/ TI = 0). Nevertheless, the complexity of the overall systems is almost comparable, as only hardware-based applications are substituted by software-based services (SOTA = 12/TI = 10).

9.2 DHA installation and startup

The rule-based authorization management of the TI 2.0 can also optimize the necessary registration and activation dialogs in the DHA, for example, by logging in with the health ID or by an automated activation and billing of the prescribed DHA *via* the identity provider (iDP) of the health insurance company apps. While the current implementations require manual data entry (SOTA = 10) for registration and verification of a user account, porting to TI 2.0 eliminates a large part of the manual entries for registration or the creation of user accounts and entry of personal data for the initial configuration and personalization of a DHA (TI = 1).

9.3 Ordering of sensors and medical devices

The fact that patients can also provide manufacturers authorization to forward personal address data (e.g., *via* the iDP of the health insurance company) eliminates duplicate and manual data when using TI 2.0 services (SOTA = 2/TI = 0). Ordering processes can be initiated automatically when the prescription is approved by the health insurance company.

9.4 Startup and coupling of sensors and medical devices

As these are local interactions between DHA and sensors or medical devices, the TI 2.0 infrastructure offers no further advantages compared to current implementations. Pairing the DHA with sensors and medical devices is based on the standardized Bluetooth protocol. This means that the individual process steps are almost identical.

9.5 Assessment of health status

All metrics for the current implementations or the processes modeled on the TI 2.0 are comparable. The advantage of the TI does not have such a strong impact, as it mainly involves local data entries and interactions with the DHA. The questionnaires, diaries, and medication details are entered *via* button clicks in both applications, so they were not counted as manual entries (SOTA = 1/TI = 0).

A comparable number of concepts for recording health status (e.g., questionnaires, symptom diary, and medication data) also mean a comparable number of data transfers to proprietary servers or to the ePA backend (SOTA = 2/TI = 5). The higher number of data transmissions with the TI is merely due to the fact that the data is transmitted sequentially.

9.6 Measurement of vital data

This is also mostly a local or application-specific process. Vital data is transmitted in both care scenarios *via* the Bluetooth interface to the DHA app and into the corresponding backend. The only advantage of TI 2.0 compared to the current status is that recorded vital data can be transferred to the ePA *via* the backend interface § 374a and thus be further processed by other TI 2.0 applications.

The large number of digital applications and sensors, which have to interact during vital data measurement, illustrates how complex the telemonitoring systems are to operate (SOTA = 11/TI = 10).

9.7 Patient information

In addition, the number of different media through which the patient receives information related to the DHA once again demonstrates the complexity of telemonitoring applications during installation and use. Patients have to perceive a variety of administrative, technical, and disease-related information (e.g., prescription information, instructions for use, questionnaires, presentation of results, knowledge content or instructions for measurement procedures). No significant difference between current implementations and TI services could be found (SOTA = 20/TI = 17).

9.8 Remote management

The communication processes for remote care also heavily depend on the interaction between patients, medical staff, and doctors and the implemented functional scope of the DHA.

In future, a secure messenger service (TIM) is to be provided on the TI 2.0. As extracts of vital data and appointment requests can also be sent *via* TIM, this will increase the number of digital data transmissions and the necessary verification steps in contrast to the current implementation status, which only provides for contact and consultation by telephone (SOTA = 0/TI = 8).

9.9 Doctor-patient conversation

Porting the current applications to TI 2.0 will significantly reduce manual data entry when making appointments for doctor-patient consultation through semi-automatic appointment allocation *via* TIM, which only requires confirmation by the doctor (SOTA = 6/ TI = 2). Media disruptions can also be reduced, as the appointment request by telephone and the subsequent entry of the appointment in the PVS or the reprinting of the prescription are no longer necessary (SOTA = 5/ TI = 0).

To access the data during the consultation, several IT services must be connected in order to transfer treatment data to the PVS. Again because of the decentralized, zero-trust architecture, the complexity of the overall system increases accordingly by porting the DHA to the TI 2.0 infrastructure (SOTA = 8/TI = 12).

10. Discussion

In this chapter, we developed a model-based approach for assessing and analyzing technically supported care processes. The approach in this report focused on quantifying both the activities of users (patients/medical staff) and technical systems and their interactions. Therefore, we developed and used the DiGA.Pro metamodel that enabled us to categorize activities and assign these activities to actors. By modeling from the user's perspective, we wanted to capture and visualize the individual process steps and information flows, ranging from prescription of a DiGA, installation, and usage all the way to the next doctor-patient consultation. Our process models should therefore reflect the reality of users as directly as possible.

The application of the metrics produced useful, comparable, and insightful outcome, although the models do not represent the detailed information about technical implementation details. The outcome is traceable and represents "hard facts" and helps to put hard numbers on the potential of optimizations. The insights gained through the metric results are traceable back to the model for a better understanding through "visual impression." Patterns and process groups could be identified during the process of modeling, allowing further analysis into optimization (through, e.g., the introduction of new common services for the TI 2.0).

To differentiate the application context of telemonitoring applications, we first provided an overview of current products and projects with telemonitoring components in medical care and research and identified different forms of application. Based on the overview and the interviews conducted, we were able to identify the central process and architecture patterns for the implementation of care processes with telemonitoring and developed an information table of the process steps.

The exemplary modeling of the two care scenarios was then carried out in BPMN notation on the basis of the interviews and with the aid of further system documentation. The modeling of four medical care processes from prescription and usage to remote care and the final doctor-patient conversation was carried out with a focus on the direct interaction of users with the technical systems. The state of implementation (SOTA) was supplemented by modeling the same application on the German Telematics Infrastructure (TI 2.0).

By applying the established metrics to the modeled care processes, the findings could be quantified, and options presented as to how the existing telemonitoring application could be migrated to TI 2.0. At the same time, the metrics helped to identify optimization potential in the respective implementation of the telemonitoring application. Based on the metrics, the following main results were quantified right down to the subprocess level:

The number of TOM process steps in both care scenarios is similarly distributed regardless of the different indications, which suggests that the care processes of telemonitoring applications with reduced monitoring requirements are comparable and possibly also generalizable.

Porting the telemonitoring applications to the TI 2.0 can reduce the number of necessary human activities across the entire care process (SOTA = 142/ TI = 112) and leads to a significant reduction in manual data entries (SOTA = 27/TI = 5).

The number of media disruptions can be halved by porting the applications to TI 2.0 (SOTA = 42/ TI = 19), and the number of paper-based interactions can even be reduced to zero (SOTA = 19/TI = 0).

The complexity of the systems and the number of data transfers on the TI 2.0 increase slightly due to its zero-trust architecture and the more modular system architecture of separable services such as ePA, eML, EMP, and TIM. (SOTA = 56/ TI = 63). This finding also correlates with the increasing number of authentication and authorization steps on the TI 2.0 (SOTA = 20/TI = 43).

The accompanying optimizations by migrating the telemonitoring applications can be identified primarily in the secondary processes such as prescription, installation, ordering processes of aids or medical devices, appointment allocation, remote communication, and less in the actual use, since the usage of the DHA is based on its local application logic (e.g., sensor coupling or assessment of the state of health, vital data measurements).

Some metrics such as "time for data entries" or "number of interactions between human and technical system" could not be implemented due to the high degree of abstraction of the models. However, this or the detailing of the models could be realized in subsequent work, for example, on the basis of simulations or empirical values.

From the technical metrics (device quality, availability, reliability, safety, and security), only the metric for determining security could be implemented to some extent. Here too, there was a lack of information at model level about the specific implementation of these requirements at system level.

11. Limitations and lessons learned

We have derived the following lessons learned from the chosen procedure in the DiGA.Pro project:

The chosen approach, consisting of a combination of interviews and the study of existing documents as the basis for modeling the technically supported care processes, was successful. This allowed modeling the telemonitoring applications to a sufficient level of detail and applying the selected metrics to the models. The models also helped to understand the telemonitoring applications and their processes in detail.

Our metamodel can be used to model clinical pathways and decision-making situations during clinical processes. These processes in clinical pathways always consist of interaction and communication with technical systems, people, and institutions. The comparative modeling of different technically supported care processes can lead to harmonization and standardization of care processes and environmental parameters and helps to understand the workflows. In addition, BPMN process models could also be used as a tool for modeling medical guidelines and establishing shared protocols between doctors and patients [41].

It should be mentioned that we only applied SW-specific metrics for capturing and analyzing acceptance, usability, and security. This approach can be supplemented by measuring the quality of use *via* questionnaire-based assessments, as commonly used in usability evaluations [28, 42, 43]. By applying the metrics, we did not focus on visualizing business process optimizations or effects nor on aspects of quality improvement in care processes [23]. For these analytical questions (e.g., profitability, efficiency increase), we would have had to develop other metrics. Our metrics only reveal where the interaction between users and systems can be improved. However, since decision model and notation (DMN) [44] can also be used to model and execute decision-making processes, we would like to point out that it may be necessary to discuss the ethical implications and possible risks of automated process chains for patients and doctors [31].

BPMN provides a comprehensible set of graphical notation elements. In our modeling process, a common level of abstraction was found that helped to compare the two telemonitoring applications. Patterns and process groups could be identified during the process of modeling, allowing further analysis into optimization (through, e.g., the introduction of new common services for the TI 2.0). The intensive discussions about how to model a process step also helped to identify similar process steps in both applications and to model them in a comparable way.

Nevertheless, during our modeling efforts, we realized that we need a common understanding of how to model the individual process steps and name them so clearly that even others without in-depth process knowledge can quickly grasp and understand them. The problem of process comparability can arise if identical process steps are modeled differently. For future work, it is therefore necessary to establish modeling guidelines to harmonize and, if necessary, standardize the way processes are modeled in the healthcare sector. Also, a standardized naming of process steps in medical care processes and their definition in taxonomy could help to integrate and harmonize the various existing concepts [45].

The modeling process was very time consuming, and the models were frequently adapted. This requires a high level of willingness to reconsider and change models that have already been created. Due to the limited time available, we had to freeze the models for analysis at a certain point. The models could therefore be further detailed, and the granularity of the models could be further harmonized. The accuracy and correctness of the modeling are the foundation for the application of the metrics. In our project, we ensured the quality assurance of the modeling using a 4-eyes principle. In the future, however, the application of quality metrics to BPMN modeling could also help to achieve models that are as reliable and reusable as possible [46, 47].

During modeling, we also faced the problem of finding the right level of abstraction. Although we conducted preparatory interviews for the modeling and analysis with the application experts, we discovered during the modeling that we were missing certain pieces of information (lack of information). For this reason, we have to point out that our models may deviate from reality to some extent.

12. Conclusion and outlook

Finally, we would like to give the following conclusion and prospect for further work.

In our opinion, the visualization of processes can help to illustrate the complex human, technical, and organizational interrelationships in care processes and thus increase acceptance of these processes. Combining an analysis of business processes with a focus on the user experience (UX) seems to be a suitable approach to gain insights into how digital technologies are used in everyday life.

The balance of metrics for technical, organizational, and human activities is a good measure to determine which activities predominate in the process and may need to be adjusted from a users' perspective. The detailed analysis of TOM activities at the level of the individual swim lanes can provide information on where there may be an overload of human or organizational activities and where a higher level of technical activities can lead to greater automation and finally to better usability and acceptance from the user's and participating institutions' point of view.

In addition, the separate evaluation of human activities is a good measure for recognizing possible acceptance problems, for example, due to too frequent manual input or for describing the complexity of a technical system (too many interactions required for use).

With its standardized notation of processes, BPMN provides a basis for the integration and harmonization of different processes, analysis approaches, and quality metrics in the healthcare sector [48–50]. To integrate these different concepts, it would certainly be of interest to consider semantic technologies such as ontologies or semantic data repositories [51].

However, if the existing limitations of this study are eliminated, a reference model for generalization of telemonitoring applications based on the DiGA.Pro models could be created as follow-up work. The individual process and architecture models for interaction and communication, data exchange, and data storage are already available in their initial stages.

Acknowledgements

This work was supported by the DiGA.Pro project funded by the German Federal Ministry of Health on the basis of a decision of the German Federal Parliament (Bundestag) under funding ID ZMI5-2521FSB010. We would like to thank the sponsors and our interview partners for their support in making this publication possible.

Author details

Michael John*, Juan Vito-Antonio Held, Nele Sassor and Michael Wagner
Fraunhofer Institute for Open Communication Systems, Berlin, Germany

*Address all correspondence to: michael.john@fokus.fraunhofer.de

References

[1] OECD. Health at a glance 2023. OECD Indicators. 2023. Available from: https://www.oecd.org/health/health-at-a-glance/ [Accessed: November 07, 2023]

[2] gematik: TI-Atlas. Wo steht die Digitalisierung des Gesundheitswesens?. Available from: https://www.gematik.de/telematikinfrastruktur/ti-atlas

[3] Heiden I, Bernhard J, Otten M. Wissenschaftliche Evaluation des Produktivbetriebs der Anwendungen der Telematikinfrastruktur 2023. Berlin: Studienbericht für die gematik GmbH; 2023. Available from: https://www.gematik.de/media/gematik/Medien/Telematikinfrastruktur/TI-Atlas/IGES-Studie_Wissenschaftliche_Evaluation_des_Produktivbetriebs_der_Anwendungen_der_TI_2023.pdf

[4] Kassenärztliche Bundesvereinigung (KVB). Videosprechstunde. Telemedizinisch gestützte Betreuung von Patienten. Stand. 2024. Available from: https://www.kbv.de/html/videosprechstunde.php

[5] Evers-Wölk M, Sonk M, Oertel B, Kahlisch C. Wie bewerten Bürger/innen die Telemedizin? Ergebnisse einer Repräsentativbefragung, TAB-Sensor Nr. 4. Available from: https://www.tab-beim-bundestag.de/news-2022-01-25-wie-bewerten-buerger-innen-die-telemedizin.php, S.9-11

[6] Doctolib Digital Health Report 2023. Digitalisierungsstrategie im Reality-Check – wo stehen wir, wo wollen wirhin? Stand Mai. 2023. Available from: https://media.doctolib.com/image/upload/mkg/file/Doctolib_Digital_Health_Report_2023.pdf

[7] Zandt F. Digitale Gesundheitsversorgung. Welche digitalen Gesundheitsdienste nutzen die Deutschen? Statista. 2023. Available from: https://de.statista.com/infografik/16205/nutzung-von-digitalen-services-von-aerzten-in-deutschland/

[8] gematik: Feinkonzept Zero Trust Architektur für die Telematikinfrastruktur. Available from: https://fachportal.gematik.de/fileadmin/Fachportal/Downloadcenter/gemKPT_Zero_Trust_V1.0.0.pdf, S.7

[9] Bundesministerium für Gesundheit (BMG). Digital-Gesetz (DiGiG). Gesetz zur Beschleunigung der Digitalisierung des Gesundheitswesens. Laufendes Verfahren. 2023. Available from: https://www.bundesgesundheitsministerium.de/service/gesetze-und-verordnungen/detail/digital-gesetz.htmlund

[10] Bundesministerium für Gesundheit (BMG), Gesundheitsdatennutzungsgesetz (GDNG). Gesetz zur verbesserten Nutzung von Gesundheitsdaten. Laufendes Verfahren. 2023. Available from: https://www.bundesgesundheitsministerium.de/service/gesetze-und-verordnungen/detail/gesundheitsdatennutzungsgesetz.htmlund

[11] Bundesministerium für Gesundheit (BMG), Krankenhauszukunftsgesetz (KHZG). Gesetz für ein Zukunftsprogramm Krankenhäuser. 2022. Available from: https://www.bundesgesundheitsministerium.de/krankenhauszukunftsgesetz

[12] Bundesministerium der Justiz (BMJ). SGB V, § 374a: Integration offener und standardisierter Schnittstellen in Hilfsmitteln und Implantaten. Available from: https://www.gesetze-im-internet.de/sgb_5/_374a.html

[13] Kassenärztliche Bundesvereinigung (KVB). DiGA Toolkit 1.0.0. Available from: https://mio.kbv.de/display/DIGA1X0X0/DiGA+Toolkit+1.0.0

[14] Fraunhofer FOKUS, DiGA. Pro. Integration von Digitalen Gesundheitsanwendungen und weiteren digitalen Diensten zu übergreifenden, patientenzentrierten Prozessen in der Versorgung. Available from: https://www.digapro-projekt.de/

[15] Bundesinstitut für Arzneimittel und Medizinprodukte (BfArM). DiGA-Verzeichnis nach § 139e SGB V. Available from: https://diga.bfarm.de/de

[16] Gemeinsamer Bundesausschuss (G-BA). Innovationsausschuss, Förderprojekte. Available from: https://innovationsfonds.g-ba.de/projekte/

[17] gematik GmbH, Arena für digitale Medizin. Whitepaper Telematikinfrastruktur 2.0 für ein föderalistisch vernetztes Gesundheitssystem, Berlin. 2020. Available from: https://www.gematik.de/media/gematik/Medien/Telematikinfrastruktur/Dokumente/gematik_Whitepaper_Arena_digitale_Medizin_TI_2.0_Web.pdf

[18] Dori D. Model-Based Systems Engineering with OPM and SysML. Springer; 2016. ISBN: 978-1-4939-3294-8

[19] Braspenning NCWM, van de Mortel-Fronczak JM, Rooda JE. A model-based integration and testing method to reduce system development effort. Electronic Notes in Theoretical Computer Science. 2006;**164**:13-28

[20] Barbarito F, Pinciroli F, Mason J, Marceglia S, Mazzola L, Bonacina S. Implementing standards for the interoperability among healthcare providers in the public regionalized healthcare information system of the Lombardy region. Journal of Biomedical Informatics. 2012;**45**(4):736-745

[21] Malhotra S, Jordan DA, Shortliffe EH, Patel VL. Workflow modeling in critical care: Piecing together your own puzzle. Journal of Biomedical Informatics. 2007;**40**(2):81-92

[22] Schweitzer M, Lasierra N, Oberbichler S, Toma I, Fensel A, Hoerbst A. Structuring clinical workflows for diabetes care: An overview of the OntoHealth approach. Applied Clinical Informatics. 2014;**5**(2):512-526

[23] Pufahl L, Zerbato F, Weber B, Weber I. BPMN in healthcare: Challenges and best practices, Information Systems. 2022;**107**:102013. DOI: 10.1016/j.is.2022.102013. ISSN 0306-4379

[24] Bowles J, Czekster RM, Webber T. Annotated BPMN Models for Optimised Healthcare Resource Planning. In: Mazzara M, Ober I, Salaün G, editors. Software Technologies: Applications and Foundations. STAF 2018. Lecture Notes in Computer Science. Cham: Springer; 2018;**11176**. DOI: 10.1007/978-3-030-04771-9_12

[25] De Ramón A, Fernández DR, Fernández, and Yolanda Sabuco García. Business process management for optimizing clinical processes: A systematic literature review. Health Informatics Journal. 2020;**26**(2):1305-1320. DOI: 10.1177/1460458219877092

[26] Muller R, Fischer J. BPMN as an enabling technology for resource-aware software processes. Software and Systems Modeling. 2011;**10**(4):491-515

[27] Zerbato F, Oliboni B, Combi C, Campos M, Juarez JM. BPMN-Based Representation and Comparison of Clinical Pathways for Catheter-Related

Bloodstream Infections. In: 2015 International Conference on Healthcare Informatics, Dallas, TX, USA. 2015. pp. 346-355. DOI: 10.1109/ICHI.2015.49

[28] Rolón E, Chavira G, Orozco J, Soto JP. Towards a Framework for Evaluating Usability of Business Process Models with BPMN in Health Sector. Procedia Manufacturing. 2015;**3**:5603-5610. DOI: 10.1016/j.promfg.2015.07.748. ISSN 2351-9789

[29] Leopold H, Mendling J, Günther O. Learning from Quality Issues of BPMN Models from Industry. In: IEEE Software, Vol. 33. July-Aug 2016. pp. 26-33. DOI: 10.1109/MS.2015.81

[30] Sadowska M. An approach to assessing the quality of business process models expressed in BPMN. E-Informatica Software Engineering Journal. 2015;**9**(1):57-77. DOI: 10.5277/e-Inf150104

[31] Braun R, Schlieter H, Burwitz M, Esswein W. Extending a business process modeling language for domain-specific adaptation in health- care. Wirtschaftsinformatik Proceedings. 2015;**32**:468-481. Available from: https://aisel.aisnet.org/wi2015/32

[32] Object Management Group®. About the business process model and notation specification version 2.0. Available from: https://www.omg.org/spec/BPMN/2.0/About-BPMN

[33] Camunda Services GmbH. Camunda modeler. Available from: https://camunda.com/de/download/modeler/

[34] Witte F. Goal question metric. In: Metriken für das Testreporting. Wiesbaden: Springer Vieweg; 2018. DOI: 10.1007/978-3-658-19845-9_22

[35] Bundesministerium für Gesundheit (BMG). Referat 524 "Nationales Gesundheitsportal", gesund.bund.de. Verlässliche Informationen für Ihre Gesundheit. Available from: https://gesund.bund.de/telemonitoring

[36] Gesundheit Digital. Telemonitoring. Available from: https://gesund.bund.de/telemonitoring

[37] Kassenärztliche Bundesvereinigung (KVB), Praxisnachrichten. Neues Versorgungsangebot startet: Telemonitoring bei Herzinsuffizienz. 2022. Available from: https://www.kbv.de/html/1150_57669.php

[38] Deutsche Hochdruckliga e.V. (DHL), Pressemitteilung. Ärzte sollen mit den Daten von Blutdrucküberwachungs-Apps arbeiten können. 2019. Available from: https://www.hochdruckliga.de/pressemitteilung/aerzte-sollen-mit-den-daten-von-blutdruckueberwachungs-apps-arbeiten-koennen

[39] Bundesinstitut für Arzneimittel und Medizinprodukte. Verzeichnis für digitale Gesundheitsanwendungen (DiGA). Available from: https://diga.bfarm.de/de/verzeichnis

[40] Gemeinsamer Bundesausschuss. Innovationsauschuss, Förderporjekte -Neue Versorgungsformen. Available from: https://innovationsfonds.g-ba.de/projekte/neue-versorgungsformen/

[41] Ferrante S, Bonacina S, Pozzi G, Pinciroli F, Marceglia S. A design methodology for medical processes. Applied Clinical Informatics. 2016;**7**(1):191-210. DOI: 10.4338/ACI-2015-08-RA-0111

[42] Davis FD, Bagozzi RP, Warshaw PR. User acceptance of computer technology: A comparison of two theoretical models. Management Science. 1989;**35**(8):982-1003

[43] Venkatesh V et al. User acceptance of information technology: Toward a unified view. Management Information Systems Quarterly. 2003;**27**(3):425-478

[44] Object Management Group. Decision model and notation™ (DMN™). Available from: https://www.omg.org/dmn/

[45] Carmody LC, Gargano MA, Toro S, Vasilevsky NA, Adam MP, Blau H, et al. The Medical Action Ontology: A Tool for Annotating and Analyzing Treatments and Clinical Management of Human Disease. medRxiv [Preprint]. 13 Jul 2023:2023.07.13.23292612. DOI: 10.1101/2023.07.13.23292612. Update in: Med. 2023 Nov 9; PMID: 37503136; PMCID: PMC10370244

[46] Dijkman R, Dumas M, van, Dongen B, Käärik R, Mendling J. Similarity of business process models: Metrics and evaluation. Information Systems. 2011;**36**(2):498-516. DOI: 10.1016/j.is.2010.09.006

[47] Vanderfeesten I, Cardoso J, Mendling J, Reijers HA, van der Aalst WMP. Quality Metrics for Business Process Models. In: Fischer L, editor. BPM and Workflow Handbook. Florida, USA: Future Strategies Inc.; 2007. pp. 179-190

[48] Blumenthal D, McGinnis JM. Measuring vital signs: An IOM report on core metrics for health and health care progress. Journal of the American Medical Association. 2015;**313**(19):1901-1902. DOI: 10.1001/jama.2015.4862

[49] Perleth M et al. Health Technology Assessment. Konzepte, Methoden, Praxis für Wissenschaft und Entscheidungsfindung. 2nd ed. Berlin: Medizinisch Wissenschaftliche Verlagsgesellschaft; 2014. ISBN 978-3-941468-71-9.

[50] Shroyer ALW, Carr BM, Grover FL. Health Services Information: Application of Donabedian's Framework to Improve the Quality of Clinical Care. In: Sobolev B, Levy A, Goring S, editors. Data and Measures in Health Services Research. Health Services Research. Boston, MA: Springer; 2015. DOI: 10.1007/978-1-4899-7673-4_7-1

[51] Tiwari S, Abraham A. Semantic assessment of smart healthcare ontology. International Journal of Web Information Systems. 2020;**16**(4):475-491. DOI: 10.1108/IJWIS-05-2020-0027

Chapter 5

Integrating Smart Meter Load Profiling for Enhanced Data Insights and Patient Care

Amleset Kelati, Juha Plosila and Hannu Tenhunen

Abstract

The utilization of smart meter data has opened new frontiers in the healthcare sector by enabling the detection of health status and daily life activities. A new methodology has been proposed to differentiate between normal and abnormal energy consumption, which can be leveraged to determine the health status of consumers by analyzing load profiling. By visualizing human activities based on electricity usage, there is a growing interest in using smart meter data for detecting health status and Activities of Daily Living (ADLs). The chapter discussed, this innovative approach utilizes the K-Means algorithm to classify the data and identify patterns in the energy usage of individuals. By analyzing this data, potential health issues can be indicated, thereby assisting the healthcare sector in addressing the needs of the elderly population more effectively. This technology has the potential to revolutionize healthcare by providing a non-invasive and cost-effective way to monitor the health of individuals and enable early intervention in case of any health issues.

Keywords: smart meter, data mining, machine learning, smart health, pattern clustering, activities of daily living

1. Introduction

The escalating population of elderly individuals and the accompanying surge in healthcare needs necessitate innovative approaches to address the challenges faced by the healthcare sector. Structural health-monitoring systems offer a potential solution by utilizing data from smart meters, which provide granular consumption details. By analyzing electricity usage patterns, these systems can offer insights into the health status of individuals. This chapter presents a methodology to determine abnormal behavior in electricity consumption significantly related to potential health issues. As the global population of elderly individuals rapidly grows, the healthcare sector faces unprecedented challenges in meeting the increasing demand. A structural health-monitoring system that leverages smart meter data to analyze consumers' electricity usage patterns can provide valuable insights into supporting the healthcare sector. This chapter explores the application of load profiling to differentiate normal and abnormal energy consumption, aiming to determine the health status of consumers.

The smart grid differs from the traditional grid due to its inclusion of peripherals for signal processing, hardware and software blocks of communications standard and management. The concept behind the smart grid involves the use of embedded computers to monitor energy generation and transmission, with the smart meter serving as a crucial peripheral device.

The integration of information technology in the smart grid has revolutionized the communication of electricity from power plants to end users. The smart meter plays a vital role in addressing the challenges associated with the rapid increase in electricity demand, while also supporting additional functionalities.

The application of the smart grid extends beyond the realm of energy management, with potential benefits in areas such as Ambient Assisted Living (AAL), healthcare, agriculture, and education. When used for health monitoring, smart grid technology can offer distinct advantages over traditional wearable devices. The smart meter serves as a key device in this context, collecting valuable information that enables elderly individuals or patients requiring special care to remain comfortably in their own homes, while receiving real-time assistance from caregivers and doctors.

The healthcare industry has been actively exploring the use of smart meter data to detect any changes in an individual's activities of daily living (ADLs) for healthcare applications. ADLs, which are considered to be fundamental self-care tasks, are necessary for an individual to live independently and maintain their overall healthcare and well-being. These tasks include bathing, dressing, grooming, toileting, eating, and mobility, all of which are crucial to ensuring an individual's health and independence. By closely monitoring changes in an individual's ADLs over time, healthcare providers can identify any declines in mobility or independence and take proactive measures to prevent further functional decline. This approach can be particularly useful for older adults, people with disabilities, and individuals recovering from illnesses or injuries that may affect their daily activities. By leveraging advanced technology such as smart meters, healthcare providers can monitor and analyze changes in ADLs and provide personalized care plans to ensure the best possible outcomes for their patients. This way, healthcare providers can improve the quality of life for their patients and help them maintain their independence, even when facing health challenges.

This chapter aims to analyze the application of smart meters within a cost-effective smart grid system that can monitor end user energy management by predicting behavioral patterns based on consumer habits and lifestyle. The overall objective of this approach is to reduce costs through energy savings and load proofing, while also monitoring the health status of consumers within their homes. The contributions of this work include: (1) a discussion of the principles of the smart grid and the new health monitoring options provided by smart grid technology features, including the integration of smart meter load profiling for monitoring patient vital signs at home; (2) an investigation of electricity usage in homes, incorporating information on usage duration and energy consumption to analyze and monitor normal and abnormal behavior; and (3) the development of a data mining model for load profiling energy usage, enabling the characterization of normal and abnormal consumer behavior.

This work is an extension of our previous paper [1], and this article is organized into several sections for a clear and organized presentation of information. The second section, labeled as 2, will delve into a discussion of related work, providing context for the research presented in the paper. In the third section, labeled as 3, the background information related to the Smart meter will be described in detail, outlining the underlying principles and technologies used. The fourth section, labeled as 4, will present a proposed load profiling method, which will be discussed in connection with both normal and abnormal behavioral characterization. Additionally, this section will include an in-depth analysis of the results obtained from this method. Finally, the paper will conclude with a discussion of future directions for research in Section 5, providing insights into where the field may be headed and what areas of investigation may be most fruitful in the coming years.

2. Related work

The theoretical background of this text is focused on the use of smart meters for load profiling in an e-health monitoring system. The text discusses how the data collected from smart meters can be used to support the healthcare sector by analyzing energy consumption patterns. The data analysis involves grouping the data, reducing it using matrix-based analysis, and using the K-Means algorithm for data mining clustering. The goal is to determine normal or abnormal behavior in electricity usage and relate it to the consumer's health status. The text also mentions the use of smart grids and smart meters in the healthcare, agriculture, and education sectors. Our resource, highlights related work on smart grids, load monitoring, and smart meter data analysis.

The study presents several key characteristics of smart grids that enable active consumer participation in marketing and service provision [2]. The researchers have examined and summarized the automation, monitoring, and remote-control capabilities of smart grids and smart meters [3]. The implementation of an Internet of Things (IoT) based smart grid system allows for communication control commands to be sent with scheduling responses, resulting in reduced response times and real-time monitoring [4].

The research emphasizes the use of load monitoring to assess the activity of patients in elderly homes. Smart meter data collection of daily living activities offers a cost-effective solution [5]. Specifically, this paper proposes an Early Intervention Practices (EIP) method that utilizes smart meter data to enable detailed real-time monitoring of energy consumption and user interactions with electrical devices [6]. The approach involves connecting the remote patient monitoring system directly to the patient's smart meter and analyzing the collected data to identify any behavioral anomalies using machine learning techniques.

Another work by the same author focuses on profiling users in the smart grid. By implementing smart meters, real-time energy usage of customers can be obtained [7]. The proposal involves analyzing smart meter data and using classification techniques to identify irregular energy usage patterns. In another paper, the same author discusses the monitoring of consumer electricity usage with high accuracy. Each device records consumer data at regular intervals, allowing for the identification and profiling of routines and habits [8]. Sudden abnormal changes in behavior can be detected based on the analysis of regular activities performed by consumers throughout the day. Advanced metering infrastructure is utilized to monitor electricity usage and distinguish between normal and abnormal usage [9].

The application of smart meters is also beneficial for identifying emerging abnormal behaviors and trends in individuals living alone with various health conditions. Load profiling and detection methods are employed to identify sudden changes in behavior related to illnesses such as depression and Alzheimer's [9].

Smart meters have the ability to detect behavioral changes and determine if a house is vacant or not [10]. Authors in this context utilize Non-Intrusive Load

Monitoring (NILM) to disaggregate a household's aggregated energy consumption into individual appliances [11].

The main research question in this study is how to use smart meter data to support the healthcare sector by load profiling normal or abnormal energy consumption. The hypothesis is that clustering the data using the K-Means algorithm can identify normal and abnormal behavior of electricity usage, which can be indicative of the consumer's health status.

Our proposed solution addresses the challenges faced in previous studies by presenting a suitable method for distinguishing patterns in consumer energy usage. This paper introduces a monitoring technique for individuals with health limitations, allowing them to live independently in their own homes for a longer period based on their individual needs and conditions. The proposal involves analyzing energy usage, smart meter data, and employing data mining, clustering, and classification techniques to identify normal and abnormal energy consumption.

3. Research method

The objective of this study is to explore the potential application of smart meters in load profiling and its impact on consumer behavior. The data obtained from smart meters is analyzed using disaggregation algorithms and machine learning tools to identify individual usage patterns. These patterns are then used to analyze and understand normal and abnormal household energy consumption patterns.

Figure 1 illustrates the overall architecture of our proposed load profiling system for e-health monitoring, which is based on the principles of smart meters and power consumption measurements on the smart grid. The system utilizes cloud

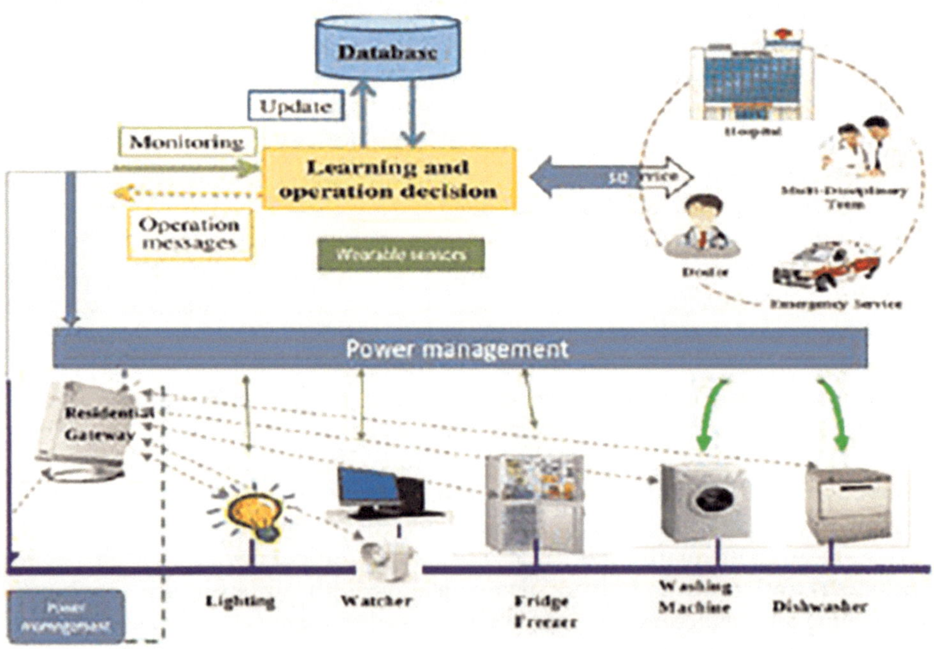

Figure 1.
The proposed smart meter load profiling architecture.

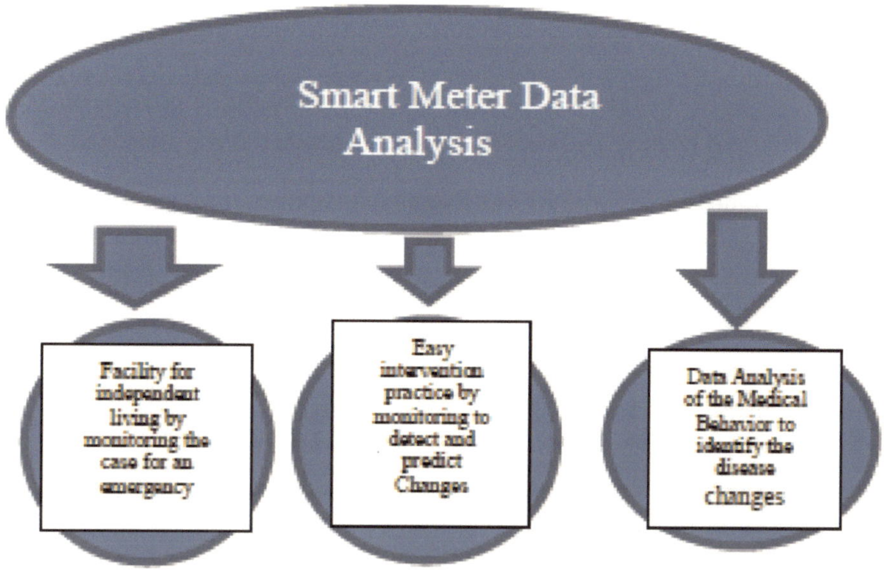

Figure 2.
Smart meter application for e-health monitoring.

infrastructures to provide comprehensive monitoring services and is capable of classifying normal and abnormal behaviors. This figure depicts the proposed architecture for smart meter load profiling.

A smart meter is a sophisticated tool used in smart grids for data collection and measuring electricity usage. It is equipped with features that enable real-time collection of energy consumption data from various households and appliances.

Figure 2 presents the key components involved in the analysis of smart meter data for e-health monitoring.

The methodology used in this research involves analyzing the electricity consumption data collected from smart meters in 12 households. The data, collected at one-hour intervals for one month, is grouped and reduced using matrix-based analysis. The K-Means algorithm is then applied to classify the data and determine normal or abnormal energy consumption patterns. The Sum Square Error (SSE) is used to assess the clustering results. The goal of this methodology is to support the healthcare sector by profiling the energy consumption patterns and detecting any abnormal behavior that may indicate changes in the health status of the consumers.

To evaluate the proposed methodology, a measured dataset from 12 households was collected using smart meters. The data spans a month and is sampled every hour. The dataset is processed by grouping it according to characteristic patterns, and then reduced using matrix-based analysis. The K-Means algorithm, a data mining clustering technique, is employed to classify the data.

4. Smart meter data analysis

In order to establish the feasibility of our study, we obtained energy consumption data from smart meters installed in 13 houses that rely on Swedish Energy for their power supply. The power consumption levels were recorded at

60-minute intervals over a one-month period in October 2017. However, one of the houses had to be excluded from the analysis due to insufficient data availability. Consequently, we were left with a total of 8940 smart meter datasets from 12 houses, which were utilized to identify patterns of normal and abnormal electricity usage. Each house featured heating and cooling systems, lighting, and a variety of similar appliances.

Upon examining the weekly and daily load, as depicted in **Figures 3** and **4** provide, we observed that, for all 12 houses, the peak energy consumption occurred in the morning and evening on a daily basis throughout the entire month. However, it is

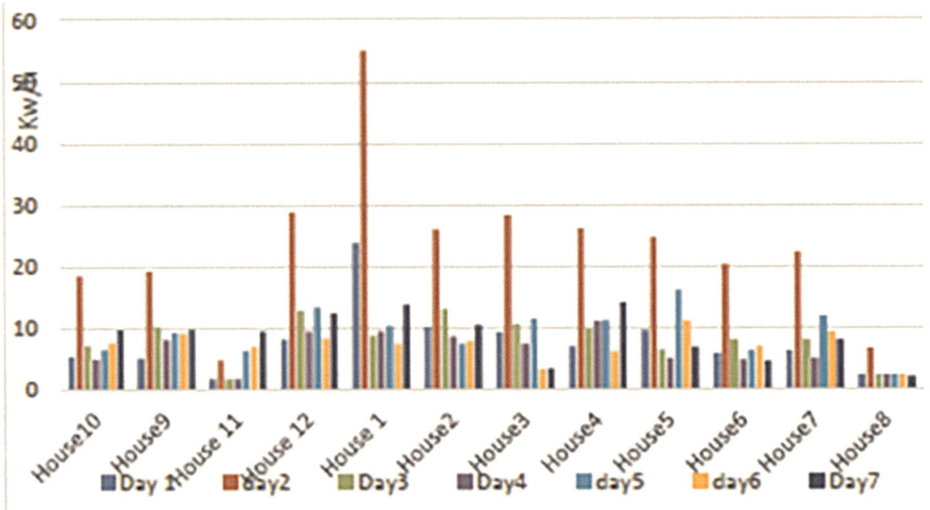

Figure 3.
Weekly electricity load consumption for visualization.

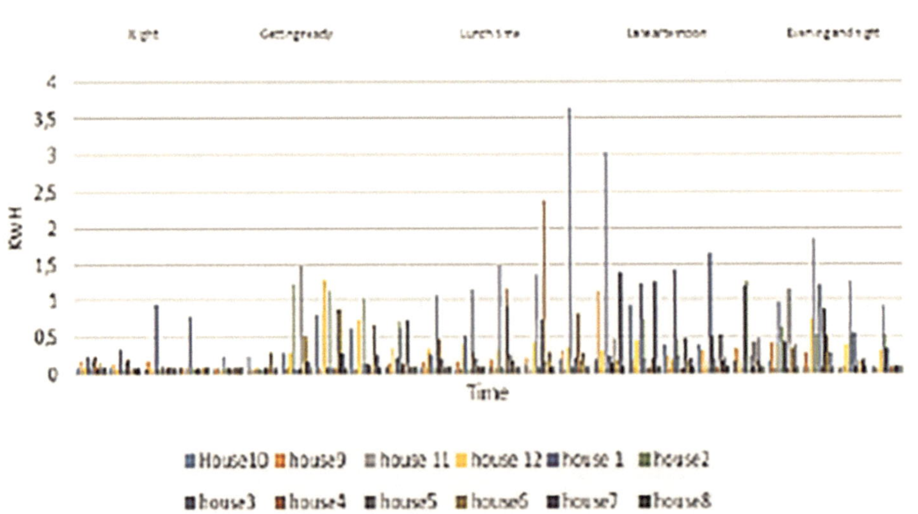

Figure 4.
The 24-hour power consumption of all the houses.

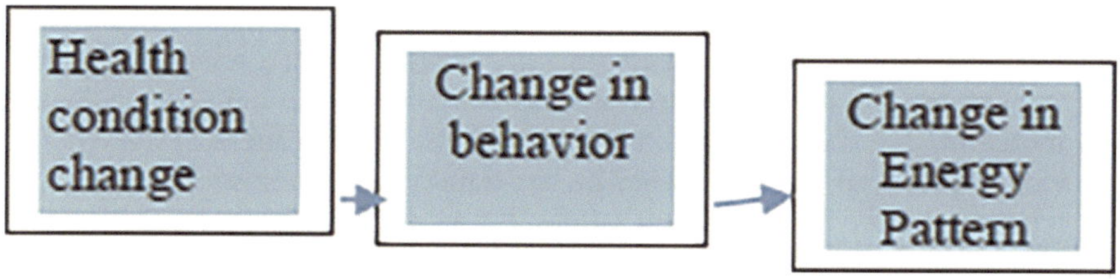

Figure 5.
The corresponding trend in behavioral change due to energy consumption.

worth noting that there were five houses that exhibited distinct trends in either low or high energy consumption levels over the course of the month, suggesting the presence of abnormal usage patterns.

Figure 1 illustrates the correlation between behavioral change and energy consumption. To observe variations in electricity usage among households, the mean and standardization of power consumption measurements were calculated. Additionally, **Figures 3** and **5** provide a clear visualization of the peak loads for each house on a daily and weekly basis.

4.1 Load profiling in relation to household behavior

Based on the analysis of the collected data, abnormal energy usage patterns have implications for the user's health. We propose that these patterns can be categorized into various behavioral health conditions, as shown in **Table 1**.

The relationship between energy usage patterns and health events demonstrates a trend where changes in health lead to changes in energy consumption. This process of behavioral change is depicted in **Figure 5**.

4.2 Data analysis

The energy usage during daily activities in the 12 houses was measured over a 24-hour period. The trend of peak loads remains consistent throughout the month. The figure allows for easy identification and visualization of periods when consumers are sleeping, at home, or when no one is home. Most houses exhibit an increase in energy consumption at specific times.

The mean and the standardization of measurements of the power consumption is calculated in order to observe the different home usage of electricity.

The weekly and a daily electricity load can clearly also lead to visualize the peaks load of each house for each day separately as shown in **Figures 3** and **4**.

The process of analyzing smart meter data for power consumption in 12 houses involves several steps. Firstly, the load pattern data of each household is measured under specific loading conditions. Secondly, representative features are selected from

Category	Energy usage category	Abnormal indication assumption
A	High energy during late hours (night and evening)	Related to (Alzheimer)
B	Low Energy in the morning	Sick or depressed (lone hours in bed)

Table 1.
Energy usage and behavioral category.

the data. Thirdly, the load pattern data is processed to create a matrix input for the specified loading condition. Finally, clusters are formed using a selected algorithm, considering the composition of household classes and time-domain data. Clustering validity indicators are then computed to evaluate the effectiveness of the clustering.

The accuracy of load profiling relies on the data collection module, the description of time stamps, and the measurement values. Signal processing and machine learning algorithms are employed to profile and characterize the measured data.

In terms of features, smart grids have the capacity to generate extensive datasets through smart meter measurements. However, visualization techniques may not always provide a straightforward means of distinguishing between different types of energy usage behavior. Therefore, the first step in dataset analysis is to extract the feature patterns and classify them using selected classification algorithms [12].

4.3 Features

The features extracted from smart meter data can be categorized into four groups based on feature selection theory described in [13]. Firstly, there are features related to maximum or minimum energy consumption, which depend on the energy usage at different times such as day or night, weekdays or weekends, etc. Secondly, there are features that represent the ratios between maximum or minimum energy consumption values. Thirdly, there are features that capture the statistical variability of power consumption, including measures such as standard deviation, sum of absolute differences, variance, auto-correlation, and other statistical values within the range of maximum and minimum. Lastly, there are temporal features of power consumption that resemble patterns, including consumption levels, peaks, and significant moments. These temporal features can indicate household activity or inactivity in terms of electricity usage.

The data in question pertains to the first group, which has seven features per consumer, resulting in a total of 84 features. These 84 features are used to identify the maximum and minimum energy consumption of each household. Additionally, the cross-correlations of the pattern data can be used to detect whether the energy consumption of a household is related to others by comparing the average energy consumption of all the houses.

There is a total of 12 houses, each with 744 instant measurements. Among these, eight have normal measurement readings, while four have abnormal readings. Further, two of the houses have low energy consumption, while two have excessive energy consumption. This excessive consumption can be indicative of a consumer's health status.

To distinguish between normal and abnormal electricity usage, one of the most effective visualization methods is through representation. In this case, the original Electricity Load can be visualized using a Matrix M, where I = 744 and N = 12. The Matrix M represents the total instant measurements for each house, allowing for a clear and detailed visual representation of electricity usage patterns.

$$M = \begin{vmatrix} A_{11} & A_{12} & \dots\dots\dots\dots\dots\dots\dots A_{112} \\ \vdots & \vdots & \vdots \\ A_{7441} & A_{7442} & \dots\dots\dots\dots\dots\dots\dots A_{74412} \end{vmatrix} \tag{1}$$

The Matrix M744 denotes the power consumption of house number 12 over the course of 744 measurements throughout the month. The matrix consists of 744 rows, representing the attributes, and 12 columns, representing the instances. The data in matrix M is transposed, with rows indicating instances and columns indicating attributes.

$$M' = \begin{vmatrix} A_{11} & A_{12} & \dots\dots\dots\dots\dots\dots\dots A_{1744} \\ \vdots & \vdots & \vdots \\ A_{121} & A_{122} & \dots\dots\dots\dots\dots\dots\dots A_{12744} \end{vmatrix} \tag{2}$$

Dimension reduction is performed on the dataset due to the excessive number of attributes. The process involves the following steps:

Firstly, we select the duration of time for one month, specifically October 2017, and consider the electricity consumption of 12 instances (houses).

Secondly, we aggregate the electricity needs for each group time of the day throughout the entire month. This aggregation is carried out by summing the electricity consumption data.

It is important to note that the dataset's information is recorded in Swedish time, and the electricity consumption of the houses is categorized into five time periods during the day, as indicated in **Table 1**.

As a result of the dimension reduction, each house (instance) is represented by five attributes, which are presented in the following matrix representations:

$$Mnew_{reduced} = \begin{vmatrix} x_{11} & A_{12} & A_{13}A_{14} \\ \vdots & \vdots & \vdots \\ A_{121} & A_{122} & A_{123}A_{124} \end{vmatrix} \tag{3}$$

$$Mnew_{reduced} datasetisusedvisualization \wedge clustering \tag{4}$$

5. Results and discussions

5.1 Results

The example dataset resulting from the dimension reduction process is shown in **Table 2**.

The following information depicts **Table 2**, which contains an unprocessed dataset of households along with their unique identification numbers and their respective electricity consumption during various time zones. This dataset outlines the quantitative data for households' electricity usage, which can be analyzed and interpreted for research or analytical purposes.

House	Night	Morning	Lunch	Late Night	Evening
#1	31	58,22	62,66	71,66	108,81
#2	20,31	59,44	46,18	46,68	87,6
#3	30,04	43,5	45,27	61,63	80,75
:	:	:	:	:	:
:	:	:	:	:	:
#12	38,6	69,21	81,14	83,18	113,03

Table 2.
The reduced dataset of the 12 houses power consumptions according to the time using $\mathrm{Mnew}_{\mathrm{reduced}}$.

5.2 Data visualization, figures representation

The graph depicted in **Figure 6** illustrates the relationship between household and electricity consumption in kW/h. The x-axis represents the households and the y-axis represents the electricity consumption. Upon analyzing the graph, it can be observed that the majority of households consume less than or equal to 100 kW/h of electricity throughout the day. However, there are a few exceptions to this trend. House #7 and House #8 have significantly low power consumption, whereas House #1 and House #12 have a higher electricity consumption rate. These variations in consumption patterns can be correlated with the abnormal health conditions mentioned in **Table 1**. Additionally, there seems to be a trend in behavioral change due to energy consumption on the smart grid, which is contributing to the consumption patterns observed in the graph.

In order to verify the similarity in specific time and power consumption between households, it is recommended to use a data mining classification method. This method is effective in identifying the similarities and differences between different households based on their energy consumption patterns. Specifically, the K-Means algorithm can be employed to cluster the dataset into different classifications, which can help to identify households with similar energy consumption patterns.

By analyzing the consumption patterns, it is possible to identify households that consume either more or less electricity than a normal household would consume. This abnormal usage can be indicative of various issues, such as faulty electrical appliances or inefficient energy usage. Therefore, by identifying these households, it may be possible to take corrective actions to improve energy efficiency and reduce energy consumption.

Overall, the use of data mining classification methods and the K-Means algorithm can be an effective way to identify abnormal energy consumption patterns in households, which can help to improve energy efficiency and reduce energy consumption. To verify the similarity in specific time and power consumption between households, a data mining classification method should be used. The K-Means algorithm can be employed to cluster the dataset into different classifications. The analysis of the consumption pattern suggests that some homes consume more or less electricity than a normal household, which indicates abnormal usage.

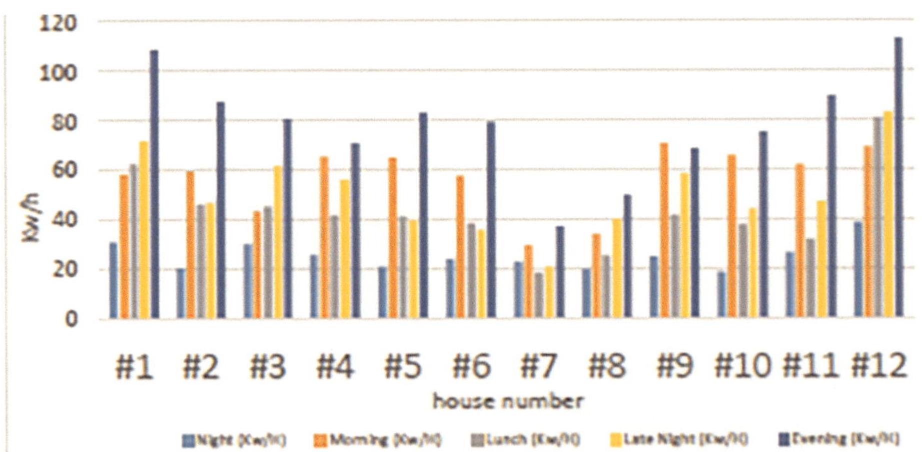

Figure 6.
The comparison graph of the total electricity consumption between the five-time periods during the day.

5.3 K-means algorithm

The k Nearest Neighbor (KNN) algorithm is a supervised classifier that is widely used for clustering and classification of large datasets. One of the most popular clustering algorithms is the k-Means algorithm, which is preferred due to its simplicity of implementation and frequent application in fields similar to electricity consumption datasets. It has been listed as one of the top 10 data mining algorithms [14] and is used to group data based on the similarity of data characteristics.

To obtain the cluster label of the data, the main parameter is to compute the distance of the data from the neighborhood data, compare the distance, assign the clusters and visualize the cluster points. This is done using different distance calculation methods, such as the Euclidean distance calculation method. The user defines the K-Means method to classify the given dataset into K clusters, where K is the number of clusters. The clustering algorithm minimizes the sum of squared distances between all points and the cluster center. The calculation and approach to determine the k function clustering have the following steps as indicated in [15].

$$D(x,y) = \sum_{i=1}^{n}(xi + yi) \tag{5}$$

The clustering algorithm uses the input dataset and computes the distance to cluster centers (usually Euclidean distance) between an instance and all instances of the training set in the matrix. By comparing the distance between the data points, the algorithm assigns each data point to its nearest cluster center. This process is repeated until the algorithm converges to a stable solution. The resulting clusters are then visualized to gain insights into the data. Overall, the k-Means algorithm is a powerful tool for clustering and classification of large datasets, and it has been widely used in various fields for its simplicity and effectiveness.

The following text describes the process of clustering data using the agglomerative algorithm. This algorithm starts with n clusters, where each cluster contains a single sample or point. It then merges two clusters that have the closest similarity between them, and this process is continued until the number of clusters becomes 1 or is specified by the user.

To determine the algorithm for n samples, the k-nearest neighbors are distinguished. The datasets are used to obtain clusters, and the two closest clusters are merged. The new cluster center is computed, and the distance is again calculated. This process is repeated until all the cases have been merged into one. The sum square error (SSE), which describes the standard deviation of each cluster to the data center, is calculated using the formula below during the clustering process:

$$\mathrm{SSE} = \sum (\mathrm{xi}\text{–}\bar{\mathrm{x}})^2 \tag{6}$$

Here, xi represents the data point and $\bar{\mathrm{x}}$ represents the mean of the data points.

The input data for this clustering process includes the measurements of all 12 houses. The process segments the data from one to five clusters to measure the SSE and the number of iterations in each. The largest SSE is obtained when clustering with 1 cluster (all the members of the house are included). However, the SSE has better performance with 5 clusters (the members of the houses are classified according to k-Means with 5 clusters). The SEE result is shown in **Table 3**.

clusters	1	2	3	4	5
SSE	13.352	10.827	6.801	4.225	2.462

Table 3.
Results from the clustering.

Cluster number	Number of cluster members	Average Night (kw/H)	Average morning (kw/H)	Average lunch (kw/H)	Average Late Night (kw/H)	Average Evening (kw/H)
1	18.34	18.34	65.52	38.01	44.35	75.77
2	21.22	21.22	31.80	21.71	30.56	43.41
3	25.04	25.04	68.08	41.78	57.43	69.74
4	22.81	22.81	61.15	39.34	42.19	85.04
5	33.21	33.21	56.98	63.02	72.16	93.58

Table 4.
Clustering result for 5 clusters.

Table 4 shows the results of the 5 clusters. In the normal case, electricity usage is highest during the evening. However, the analysis from the SSE result indicates that, for some members of the cluster, the lowest power consumption is during the night.

There are also abnormality indications for the member of the cluster that has abnormal power consumption during the 24 hours of the day.

Figure 7 and **Table 4** show the clustering results that identify the houses with very high and very low electricity usage, including the corresponding 24-hour power consumption measurements.

Initially, it was expected that the feature set 4 households have abnormalities in power consumption compared with the others. However, the analysis of the k-Means clustering algorithm demonstrates that the prediction on the pattern clusters of the households can detect abnormal energy usage behavior. The result of the status of each house is described as follows:

The houses with high power consumption are household #1 and household #12. These conditions remain true even during the evening and late-night hours.

The houses with low power consumption are household #7 and household #8. These conditions also remain true even during the morning (wakeup time), lunch, and most of the day.

5.4 Discussions

Technology has greatly influenced human civilization throughout history, from the invention of tools to the creation of the internet. It has brought numerous benefits and advancements but also raised concerns and challenges that need to be addressed. The internet and digital communication have transformed the way we connect and interact with one another, revolutionized the workplace, and created new opportunities. However, the rapid pace of technological advancement has raised concerns about the digital divide, privacy, and data security.

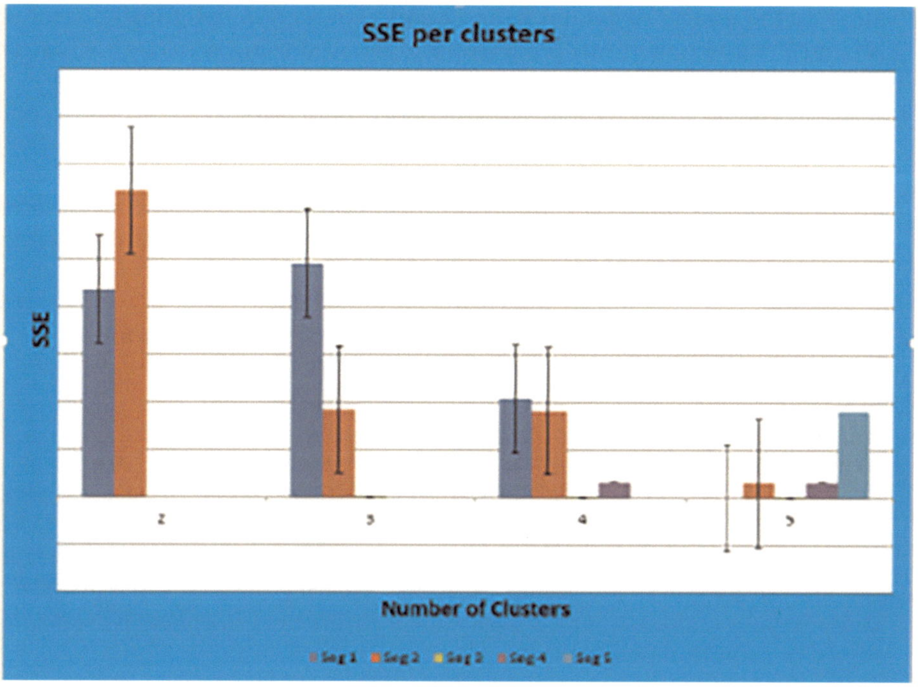

Figure 7.
Comparison of SSE for each segment of houses.

As the population of elderly individuals continues to grow, the healthcare sector is facing unprecedented challenges in meeting the increasing demand for healthcare services. To address these challenges, a structural health monitoring system that uses smart meter data to analyze consumers' electricity usage patterns has been proposed. This system can provide valuable insights into supporting the healthcare sector by analyzing the electricity usage patterns of elderly individuals.

This study explores the use of load profiling to identify abnormal energy consumption and potential health issues. Data was collected from 12 households using smart meters and analyzed using the K-Means clustering algorithm. The results showed a clear connection between abnormal energy usage and potential health issues, which can assist the healthcare sector in addressing the needs of the elderly population more efficiently. Overall, this article presents a novel approach for utilizing structural health monitoring systems to support the healthcare sector for ADL in meeting the needs of the rapidly growing elderly population.

1. Research the global population of elderly individuals and the challenges faced by the healthcare sector in meeting their increasing demand.

2. Learn about structural health monitoring systems and their potential to leverage smart meter data for analyzing electricity usage patterns.

3. Understand the concept of load profiling and how it can differentiate normal and abnormal energy consumption.

4. Study the methodology presented in the paper for evaluating abnormal behavior in electricity consumption significantly related to potential health issues.

5. Analyze the measured dataset from 12 households collected using smart meters and understand how it was processed and reduced using matrix-based analysis.

6. Learn about the K-Means algorithm, a data mining clustering technique, and how it was employed to classify the data.

7. Study the clustering results and their connection with the normal or abnormal behavior of electricity usage, which enables the determination of potential health issues for the consumer.

8. Understand how the clustering results can be compared to known health conditions to assume the consumer's health status and AAL in the category of ADL

9. Evaluate the novel approach presented in the paper for utilizing structural health monitoring systems to support the healthcare sector for ADL.

10. Identify future work that should focus on validating the methodology on a larger dataset and incorporating additional parameters to enhance the accuracy of health condition predictions.

6. Conclusion

The Article has shown that smart meters can play a crucial role in providing valuable insights into the daily routine changes or ADL of individuals, particularly for healthcare applications. This is a significant development in the healthcare industry as it can help in early detection and timely intervention, which can significantly improve the quality of life of patients while reducing healthcare costs. Smart meters can collect data on various aspects of an individual's life, including sleep patterns, energy consumption, and mobility. This data can be analyzed to identify changes in daily routines, which can indicate early signs of illness or injury. By studying this data, healthcare professionals can provide timely support and care to individuals, potentially preventing the need for expensive hospitalizations and other medical interventions. The use of smart meters for health care and ADL detection is an exciting area of research with promising implications for the future of healthcare.

The data collected from smart meters can help healthcare providers to identify patterns and trends in the daily routine changes of individuals, which can be used to prevent or manage chronic diseases such as diabetes, hypertension, and cardiovascular diseases. In conclusion, the use of smart meters for healthcare applications is a significant advancement in the healthcare industry. It has the potential to improve the quality of life of patients while reducing healthcare costs. By providing early detection and timely intervention through the analysis of smart meter data, healthcare professionals can help individuals live healthier, happier lives.

Our upcoming research will focus on ensuring efficient and secure data management in smart meters suitable for healthcare applications. We aim to address security concerns by exploring encryption technologies, including advanced encryption algorithms that provide end-to-end encryption, to ensure secure data transmission between the smart meter and the utility provider. Our next phase of this research will

DOI: http://dx.doi.org/10.5772/intechopen.1004777

focus on developing algorithms that are tailored to specific healthcare applications to determine the most appropriate anonymization method. This way, sensitive data can be stored securely and only authorized individuals can access it.

In conclusion, smart meters are promising technologies that can improve AAL and support healthcare applications. However, we must address data security and privacy concerns before their implementation. Our approach involves developing more advanced encryption algorithms and anonymization methods that prioritize data security and user privacy without compromising system efficiency and cost-effectiveness.

Acknowledgements

This section of your manuscript may also include funding information.

Acronyms and abbreviations

AAL	Ambient Assisted Living
ADLs	Activities of Daily Living
IoT	Internet of Things
NILM	Non-Intrusive Load Monitoring
SSE	Sum Square Error

Author details

Amleset Kelati*, Juha Plosila and Hannu Tenhunen
Department of Computing, University of Turku (UTU), Turku, Finland

*Address all correspondence to: amlkel@utu.fi

References

[1] Kelati A, Plosila J, Tenhunen H. Smart meter load profiling for e-health monitoring system. In: 2019 IEEE 7th International Conference on Smart Energy Grid Engineering (SEGE). Oshawa, ON, Canada: IEEE; 2019. pp. 97-102. DOI: 10.1109/SEGE.2019.8859936

[2] Enose N. Advanced technologies implementation framework for a smart grid. Journal of Clean Energy Technologies. 2014;**2**(1):88-94

[3] Lobaccaro G et al. A review of systems and technologies for smart homes and smart grids. Energies. 2016; **9**(5):348. DOI: 10.3390/en9050348

[4] Tanyingyong V et al. IoT-grid: IoT communication for smart DC grids. In: 2016 IEEE Global Communications Conference (GLOBECOM). IEEE; 2016. DOI: 10.1109/glocom.2016.7841917

[5] Xiao CD, Xue Y, Zhang XL, Zhang PH. Modeling and Simulation of Smart Meters Based on Matlab/Simulink Software2013. DOI: 10.4028/www.scientific.net/AMR.846-847.760

[6] Chalmers C, Hurst W, MacKay M, Fergus. Profiling users in the smart grid. In: Emerging 2015: Seventh International Conference on Emerging Networks and Systems Intelliegence. (EMERGING 2015: Seventh International Conference on Emerging Networks and Systems Intelliegence, 19th - 24th July 2015, Nice, France). EMERGING 2015

[7] Chalmers C, Hurst W, Mackay MI, Fergus P. Smart monitoring: An intelligent system to facilitate health care across an ageing population. In: EMERGING 2016, the Eighth International Conference on Emerging Networks and Systems Intelligence. pp. 34-39. (The Eighth International Conference on Emerging Networks and Systems Intelligence, 09 October 2016 - 12 October 2016. Venice, Italy: Think Mind

[8] Chalmers C, Hurst W, Mackay M, Fergus P. Smart health monitoring using the advance metering infrastructure. In: Computer and Information Technology; Ubiquitous Computing and Communications; Dependable Autonomic and Secure Computing; Pervasive Intelligence and Computing (CIT/IUCC/DASC/PICOM) 2015 IEEE International Conference on. Liverpool, UK: IEEE; 2015. pp. 2297-2302

[9] Chalmers C, Hurst W, Mackay M, Fergus P. A smart health monitoring technology. In: Huang DS, Bevilacqua V, Premaratne P, editors. Intelligent Computing Theories and Application. ICIC 2016. Lecture Notes in Computer Science. Vol. 9771. Liverpool, UK: Springer; 2016. DOI: 10.1007/978-3-319-42291-6_82

[10] Zhang Y, Chen W, Black J. Anomaly detection in premise energy consumption data. In: Power and Energy Society General Meeting, 2011. IEEE; 2011. pp. 1-8

[11] Alcalá JM, Ureñá J, Hernández A, Gualda D. Assessing human activity in elderly people using non-intrusive load monitoring. Sensors. 2017;**17**(2):351

[12] Duda RO, Hart PE, Stork DG. Pattern Classification. 2nd ed. New York: John Wiley & Sons Ltd.; 2001. pp. 202-220

[13] Kelati A. Data-driven Implementations for Enhanced Healthcare Internet-of-Things Systems (Doctoral dissertation, KTH Royal Institute of Technology). 2021

[14] Beckel C, Sadamori L, Santini S. Towards an automatic classification of private households using electricity consumption data. In: Pappas GJ, editor. Proceedings of the Fourth ACM Workshop on Embedded Sensing Systems for Energy-Efficiency in Buildings. Toronto: ACM; 2012. pp. 169-176

[15] Davò F, Vespucci MT, Gelmini A, Grisi P, Ronzio D. Forecasting Italian electricity market prices using a neural network and a support vector regression. In: Proceedings of the 2016 AEIT International Annual Conference (AEIT); 5–7 October 2016; Capri, Italy: IEEE; 2016

Chapter 6

City Competent Model to Implement Care at Home

Francesca Cioffi, Daniela Sgroi, Tiziana Chiriaco, Marina Cerbo and Francesca Milito

Abstract

The Local Health Unit, called ASL Roma 3, is focused on the best organizational and technological solutions that allow citizens, especially those with greater fragility and disabilities, to benefit from assistance at home. To facilitate both the collaboration between operators and citizens and the provision of telemedicine, ASL Roma 3 recently introduced Participative Art as an innovative model to empower citizens and strengthen the use of telemedicine services, modernizing its approach. Here, we describe how participative art facilitates the new model of relation between Institutions and empowered citizens, called City Competent. IPACS, Institutional & Public Coaching Services supported ASL Roma 3 with coaching and participative art to achieve change in homecare culture and positive relationships between institutional operators and citizens. As a result of upskilling in communication, negotiation, and decision making, the diffusion of telemedicine services increases, strengthening home care and remote collaboration between professionals facilitated by the City Competent Model.

Keywords: telemedicine, homecare, participative art, city competence, competence economy

1. Introduction

The NRRP [1] Mission 6 - Health - aims to strengthen and reorient the National Health Service (NHS) to improve its effectiveness in responding to people's care needs, also considering critical issues emerged during the pandemic emergency, and is divided into two components:

- Component 1: Proximity networks, intermediate structures, and telemedicine for territorial assistance.
- Component 2: Innovation, research, and digitalization of the National Health Service.

IntechOpen

Component 1 aims to strengthen the services provided in the area thanks to the improvement of territorial structures and facilities (such as Community Houses and Community Hospitals), the reinforcement of home care, the development of telemedicine, and more effective integration of all social and health services.

Telemedicine, or the provision of remote health services, represents a pillar for the innovation of health services, as it facilitates collaboration between professionals and citizens; in this view, strengthening of telemedicine services has become one of the "enabling" interventions within the NRRP to bolster digital public services and modernize the National Health Service.

The European Commission has attributed particular importance to the topic of telemedicine for over a decade.

With the European Communication "Telemedicine for the benefit of patients, health systems and society," of November 4, 2008, a series of actions were identified that involve all levels of government, in the both community and individual Member States, to encourage greater integration of telemedicine services into clinical practice, removing the main barriers that hinder their full and effective application.

For a systematic use of telemedicine within the National Health Service and to implement European Communication, the Technical Table on telemedicine was established at the Superior Council of Health, which has drawn up specific national guidelines for:

- place the priority areas of application of telemedicine.
- analyze models, processes, and methods of integrating telemedicine services into clinical practice.
- define common taxonomies and classifications.
- define the aspects concerning the legislative and regulatory profiles and the economic sustainability of telemedicine services and performances.

Being the world-leading continent toward a truly democratic future engaged with Care at Home, the European Union faces a series of needs. In line with the 2030 Agenda—which has also been reaffirmed by Next-Generation EU—the care at home needs to be accompanied by the digital transition, which may be viewed as providing important operational support to both professionals and citizens. It is a bottom-up approach where individuals can be educated and motivated to intelligently collaborate with public sector institutions and the various levels of government. Educating and motivating such intelligent bottom-up collaboration is exactly the prerogative of the City Competent persons who result from the Competence Economy Project (www.competenceconomy.it).

In 2018, IPACS (www.ipacs.it) intercepted, with a regional survey of 30 Italian Local Health Authorities (LHA), two essential needs not satisfied in the political-institutional field: (1) developing the ability to interact and forming an alliance between the institutions and the citizens; and (2) developing attitude to work with an interdisciplinary approach, as informal leaders in action, to manage complex contexts and adapt the organization to rapid changes.

In June 2019, in an institutional event, with the patronage of the Ministry of Health and the Ministry of Cultural Heritage, IPACS validated and launched the use of Participatory Art, as a *learning strategy*, to *accelerate* the process to work with *interdisciplinary perspective* in action, as well as to *develop policies, such as bringing telemedicine to citizens*" [2–5].

Competence Economy think tank (www.competenceconomy.it) introduces the new organizational and learning model that connects territorial operation centers (COT) with the hospital operation center (COO), empowering the main skill called "emotional intelligence," essential to achieve social objectives (such as those of NRRP) and inclusiveness in a short period of time, and measuring the related impact on social economy.

During 2022 and 2023, ASL Roma 3 has carried out several activities of training for representatives of all the operational units and clinical services for the use of the digital and telemedicine systems, besides the definition of institutional procedures for telemedicine.

Moreover, in ASL Roma 3, there is an institutional office that deals with the coordination of telemedicine services with monthly meetings to manage process and applicative problems and for proposals regarding service improvement. A service center for support and resolution of IT problems is also set up.

To support the access to tele visits by patients, doctors and nurses involved in tele visit activities provide guidance and indicate to patients/caregivers how to access the system and the European Social Fund (ESF). The information is also accessible on the company website and posted in the clinics to increase citizens' access to the ESF.

Currently, the present and future challenges for national and local institutions are to achieve the best use of the NRRP resources to strengthen telemedicine services, encourage the digitalization and reorganization of the management processes, and renovating the mode of interaction between LHA and patients, reducing distances, and increasing their digital and self-care skills.

2. Methodology and steps

The methodology implemented in ASL Roma 3 is based on the intention of intercepting citizens eligible to become City Competent leaders who help communities and institutions to give practical solutions and implement plan of action to address unmet social needs, specifically concerning the implementation of Care at Home and Telemedicine.

The expected impact of potential City Competent leaders will be: (1) developing the ability to interact and create alliances between institutions and the communities to reduce access inequalities to telemedicine; (2) developing an "informal leadership," among citizens and institutions to manage complex contexts of remembrance and adapt to rapid changes of Care at Home. We are in the trend called "empowerment of the citizen" and in the OECD guideline "lifelong adult learning." After step 1, where the potential City Competent are selected from the whole population, citizens are placed in a learning and evolution art and coaching pathway (step 2), together with the managers of public administration, to achieve the common system objective. The aim is to build communities by activating at least n.10 additional citizens for each City Competent empowered (in a ratio of 1:10). Step n.3 is aimed at certifying City Competent, putting them in a reputational list, and involving them in further system objectives useful to communities and institutions.

Adhering to the City Competent Model, citizens are allowed to access the following four benefits:

IPACS is a Social Enterprise Ltd who aims to empower citizens, including managers of the Public Administration in soft skills useful for developing policies, through a skills-based economy model, which connects the system objective with the soft skills functional to it. Its mission is to perform social research, starting from the concreteness of the experience of "Competence Economy" (www.competenceconomy.it), to measure results of empowerment on individuals and target communities, after providing a learning experiential pathway, integrated with coaching and participatory art, lasting about 6 months (research protocol). Participatory art helps citizens to find common goals and benefits, to develop critical and creative thinking; coaching supports citizens to develop creative solutions to system constraints.

Table 1.
IPACS's vision and mission.

Citizens are certified as "City Competent" able to implement telemedicine, and are listed on a specific reputation ranking list.

Citizens will be part of a community recognized nationally and internationally as facilitators of "Social, Economic and Healthcare Innovations."

Citizens will be strengthened in the meta-skills identified as strategic for their community and territory. The results will be measured with an assessment pre and post the IPACS' integrated pathway. Results are measured as well in terms of progress in system objective plans (e.g., number of activities put in place).

The participatory Art method will ensure intergenerational and interdisciplinary exchange of experiences, practical knowledge, achievements, resources, values, mindset, and perspective.

The level of skills acquired influences people's well-being and opens opportunities that would otherwise be precluded; on the other side, lifelong learning is useful for building and participating in contemporary society. In a society where a low level of trust in politics and democratic institutions is replaced by an innovative approach with Participative Art, which deconstructs people's beliefs and builds a bridge between institutions and citizens, among citizens of a community, to reach specific common objectives, working, and co-creating together. We would like to emphasize that our innovative methodology starts with an analysis of the social and cultural issues, opportunities, and social needs, upon which we will build a survey to list activities and behaviors to be implemented through the empowerment of meta-skills. The IPACS' vision, mission, and scientific results are pointed out in **Table 1** and **Appendix B**.

3. The context in which the city competent model is applied

The resident population in the territory of the Local Health Institution ASL Roma 3 is equal to 575,585 people, of which 9.8% are affected by two or more pathologies. These patients, mostly elderly, require multi-professional and multidisciplinary assistance to prevent further complications, guaranteeing, where possible, permanence in the socio-family environment, with a respectful approach that protects the dignity of life of the person and the family.

Inspired by the principles of equality and fairness, the ASL Roma 3 has for years been engaged in researching the best organizational solutions that allow citizens, especially those with greater fragility and disabilities, to benefit from assistance at home.

Telemedicine, or the provision of remote health services, represents a pillar for this organizational innovation of health services, as it facilitates collaboration between professionals and their relationship with citizens, and the strengthening of telemedicine services has become one of the "enabling" interventions within the NRRP to strengthen digital public services and modernize the National Health Service.

Currently, the present and future challenges for our institution are to achieve the best use of the NRRP resources to strengthen Telemedicine services, and encourage the digitalization and reorganization of the management processes and a new mode of interaction between ASL and patients, reducing distances, and increasing their digital and self-care skills.

The ASL Roma 3 has a territorial area of 517 square km, which corresponds to the Municipalities of Rome and the territory of the Municipality of Fiumicino.

It has a catchment area of 604,787 inhabitants divided into four districts, coinciding with the mentioned municipalities.

Of the 604,787 [6] residents in the Asl's territory, 52.39% are female and 47.61% are masculine. The demographic structure is characterized by a significant share of the elderly population (22.6% of those over 65) but with a value that does not differ from the regional average (equal to 22.8%).

The analysis of the demographic structure of the population highlights a certain lack of homogeneity in the company territory. In fact, urban areas are characterized by an older population, in particular Municipality XII, in which the fraction of people over 65 is equal to 25.7%, and of these, over half are over 75 years old.

In contrast, the coastal areas are characterized by a younger population, in particular, the Municipality of Fiumicino, in which the fraction of people over 65 is equal to 17.9%.

The ASL old age index is equal to 164.9, lower than the regional average [7], but with significant differences between the different districts, in fact in Municipality XII, the old age index is equal to 212.9, while in the Municipality of Fiumicino is 118.7.

The dependency ratio also shows how the aging population "weights" on active population, once again remaining higher in the two Roman districts (average regional 55.5 [7]).

The resident foreign population stands on average at 11.3% compared to a regional average of 10.8%, with a greater presence of immigrants regularly registered in Municipality XI.

The trend in mortality of residents in the Company, in the last decade, shows a trend decreasing, with a standardized rate of 817.1 per 100,000 in 2019, in line with the average regional.

Cardiovascular diseases, in line with the regional average, represent the leading cause of death in both women and men, followed by malignant tumors (with a slightly higher percentage than the regional figure) and respiratory diseases. Also, for other causes of death, we observe an overlap with regional data.

The analysis conducted by the Department of Epidemiology of the Lazio Regional Health Service – ASL Rome 1 (DEP Lazio) in 2021 [7] on the estimate of the healthcare needs of the ASL population highlights that 9.8% suffer from at least two chronic pathologies (2.3% of cases are characterized from high complexity), takes polypharmacological therapy, and presents, in 17.6% of cases, a socio-economic vulnerability.

The epidemiological, social, and demographic context described above, as well as the economic impact of multichronicity in the Health Service, have led the ASL to adopt an approach to chronic and multi-chronic population centered on the Case Management and Transitional Care model through the definition of personalized care paths aimed at avoiding fragmentation of care and ensuring, as far as possible, that the patient remains at its own home. This approach is consistent with the interventions envisaged by Component 1 of Mission 6, "Networks of proximity, structures, and telemedicine for local healthcare" of the NRRP [1], and materializes in a series of actions, some already carried out and others in the implementation phase inspired by the following principles:

Equity and universality: guaranteeing healthcare services to all citizens without distinction of individual, social, and income conditions.

Centrality of the person: pursuing "global" care of the person, and in particular of the person with fragility and chronicity, activating the appropriate health and social-health interventions according to the paradigm of proximity, accessibility to care, and integration between services hospital and local, with the contribution of telemedicine services.

Participation: promote the participation of citizens, associations, and the community.

Initiative healthcare: prevention and improvement of chronic disease management in every stage, from primary prevention to early diagnosis, to clinical and healthcare management, to the prevention of complications, through proactive follow-up also supported by telemonitoring and teleassistance tools, for the global management of multimorbidity.

4. Sustainability and innovative management of human resources through the creation of mixed groups composed of local health authority employees and competent citizens

The Ministerial Decree of May 23rd, 2022, n. 77 "*Regulation containing the definition of models and standards for the development of territorial assistance in the National Health Service,*" published in the Official Gazette no. 144 of June 22nd, 2022, identifies the qualitative, structural, technological, and quantitative standards of the structures dedicated to territorial assistance and the prevention system in the health, environmental, and climate fields. The new approach involves the use of population stratification systems and the definition of functions of the professional figures already operating within the Health Institution within the new territorial services, as summarized in **Table 2**.

Working on digital skills and the well-being of your employees becomes more fundamental than ever. Digital transformation paths represent a real opportunity to put this new concept of human resources at the center of the reorganization of service strategies.

Interdisciplinary team	Main contact for
General Practitioner, Community Doctor, Service doctor	Main contact for clinical pathway, for territory planning, and Community House activities
Nurse	Main contact for global needs analysis
Specialized doctor	Main contact for diagnostic and therapeutic complexity
Pharmacist	Main contact for pharmacological therapeutic program
Psychologist	Main contact for the assessment of psychological needs
Social worker	Main contact for the assessment of social needs

Table 2.
Main contact for the new territorial services.

In this context, health institutions are called upon to promote a real corporate culture oriented toward change. It is necessary to encourage a transformation of leadership roles and styles, as well as identify the skills and professional figures necessary for the management of innovation. The final goal is to become a digital organization founded on a new managerial culture, on the valorization of people's talent and on cutting-edge digital skills. With the spread of new technologies, the complexity of the term digital competence grows today. It not only refers to a set of technological skills that go beyond the simple use of the computer but also requires flexibility and speed of learning.

A survey—carried out by Piessepi and Nomisma with the support of Gidp [8] on human resources managers belonging to a panel of leading Italian companies, which evaluated events in the last 24 months, in relation to the organization, initiatives in favor of organizational well-being and for the enhancement of digital skills—has documented that almost half of the companies involved declare having carried out technical training activities in the last 24 months, 42% have carried out soft skills training activities, and 23% have undertaken individual coaching courses that support people in their growth phase.

In fact, in addition to hard skills (such as technical-professional skills such as qualifications, experiences, and certificates), for the new health services being activated, it is necessary to evaluate additional transversal skills and aptitudes such as:

- Internal transversal skills: These are the skills through which one perceives and interacts with oneself.
- External transversal skills: these are the skills through which one perceives and interacts with others.
- Even in the healthcare sector, it is important to introduce, in addition to the evaluation of skills in the clinical and healthcare fields, methods of evaluating soft skill indicators (behavioral attitudes) for the following additional areas:
    - Adaptability
    - Cultural contribution
    - Interpersonal skills
    - Leadership
    - Growth potential
    - Time and priority management
    - Analytical skills
    - Problem solving
    - Team working
    - Multitasking
    - Passion and enthusiasm

These skills, translated as transversal skills, represent the personal qualities, or rather, attitudinal characteristics, of a candidate: character traits, personal attributes, communication skills, and a whole series of signals that could facilitate success at work.

In the context of the reorganization of territorial and hospital services in light of Ministerial Decree 77 and in the realization of the objectives of the NRRP, it is therefore crucial to increase the aforementioned skills in all professionals and identify the specific skills to guide the choice of personnel who will be dedicated to the new services, and at the same time activate new staff search methods to evaluate all the aforementioned types of skills.

4.1 Sustainability

To guarantee the sustainability of the services being activated with the NRRP, beyond the time horizon of the plan, it is important to define the framework of activities and functions of the new services in order to evaluate a company standard, in addition to the personnel standards defined by the Ministerial Decree 77/2022, to identify the professionalism to be dedicated to the Territorial Operations Centers (COT), Community Nurses, Single Access Point (PUA), Community Houses (CDC), and Telemedicine Service Centre.

For example, to define an activity benchmark for the Operations Centers, it would be appropriate to evaluate the number of activations of home, rehabilitation, and residential programs and the number of services provided in the national and regional information flows.

Furthermore, for an evaluation of the population that may need telemedicine assistance for chronic patients and home services, the stratification of the same by risk profiles, through predictive algorithms, allows to differentiate the intervention strategies for the population and for taking charge of patients based on the level of risk, health needs, and consumption of resources.

In our region, it is possible to use the stratification of the population resident in the territory carried out by the SSR Department of Epidemiology (DEP). In the territory of ASL Roma 3, we have the following population stratification summarized in **Figure 1.**

Finally, the use of digital applications in the context of the activities of management of care and assistance paths allows the evaluation of workloads, duration of activities and search for benchmarks for a series of innovative performances both in favor of patients and for the cooperation with other professionals, provided in the COT, CDC, and Telemedicine Services. In this regard, the development process of the services requires the acquisition of new professional figures and the continuous integrated training of those present through a process of continuous monitoring of the required skills and abilities.

The necessary professionals will have to carry out global responsibility tasks that will accompany the patient-user in the system and will have to govern the system itself in such a way as to limit the use of acute hospital facilities to a minimum, constantly accompanying the patient, thanks to digital tools and of telemedicine, in its healthcare needs. See the summary in **Table 3**.

Appendix A summarizes the innovative human resources management introduced by Ministerial Decree 77/2022 (DM77).

In order to put in place and combine the needs for information, training in the field of digital services, telemedicine, and new healthcare models of social

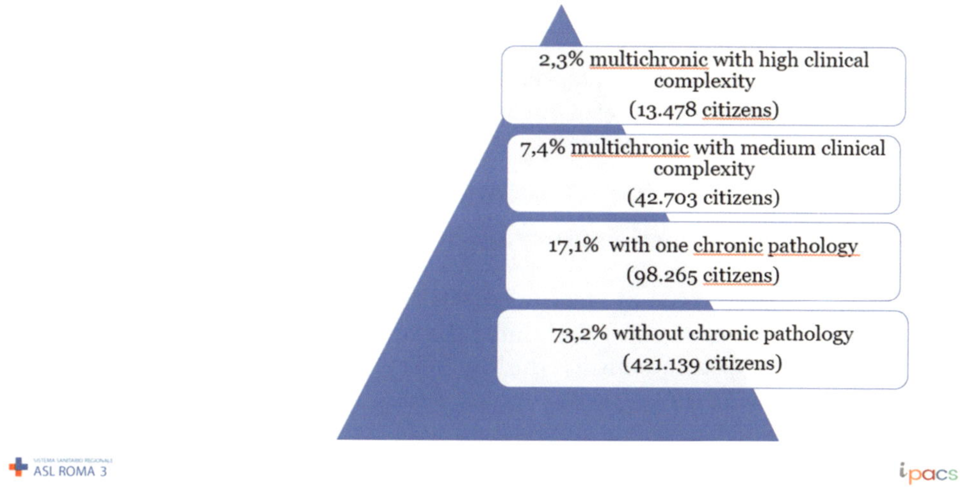

Figure 1.
ASL Rome 3 population stratification.

Community Houses	Physical and easily identifiable place to which citizens can access for health, social and healthcare needs. In the Community House all professionals work in an integrated and multidisciplinary manner for the planning and provision of health and social integration interventions.	7–11 Nurses 1 Social Assistants 5–8 Administrative—Social Operation support
Community Nurses	Reference professional figure who ensures nursing care at different levels of complexity in collaboration with all the professionals present in the community	1 community nurse every 3000 inhabitants
		1 UCA pract. and nurse) x 100.000 inhab
Continuity of Care Unit	District mobile team for the management and support of taking charge of individuals, or communities, who find themselves in particularly complex clinical-care conditions and which involve a proven operational difficulty	1 nurses coordinator, 3–5 nurses 1–2 Operation support
Territorial Operation Center	Organizational model, which carries out a function of coordination of taking care of the person and connection between services and professionals involved in the different care settings: territorial, health and socio-health, hospital activities, and dialogs with the emergency-urgency network.	7–11 Nurses 1 Social Assistant, 5–8 Operation support

Table 3.
Standard resources and services locations in ministerial decree n.77/2022.

and health integration during 2023, the ASL Roma 3 and IPACS (Institutional and Public Coaching Services) have launched the City Competent Model on Telemedicine topics, with the aim of making citizens and operators of the ASL Roma 3 literate about the new healthcare in the area, and about the digital tools available.

Making the citizens of ASL Roma 3 literate means making sure that they understand how it works and how to access the new health care in the area, how assistance works after hospitalization at home, what are the digital tools that bring citizens closer to ASL professionals, such as they are digital self-care tools.

Literalizing the internal and external operators of ASL Roma 3 means ensuring that they understand how services are integrated into the new treatment path for fragile patients, how healthcare interventions for citizens can be improved from self-care to home assistance, how to guide citizens to access health services, such as coordinating nurses on local services.

5. Role and impact of participatory art in the competent citizen model

An interdisciplinary team of economists, artists, pedagogists, coaches, and psychologists has launched since 2021 under the coordination of Prof. Francesca Cioffi (www.competenceconomy.it), the Manifest of Competence Economy to study how emotional intelligence may enhance the ability of individuals to improve change and flexibility to accept an innovation such as telemedicine. The central idea is that enhancing emotional intelligence could empower transformative participatory citizenship. Moreover, publications [9] show that higher emotional intelligence enhances happiness and flourishing, compensates for the negative effect of perceived inequality, and creates an indirect effect on happiness and flourishing by nurturing sustainable and innovative consumption such as telemedicine's services. Taking all these results together, the team envisages a possible future in which City Competent people can help nurture a more technological society where individuals become the

Milestone	Description	Date
Measure the relationship between empowered professionals and activated citizens in a specific territory and in response to the achievement of a specific system objective, such as bringing telemedicine to citizens	The research by IPACS in 2019 and 2020 on a total of 112 Public Managers (n.41 in 2019 and n.71 in 2020) showed that 112 enhanced professionals activated around 1000 citizens. The 112 professionals were strengthened in their core skills (goal orientation, networking, and teamwork communication), reaching the achievement of 80% of the action plan. The selected and achieved system objectives have shown that the empowerment of professionals determines the ability of patients and citizens to take action (i.e., adhere to HCV drug therapy and return to follow-up).	2019 2020
Relationship between empowered professionals and activated citizens confirmed	IPACS research in 2021 on a total of about 142 empowered professionals on five soft skills (the four core plus the emotional intelligence soft skill) confirmed the relationship between one empowered professional and ten activated citizens, which is maintained at a ratio of 1:10.	2021
Strengthening the set of five soft skills (goal orientation, networking, teamwork, communication, emotional intelligence) allows the achievement of the action plan	The IPACS research in 2022 on a total of 48 professionals who worked—from an interdisciplinary perspective—with 40 citizens in the same interinstitutional meetings demonstrated that the achievement of the action plan is 100% against the strengthening of the set of five soft skills (goal orientation, networking, teamwork communication, emotional intelligence).	2022
Accelerate the implementation of strategic system objectives	The City Competent Model is aimed at creating institutional interdisciplinary roundtables composed of Citizens and Public Managers to facilitate the learning and accelerate the implementation of strategic system objectives.	2023 ongoing

Table 4.
City competent model milestones.

main characters of their own future. In this chapter, we want to point out that telemedicine implementation is facilitated with the participative art methodology. The project will allow the testing of this last hypothesis, allowing the design of coaching and participative art activities that consider the main findings of the research to focus on elements that can enhance individuals' emotional intelligence.

Competence Economy and City Competent Model (Empowerment Platform and Participative Art content) are covered by copyright.

Table 4 points out milestones of the City Competent Model.

6. Description of results achieved in Italy in telemedicine, since 2012

1. The first national guidelines on Telemedicine were approved by the General Assembly of the Superior Council of Health on July 10th, 2012. On February 20, 2014, in order to guarantee the "coordinated, harmonious and coherent development of telemedicine within the National Health Service," the Agreement was signed between the Government, the Regions, and the autonomous Provinces of Trento and Bolzano on the document "Telemedicine – National guidelines."

The Agreement represents a particularly relevant result considering the need to rethink the organizational and structural model of our country's National Health Service, with respect to the fact that the diffusion of telemedicine services across the territory can constitute an important enabling factor.

The implementation of the national guidelines on Telemedicine was assessed during LEA obligations up to 2017 to verify their adoption. Since 2018, all regions have implemented the guidelines themselves with their own resolutions.

In 2019, as part of the work of the NSIS control room, the Ministry approved the establishment of a working group on telemedicine, which includes representatives of the regions Lombardia, Veneto, Emilia Romagna, Piemonte and Tuscana, as well as the National Center for Telemedicine and New Assistance Technologies of the National Institute of Health (ISS), which has created a national mapping of regional experiences and produced uniform indications across the entire national territory for the provision of remote services.

Following the State-Regions Agreement of February 20, 2014, and the Reports of the ISS COVID-19 n. 12/2020 *"Interim indications for telemedicine healthcare services during the COVID-19 health emergency"* of April 13, 2020 and n.60/2020 *"Interim indications for telemedicine healthcare services in pediatrics during and beyond the COVID-19 pandemic"* of October 10, 2020, in the meeting of the NSIS control room on July 28, 2020, the Ministry of Health and the Regions and Autonomous Provinces of Trento and Bolzano shared the need to provide uniform indications across the entire national territory for the provision of remote services, with particular attention to specialist activities, extending medical and healthcare practice beyond the physical spaces in which it usually takes place according to traditional procedures, also in relation to the initiatives launched by some regions during the Covid emergency period.

The working group on telemedicine, also integrated by experts and representatives of the national federations of health professions (FNOMCeO and FNOPI), has therefore prepared the document:

- "National indications for the provision of telemedicine services," which was approved by the NSIS control room in the session of October 28th, 2020, and was adopted with the Agreement in the State-Regions Conference of December 17th 2020 (Repertoire of documents no. 215/CSR). This document intends to provide the indications to be adopted at a national level for the provision of some telemedicine services such as tele visits, medical teleconsultation, medical-health teleconsultation, teleassistance by health professionals, telereporting, so that the possibility of using telemedicine services (e.g., tele visits for check-ups) represents a concrete element of organizational innovation in the care process.

- "Indications for the provision of telerehabilitation benefits and services by healthcare professions," which was approved by the Control Room in the session of 9 April last and was adopted with Agreement in the State-Regions Conference on November 18, 2021 (Repertory of Acts no. 231/CSR).

This document intends to provide uniform indications for the entire Italian healthcare system regarding telerehabilitation services by healthcare professionals, as well as the services that can derive from the combination of the services with each other and with other healthcare services. Just like rehabilitation, telerehabilitation also finds application in all age groups, from developmental age to the elderly, in various areas including cognitive motor, neuropsychological, occupational, communication, swallowing, behavior, cardiological, and telerehabilitation pulmonary. In consideration of their specificity, the specific aspects of the fields of cardiac and pulmonary telerehabilitation are not covered; subsequent national indication documents will be dedicated to them.

- The first National Consensus Document on telemedicine for cardiovascular diseases was published: indications for telerehabilitation and telemonitoring. The document aims to define the medical indications for performing telecardiology services: the appropriate telemedicine activities are indicated for chronic patients with heart failure, arrhythmias, atrial fibrillation, chronic ischemic heart disease, adults with congenital heart diseases, and for the prevention of pathologies cardiovascular.

For this purpose, three types of services were examined: telereporting, telemonitoring, and telerehabilitation.

As part of the NRRP's Health mission, Home as a place of care and telemedicine, the Ministry of Health has also planned the creation of a single telemedicine system, integrated with national digital health systems.

It was initiated by the notice published by Agenas as the implementing institution for the design, implementation, and management of the enabling services of the National Telemedicine Platform, as decided by the Interministerial Committee for the digital transition on December 15, 2021. The objective is to bridge the gap between territorial disparities and offer greater integration between regional health services and national platforms, through innovative solutions. The development of telemedicine is among the interventions that have made the home the first place of care. The National Telemedicine Platform is understood as the set of different services (tele visit, teleconsultation, telemonitoring, and teleassistance) which, by cooperating and interoperating in synergy, create the final services for patients and operators, guaranteeing the monitoring of the processes at the different levels of government involved.

The Organizational Guidelines containing the digital model for the implementation of Home Care (Milestone EU M6C1–4) contain the fundamental components of the telemedicine services home organizational model, with the following principal lines:

a. The home care service, which guarantees continuity of assistance in the modalities indicated by national and regional legislation.

b. The planning of home access, developed over the entire second week as provided for by the legislation, considering the clinical-care complexity of the patients.

c. The home care service integrated with remote telemedicine services.

It aims to contribute to the achievement of the following system objectives:

- Increase the number of patients cared for at home, allowing the threshold value of 10% of patients aged over 65 to be reached.
- Guarantee the entire population the same level of care and quality of care provided, improving organizational efficiency even in geographically disadvantaged contexts.
- Provide the patient with assistance that includes responses to clinical-care needs and psychological needs to reduce the negative impact of the patient's illness experience.
- Reduce access to the emergency room, hospitalization, and exposure to related risks, as well as the use of institutionalization.
- Allow a protected discharge from hospitalization facilities by ensuring home care continuity of assistance and equally effective treatments.
- Reduce day hospital visits by developing alternative responses at home.

7. Description of impact of the city competent model on telemedicine in ASL Roma 3

The 9.8% of resident population in the territory of the Local Health Institution ASL Roma 3 is affected by two or more pathologies. These patients, mostly elderly, require multi-professional and multidisciplinary assistance to prevent further complications, guaranteeing, where possible, permanence in the socio-family environment, with a respectful approach that protects the dignity of life of the person and the family.

Inspired by the principles of equality and fairness, the ASL Roma 3 has for years been engaged in researching the best organizational solutions that allow citizens, especially those with greater fragility and disabilities, to benefit from assistance at home.

In ASL Roma 3, are active multiple telemedicine services such as teleconsultation, tele visit, telemonitoring, and home teleassistance, which were also launched through projects prior to the pandemic period and which have allowed our Institution to use the skills already acquired in strengthening home care of patients and remote collaboration between professionals.

Specifically, for the management of patients in emergency procedures, a teleconsultation service has been active since 2020 between the doctors of the Emergency

Department of the Giovan Battista Grassi Hospital and the specialists of the reference Hubs hospital for the emergency networks, infectious diseases, stroke, trauma, which are at least 20 km away. Since the start of the service, approximately 2000 teleconsultations have been carried out, which confirms the importance of telemedicine as a collaboration tool between professionals involved in emergency patient care despite the territorial distance between the structures.

In line with the national and regional indications on tele visit, an institutional procedure has been adopted in our ASL, with the aim of promoting the uniform application of the rules and regulations of the legal system for the execution of tele visits for patients belonging to outpatient specialist care settings, protected discharge, local and home services, mental health outpatient services, and consultancy, and therefore to promote the improvement of the quality of the Service Healthcare.

In the outpatient setting, 12 tele visit ambulatories have been activated since 2020, at both hospital and local levels, including, since July 2020, over 5500 follow-up tele visits for follow-up and for the renewal of treatment plans for cardiological, endocrinological, and pneumological devices and drugs. Specifically for the renewal of treatment plans, the company-wide service has been active since November 2020 at the Acilia Polyclinic, and the company website "*Therapeutical plans - ASL Roma 3*" provides details to facilitate access by citizens to this service and to the Electronic Health Record.

Furthermore, for over 10 years, the Cardiology Unit of the P.O. G.B. Grassi Hospital has an active telemonitoring and teleassistance service dedicated to patients with cardiac devices (pacemakers, defibrillators, and loop recorders, with approximately 1450 telemonitoring), while at the Nephrology Unit, a teleassistance service has been active for about 3 years for 30 patients undergoing dialysis treatment at your domicile.

Finally, since March 2020, a teleassistance nursing service has been activated for more than 48.000 COVID-19 patients, under home management and for patients with chronic pathologies or in fragile conditions during the regional "Heat Waves" prevention campaign, in collaboration with the District Coordination and the general practitioners and pediatricians. In total, 80 users including doctors and nurses have been enabled for the system, with an institutional procedure. If, during teleassistance, the need for a re-evaluation for a chronic pathology or renewal of a cardiological, endocrinological, or pneumological therapeutic plan emerges, the nurses will contact the doctors of the company's territorial tele visit service.

During 2022 and 2023, this service was extended to patients at greater risk of side effects from heat according to the relevant prevention regional plan. During 2023, 6553 patients resident or domiciled in ASL Roma 3 were followed via teleassistance, as follows:

- Health District X Municipality: 2127 assisted.
- Health District XI Municipality: 1861 assisted.
- XII Municipality Health District: 1801 assisted.
- Municipality of Fiumicino Health District: 764 patients.

Furthermore, in the 2020–2021 emergency period, the Mental Health Department of our Institution has remotely followed 4272 patients (2032 aged 0–17 years and 2240 > 18 years) for a total of 11,651 services, including consultations, clinical evaluations, visits medical, interviews, psychotherapy, as well as liaison activities with the bodies involved in the individual case.

8. Results of city competent model achieved in ASL Roma 3 on telemedicine driving objectives

Based on the result analysis of the incoming and outcoming skill assessment test, summarized in **Figure 2**, we empowered the behaviors of 24 potential Competent Citizens and Local Health Authority Operators aimed at overcoming internal obstacles, in the medium term, through the result and process indicators, summarized in **Table 5** for Municipalities X, XI, XII, and Fiumicino.

Participatory Art, with the tool of dialog and feedback, used in the co-design of two landing pages, moved the team from an approach centered on themselves, on their own vision of reality, to a vision integrated with the perspectives of others. The

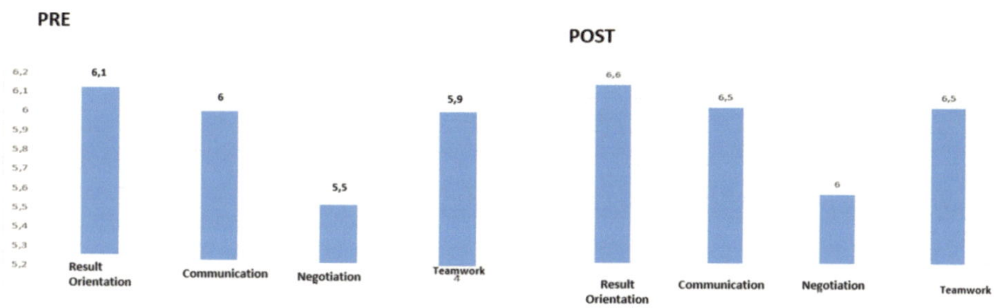

Figure 2.
Analysis of the assessment test in and out skills linked to the guiding objective.

Making the citizen of ASL Roma 3 literate means making sure that they understand how it works and how to access the new healthcare in the area, how assistance works after hospitalization at home, what are the digital tools that bring citizens closer to ASL professionals, what are the digital self-care tools
Indicators
1. Dedicated time-territory/area.
2. Number of virtuous behaviors performed (grounded in everyday life) in the role of City Competent *(e.g. suspension of judgment regarding the ideas and opinions of others, introspection, giving feedback, asking open questions, understanding one's own and others' emotions and own and others' needs, activate trust, mediate needs, mediate communications, expose oneself personally without fear of being judged, and feeling vulnerable)*
3. Number of citizens and ASL operators contacted
4. Evaluation of the doctor/specialist-patient interaction
5. Comparative assessment of the needs of the front office operator (non-empathic communication) and analysis of URP complaints
6. Exam booking report analysis
7. Number of common spaces managed with volunteers, GPs, PUA operators, district
8. Number of integrated and uniformly implemented forms
9. Reduction of complaints for failure to integrate services
Literacy of the internal and external operators of ASL Roma 3 means ensuring that they understand how the services are integrated into the new treatment path for fragile patients, how the healthcare intervention for citizens can be improved from self-care to home assistance, how to guide citizens to access health services, how citizens can be improved from self-care to home assistance, how to coordinate operators in local services.

Table 5.
Impact of the City competent process on behavior, indicators, and activities in the medium term in ASL Rome 3.

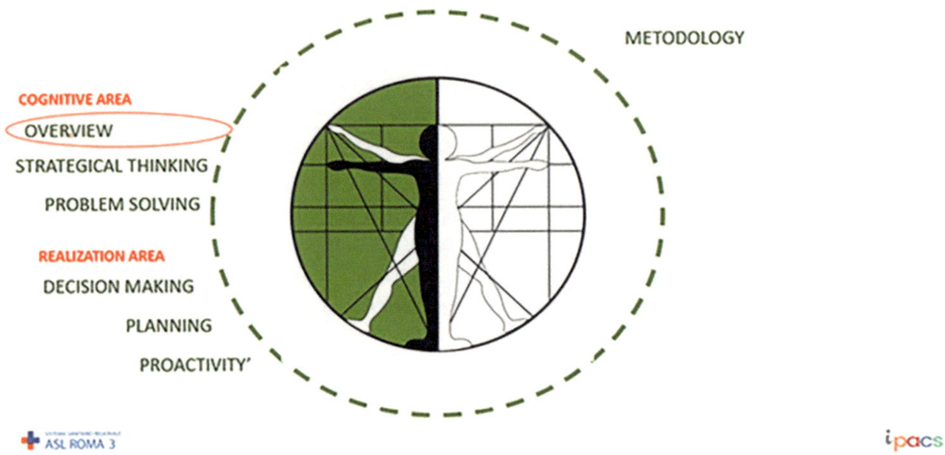

Figure 3.
Summary of the main critical issues overcome with the tool of participatory art.

development of an overall vision was preparatory for the interdisciplinary team to define a working methodology and activity planning, training both the cognitive area (strategic thinking) and the implementation area (planning). The summary is shown in **Figure 3**.

Participatory Art has trained dialog and comparison between City Competent and Institutional managers, which has facilitated City Competent to think in an analytical, strategic way and to benefit from the areas of implementation, improving planning, and decision making.

9. Discussion

To achieve the objective of implementing telemedicine services in existing care pathways is necessaire a literacy project for operators and citizens regarding the new digital and organizational tools of the NRRP, including telemedicine. It is also helpful to start a certification process for representatives of some patient associations, operating in the territory of our ASL, as competent citizens to support the realization of the socio-health objectives of the NRRP.

Participative art accelerates the community's empowerment in emotional intelligence soft skills, specifically concerning dialog and empathic communication.

Expanding on the issues addressed by the Competence Economy Model, digital transformation and telemedicine impose the need for new digital skills required. In turn, updating skills redesigns contents and teaching targets, including adult people needing permanent training. Work changes influence training dynamics: Lifelong learning processes become an enduring need for people in all sectors and roles. Today's skills will not match tomorrow's telemedicine's services, as newly acquired skills could quickly become obsolete [10]. It has been estimated that 85% of the jobs that today's citizens will have in 2030 have not yet been invented, and 90% will require digital skills. However, according to Digital Europe (2020), 44% of EU citizens still lack basic digital skills. In a ranking provided by DESI (Digital Economy and Society Index), Italy ranked 25th among the EU-28 in 2017, well below the European average: only 44% have "basic or above" digital skills (vs. the EU-28 average of 56%). Currently, 52% of the European workforce needs retraining due to changes in the labor market—it drops to 32% if we shorten the horizon to 2025 (Digital Europe, 2020). If we look at Italy, the numbers are further burdensome: We have 13 million adults with an eighth-grade level of education, and the estimate for those in need of retraining in the 25–64 range is up to 59%. These numbers justify the need to find new patterns of lifelong learning process, enabling fruitful overlapping between schools, universities, and workplaces to identify and satisfy the stakeholders' needs (e.g., employer/unemployed).

Moreover, the need for hard skills must be accompanied by the development and strengthening of soft skills, such as adaptability/learnability, cognitive flexibility, and emotional intelligence. This last one is considered the attribute that is perhaps the most influential to enable all the other soft skills (such as teamwork, communication, result orientation, and managing conflicts), which are considered more and more essential for success on the one hand and also for retraining on the other. These are the skills that are hardest to understand and systematize and the skills that give—and will continue to provide—humans an edge over robots [11]. According to Deloitte (2019), two-thirds of jobs created between now and 2030 will strongly rely on soft skills. Unfortunately, we already face significant shortages, which are forecasted to worsen.

These inequalities in skills will result in inequality in access and use of resources, exacerbating the already high disparities within and between countries that have been growing again in the last few years. Participative art is aimed at changing culture through disseminating value as dialog to overcome social inequalities [12]. As emphasized by the ILO in its updated version of the "Declaration on Social Justice for a Fair Globalization" [13], labor is not a commodity, and poverty anywhere constitutes a danger to prosperity everywhere. The persistence and growth of inequalities affect social cohesion [14], calling for strengthening social justice (it can be understood as Rawlsian primary goods or as Capabilities and Functioning by Sen and Nussbaum), which should not be underestimated. Even if the concept of justice—understood in the sense of what is considered right—is a concept that varies and evolves over time according to historical, institutional, and social conditions, societies' ambition toward instances of justice is always at work.

10. Conclusions

The access to digital medicine ensures health and health to social-economic systems, as it ensures harmony between the expectations of citizens and what is practiced is essential for stable and resilient societies. Here comes into play the role of Institutions that are called to adopt participatory patterns in promoting the capacities and skills to be productively effective in implementing telemedicine and common well-being [13]. This is of primary importance and true everywhere, even more in Europe.

The City Competent Model should be escalated to a higher part of the population to measure the impact among citizens empowered communities in realizing telemedicine system objectives.

Appendix A. Ministerial Decree n.77/2022 – multi-professional management summary

New professions. New skills translate into new digital professions, all capable of managing the complexity of new technologies. From the Data Scientist to the IoT Software Engineer, it is necessary to identify suitable figures and integrate them with those already present in the company. Furthermore, with Ministerial Decree 77/2022, transitional care management services are activated, which involve the use of multi-professional and multidisciplinary resources, with a global vision of the clinical-care pathways available and a great capacity for communication and team working relationships.
Job market. Thanks to the Legislative *Decree n. 80/2021*[1] (converted with law no. 113 of 6 August 2021), it is possible to recruit staff specifically intended to carry out the projects of the administrations for which they have direct ownership of implementation. To speed up the procedures for the recruitment of fixed-term staff for the implementation of the NRRP, it is possible for the administrations involved to stipulate fixed-term employment contracts and collaboration contracts for a total period exceeding 36 months but not exceeding the duration of implementation of the relevant projects (not exceeding 31 December 2026). Failure to achieve the intermediate and final goals and objectives envisaged by the project constitutes just cause for the administration to withdraw from the contract pursuant to art. 2119 of the civil code. Furthermore, the administrations can carry out competitive procedures relating to the recruitment of staff with fixed-term employment contracts for the implementation of NNRP projects using digital methods. To this end, the Department of Public Function has created a unique platform for recruitment in Central administrations and strategic personnel planning, with fast, transparent, and rigorous selection paths to select the technical and managerial profiles necessary for the implementation of the NRRP. The portal aims to improve the quality of public administration recruitment through an innovative digital system that simplifies and speeds up the matching of supply and demand for public jobs. To support strategic staff planning, the definition of development plans, and the identification of any training gaps, the platform will be integrated with information regarding the skills and abilities of existing staff, with the aim of valorizing the data collected through artificial intelligence and business intelligence systems. At the base, a defined set of "skills descriptors" (including soft ones, i.e., behavioral ones) to be used to compose the different professional profiles and to be used as a reference parameter for hiring policies to improve consistency between skills possessed and career paths and to design training courses starting from the actual detection of skills gaps.
To encourage the selection and rapid hiring of specialist profiles, it will also be possible to activate selection paths other than the competition, for example, through agreements with universities, higher education centers, and professional associations. The staff thus selected will be on a fixed-term contract, and the experience and skills gained may be valorized for the purposes of hiring in relation to the achievement of objectives linked to the individual projects, following a specific selection procedure.
Social Recruiting. Social Recruiting is an increasingly frequent method adopted by professionals to find work and by companies to hire new collaborators. Furthermore, through a targeted strategy on the part of organizations, it is not only possible to recruit the best candidates, but also to retain their employees.
Employer Branding. To make quality hires, the company must also be able to be chosen. For this reason, an employer branding strategy is increasingly necessary, i.e., a promotion process aimed at standing out from other organizations and attracting qualified personnel. In the context of healthcare companies, it could therefore be useful to define a social strategy aimed at finding new talent, sharing job offers, and consolidating a set of processes to promote a company as an ideal employer for a specific target that the company intends to attract, hire, and retain. In this way, it is possible to be a "great place to work," that is, to have the image of a collaborative, stimulating work environment where it is possible to achieve company objectives thanks to a common vision – an environment from which employees can therefore benefit. Collaborators and management. This results in quality hires, loyal employees, and an increase in productivity due to the satisfaction of both management and candidates.
Evaluation of soft skills and aptitudes. The evaluation of soft skills can often make a difference and be decisive in choosing the best candidate and successfully completing the entire recruitment process. It is well known that 89% of hires are wrong due to the candidate's lack of personality or motivation, often due to the lack of in-depth analysis of soft skills[2].
Analysis of soft skills

Hard skills (such as technical and professional skills such as computer skills, university diplomas, certificates, references, and experiences) represent a good starting point in the initial phase of a recruitment process, but they are not enough: intuition, empathy, ambition, emotional intelligence, tenacity to achieve professional objectives, a strong ability to organize work, exemplary behavior in a working environment, the aptitude for team collaboration, for example, represent crucial transversal skills for starting a successful professional career, in all professional environments, even the most technical.
It is not easy to quantify and identify soft skills: it can be very complicated, for example, to identify them in a group interview because they do not always emerge from aptitude or personality tests. The quality of the questions, during a structured selection process, therefore, becomes fundamental: they must be targeted and effective to achieve the final objective. The moment of the interview is therefore central, with questions aimed at evaluating the response methods that reflect the candidates' orientations in specific aptitudes.
During the interview, there are some precautions to keep in mind so as not to choose the wrong candidate and to avoid not achieving the desired result. Below is an example of red flags to pay attention to when trying to evaluate a candidate's soft skills.
When candidates give canned answers. Sometimes candidates, when faced with generic and usual questions such as "Describe your role within the team," provide standard and predefined answers. It becomes important, therefore, to add to the questions, scenarios, and hypothetical situations that take the candidate by surprise, "forcing" him to make instant reflections.
When the candidate is inconsistent. To research and satisfy a specific soft skill you do not need to focus on just one path. Comparing, for example, candidates' answers during the interview with their emails or their performance in a certain task is a good way to evaluate the consistency of the candidate's skills.
The candidate does not provide specific examples. A good resource must be able to relate his or her soft skills to real-life experiences. A candidate who never provides specific examples related to his life experiences is probably a resource not to focus on.
The candidate does not have a cultural fit. The best candidate is the one who has a background and mentality that fits perfectly with the culture, vision, and company logic. In this direction, the image communicated by the company through a perfect Employer Branding strategy becomes fundamental.
There are also selection process support systems that allow you to set up personalized evaluation forms for the role you are looking for, the assignment of tags, and video interviews.
Setting up the selection process with a structured analysis (also with the support of specialized companies) of hard and soft skills not only allows you to identify the correct figures for specific roles but also reduces time and the risk of staff impatience.
Employee well-being. A first step could be to introduce corporate welfare through non-monetary benefits, which have the aim of improving the well-being and quality of life of human resources and their families. Since they are not monetary compensation, the goods and services do not burden the employer's finances and, at the same time, favor the improvement of the productivity of collaborators and employees.
Benefits of Age Management. Another factor, important for promoting the inclusion of human resources, concerns initiatives aimed at encouraging dialog and cooperation between generations, often very different in terms of skills and working approaches. Compared to recent decades, the percentage of senior workers has increased, and conversely, the number of junior figures has decreased. Age Management initiatives are therefore becoming increasingly indispensable.
Smart Working. Smart Working refers to a flexible organizational model that links digital elements to those of personal well-being. However, doing Smart Working does not simply mean "working from home." In fact, we are talking about a real managerial philosophy, capable of bringing benefits in terms of productivity and cost reductions. Before the health emergency, only a few large companies had reaped the benefits of Smart Working. Today, however, things have changed, and other companies understand the importance of this new agile working model. Even in the healthcare sector, the areas of analysis, planning, reporting, and telemedicine activities can encourage the articulation of work even remotely, in order to promote integration between work, personal, and family activities.

Development of digital skills. Another key element of the PNRR in the field of work is the development of digital skills by Italian citizens, necessary to fully seize the opportunities offered by technological innovation, support the green and digital transition, and enhance economic growth. According to the results of the DESI Index today in Italy, only 42% of people aged between 16 and 74 have at least basic digital skills (compared to 58% in the EU), far from the 70% threshold, which the European Commission has set out to achieve by 2025. The support measures envisaged by the plan are:

- *Recognition of tax credits* to companies that invest in training activities for digitalization and the development of related skills.
- *Development of a managerial retraining model (for digital)*, focused on SMEs with ad hoc training programs, involving the involvement of trade associations and the use of dissemination models focused on digital platforms.
- *Ad hoc training programs during layoff periods*, incentivized through the (temporary) cut in the tax wedge for both the company and the worker, with a view to digital upskilling.
- *Establishment of the Digital Civil Service*, a specific area of implementation of the universal civil service to enhance the role of young people as "digital facilitators" with the task of helping approximately one million users acquire basic digital skills.
- *Strengthening professional education,* in particular Higher Technical Institutes and STEM disciplines. Greater investments planned for Higher Technical Education and infrastructural interventions, such as the preparation of learning environments connected and enriched by digital tools.

Continuous training. Most of the initiatives envisaged by the Plan are linked to active labor policies and only have a limited impact on those who are already working. However, the challenges linked to the continuous updating of skills, and the development of digital knowledge, involve the entire workforce, and corporate training takes on an increasingly strategic role for the competitiveness of companies. The doubt is that it remains limiting to talk about training almost exclusively in relation to worker mobility, relocation, and finding your first job.

In an increasingly fluid labor market like the one expected soon, the real objective will be to guarantee continuous training (lifelong learning) to all workers, and on this, the actions envisaged in the PNRR do not appear to be effective.

It is important, however, during the implementation of the interventions envisaged by the NRRP, to guarantee adequate training of staff in the use of digital systems and in the new ways of working and relating required, for example, in the management of transitional care paths or telemedicine services.

The mapping of internal skills (also within the scope of the six soft skills mentioned previously), the benchmarking with internal and external resources, and the identification of gaps, are certainly key points from which to start for the construction of more effective training paths, for activate strategic planning of new resources to be included and for the more fluid management of careers and promotions. However, to follow up on a significant change of this magnitude, administrations and staff will need coaching paths, change management programs, and specific training plans, in addition to the use of online courses and the communities of practices currently envisaged by the Plan.

In the healthcare sector, it would be appropriate to integrate the training courses already in place with the digital skills development actions and the internship in the operational realities that will be foreseen as early as 2024, such as COT, CdC, and IFEC. These integrated paths will allow entry into the world of work of personnel already oriented in the operational paths created for the implementation of the NRRP interventions. The training path should create a process of osmosis between skills also favored by the support of the technological component.

The importance of an immediate definition of integrated training paths for the creation of new professional figures (e.g., transitional care experts) in some cases, and in other cases retrained ones, becomes a critical factor in the success/failure of structural and system that are being undertaken with the NRRP. The change in roles and technological innovation would also become an element of help in this phase of structural shortage of professional figures, as well as helping to trigger useful motivational processes in professionals.

[1] *"Urgent measures to strengthen the administrative capacity of public administrations functional to the implementation of the National Recovery and Resilience Plan (PNRR) and for the efficiency of justice."*
[2] *https://www.pwc.com/gx/en/ceo-survey/2019/Theme-assets/reports/talent-trends-report.pdf.*
[3] *https://digital-strategy.ec.europa.eu/it/policies/desi.*

Appendix B. Press review of city competent model

Press Review:
1. http://www.sanita24.ilsole24ore.com/art/notizie-flash/2022-12-05/promozione-salute-e-inclusione-competence-economy-forma-cittadini-diventare-city-leader-124345.php?refresh_ce=1&uuid=AE7EMiMC
2. https://www.panoramasanita.it/2023/12/22/la-presa-in-carico-degli-anziani-fragili-e-soli-facilitata-dallarte-relazionale/#lightbox/0/

Author details

Francesca Cioffi[1]*, Daniela Sgroi[2], Tiziana Chiriaco[3], Marina Cerbo[4] and Francesca Milito[5]

1 CEO of IPACS, Institutional & Public Coaching Services, Italy

2 Health Director Local Health Authority Roma 3, Roma, Italy

3 Telemedicine and Unitary Coordination of Single Access Points Unit Manager, Local Health Authority Roma 3, Roma, Italy

4 Head of Scientific Committee of IPACS, Institutional and Public Coaching Services, Italy

5 General Manager Local Health Authority Roma 3, Roma, Italy

*Address all correspondence to: francescacioffi2@gmail.com

References

[1] NRRP Missions and Component. Update nov 2022. Available from: www.governo.it

[2] Cioffi et al. How does Emotional Intelligence act on Institutional Policies? A New Set of Behaviors to Facilitate Implementation of the Recovery and Resilience Plan (RRP) in local Health Units in Italy. 2023. Available from: https://hpr.termedia.pl/How-does-emotional-intelligence-act-on-institutional-policies-A-new-set-of-behaviors,166564,0,2.html

[3] Cioffi et al. A scientific and integrated coaching training pathway to accelerate HCV eradication and use of telemedicine for Covid 19 patients in 5 local health units in Italy. Special Report- Interdisciplinary Journal of Virtual Learning in Medical Sciences. 2022;**13**(2):137-140. DOI: 10.30476/IJVLM2022.95094.1150

[4] Cioffi et al. Tools for Developing and Measuring Skills for Clinical Innovation: The Case of Telemedicine and the Case of the Eradication of the HCV viru2021_13_FRANCOANGELI_Mecosan_118_2021.indd 133 09/07/21. 2021

[5] Cioffi et al. Testing of an inter-disciplinary model to develop institutions and policy based on the value of skills. 2019. DOI: 10.23753/htafocus2019.03.014

[6] Istituto Nazionale di Statistica (ISTAT). Open data [Internet]. 2023 [cited 2023 Dec 31]. Available from: https://www.istat.it/it/dati-analisi-e-prodotti/open-data

[7] Regione Lazio. Salute Lazio [Internet]. 2023 [cited 2023 Dec 31]. Available from: https://www.opensalutelazio.it/salute

[8] Workshop 2022 October 24. Available from: https://www.nomisma.it/press-area/competenze-benessere-organizzativo-piessepi-gidp/

[9] Cornelissen G, Pandelaere M, Warlop L, Dewitte S. Positive cueing: Promoting sustainable consumer behavior by cueing common environmental behaviors as environmental. International Journal of Research in Marketing. 2008;**25**(1):46-55

[10] World Employment Social Outlook 2019- International Labour Organization. Available from: https://www.ilo.org

[11] Kim S. Working with robot: Human resource development considerations in human-robot interaction. 2022;**21**. DOI: 10.1177/15344843211068810

[12] Ritratti. Seven Women tell their stories. May 25062019. ISBN 9788897708292ù

[13] The ILO and the future of work. The politics of global labour policy 2022

[14] OECD labour force statistics 2024. Updated Jan 2024. Available from: https://www.oecd.org

Section 3

Applications

Chapter 7

Treatment Outcomes

Suad J. Ghaben and Arimi Fitri Mat Ludin

Abstract

This chapter aims to provide guidelines on implementing treatment outcome measures (TOMs) in telemedicine. It outlines the definition and the ICF classification of TOMs and highlights the considerations for integrating TOMs in telemedicine. We identified the STEERING model, which guides toward the development of effective TM systems that have the potential to promote TOMs. Furthermore, the chapter provides a roadmap on how to administer TOMs in telemedicine, with an emphasis on facilitators and barriers to this process. Finally, the chapter provides a schematic representation of selected TM systems with and without hardware and highlights the implemented TOMs in the context of the STEERING model and the three-pronged approach.

Keywords: treatment outcome measures, patient-centered, integration, telemedicine, telerehabilitation

1. Introduction

Treatment outcomes are essential in monitoring patients' progress, tracking success, and evaluating the cost-effectiveness of physical, occupational, and recreational therapy, nursing, speech and language pathology, and psychiatry [1–4]. Additionally, treatment outcomes are meaningful for healthcare services and policymakers as they *maximize* their performance, payment potential, and reimbursement, leading to the enhancement of quality care. They also serve as a strategy for accountability [2]. Integrating TOMs into clinical settings has supported HCPs in clinical decision-making, enhanced their communication, and improved patient engagement; therefore, the adoption of TOMs has facilitated the administration of clinical trials and enhanced the evidence-based development [2, 5, 6]. The WHO has defined telemedicine (TM) as the delivery of healthcare services from remote locations by all HCPs and using Information and Communication Technology (ICT) to communicate valid data about diagnosis and evaluation, treatment and prevention, research, and education of diseases and injuries with the ultimate goal of enhancing the health of individuals and communities [7]. The TM system encompasses an interface between hardware, software and a communication channel to connect two distant locations to exchange data and enable tele-consultations [8]. Telerehabilitation (TR) is a crucial subdiscipline of TM and is just as significant as TM [9], and is ought to provide diagnosis, evaluation, monitoring, prevention, supervised interventions, education, and consultation through TR systems, which include software and hardware, through a communication channel with or without cloud [10, 11]. Thereby, the TM system will be used across this chapter to refer to both the TM and TR systems. Telemedicine, likewise, TR demonstrates a safe and convenient service delivery environment with the potential to enhance treatment outcomes, including function and QoL [10]. However, little is available about the implementation and evaluation of TOMs in TM [12], which highlights the necessity of identifying guidelines for integrating treatment outcomes in telemedicine.

2. What are the treatment outcome measures (TOMs)?

Treatment outcomes are defined as significant results following an intervention episode, which refers to aspects of measurement that healthcare professionals (HCPs) intend to enhance [5]. These measurements could relate to the patient, HCPs, process, or health care system, such as pain, function, and satisfaction. Likewise, outcome measures (OMs) are defined as procedures or tools for quantifying progress toward a particular objective [5], OMs can be published evaluations that create scores or measurement methodologies and can be replicated by HCPs [1, 5].

2.1 Reporting of TOMs

Patient-reported outcomes (PROs) are defined as any data obtained directly from the patient about the outcome of healthcare, without modifications or interpretations by HCPs [13]. Simply they reflect the patients' voice about their experience with healthcare and their ability to engage in health behaviors and activities. Raw data from PROs may be subject to variable degrees of subjectivity and biases [13, 14]. This highlights the necessity to standardize such raw data through the implementation of Patient-reported Outcome Measures (PROM), which indicates the use of a structured, standardized tool to collect data directly from the patient about his health condition, behavior, and experience with healthcare. Using such structured, standardized tools yields quantitative data that enables comparisons, and minimizes bias [13, 15]. PROMs can be either self-reported or proxy-reported. Proxy, indicating a person responds about someone else, and proxy-reported outcome refer to the collection of data from someone else who takes care of or observes the patient, such as "observer-reported measures" [14] which collect data from parents or caregivers of young children or patients who are unable to answer questions, "clinician-reported measures" is another example of proxy-reported outcomes, which are essential in case there is a need to gather complementary data. However, sometimes, it lacks accuracy [13]. Lastly, the performance measure (PM) refers to the quantification of health care quality for a hospital, health plan, nursing home, clinician, etc. [13, 15]. Careful selection of PROMs, considering the concept model, validity, reliability, responsiveness, interpretability, feasibility, variable methods of administration, cultural and language adaptations, and electronic health records, helps employ them in performance measurement, particularly quality of care [13]. Although challenged, PROMs have been increasingly incorporated into various disciplines of clinical practice and research and have resulted in identifying care gaps and unmet needs, prioritizing patients' requirements, and enhancing the quality of care [14, 16, 17].

2.2 Methods of administration of PROMs

PROMs vary in how they are administered in clinical practice; the source of data could be self-reported or proxy-reported [13, 14], and the method of administration may be paper and pencil or electronic using a computer or digital platforms such as app-based interface, web-based chatbot interface, and a speech-operated Alexa interface [13, 18]. They also vary in the mode of administration to be self-administered or interviewer-administered; the setting of administration either at home or in healthcare facilities; and finally, PROMs vary in their scoring system, which may administer raw data or probability data [13].

2.3 Barriers and facilitators of administering PROMs

In routine practice, the administration of PROMs has been challenged by factors related to the patients and caregivers, the healthcare system, and the HCPs [16, 19, 20]. Patients' and caregivers' related factors include the lack of time and understanding of the significance of PROMs, concerns about their privacy and relationship with HCPs, and difficulties using the assessment tools, either paper-based or electronic-based [16, 19]. The HCPs-related factors encompass lack of knowledge and experience in administering PROMs, lack of training opportunities, lack of time for the convenient administration of PROMs, interpretation, and integration of them into routine clinical practice, and difficulties in using the electronic-based PROMs [16, 19, 21]. System barriers include inadequate resources for implementing PROMs, lack of ICT infrastructure to administer electronic-based measures, difficulties in integrating PROs into routine clinical practice and workflow, inability to utilize PROMs data effectively, and low institutional support for implementing PROMs [16, 19, 20]. The contextual variations are crucial as well; most PROs have been developed and standardized for Western, well-resourced settings, which is unsuitable for other settings unless standardized [19].

Facilitators for administering PROMs are the identification of HCP roles, allocation of sufficient time and resources for implementing and interpreting them, enhancement of knowledge and skills related to the administration of PROMs, including training of professionals, awareness of patients and their caregivers, and consolidated evidence of PROMs role in saving time and enhancing quality care for policymakers. Additional facilitators would be integrating PROMs into clinical practice and flow through reliable procedures, and building up or making the ICT infrastructure available for HCPs [21].

2.4 Patient-centric care (PCC)

Patient-centered care is where HCPs partner with patients and their families to design and deliver individual healthcare by responding to their preferences, needs, and values. PCC has been associated with enhanced patient' experience, positive TOMs, reduced cost of healthcare, and diminished length of hospital stay and rate of readmissions [22]. Patient-centric e-health identifies the patient's focus, activity, and empowerment. However, evidence shows that the focus of e-health is the needs of healthcare providers and organizations, with consideration of patients' acceptability factors [13]. The administration of PROMs in telemedicine has the potential to enhance patient centricity by enhancing access, engagement, ongoing tracking, and patient-HCP relationships [13, 18].

2.5 The ICF classification of function

The International Classification of Function (ICF) is a dictionary that sorts terms in logical and hierarchical order. It was identified by the World Health Organization

(WHO) and underpins definitions, classifications, measurement, and policy of functions and disability of health conditions [23, 24]. The ICF identifies three levels of human performance: body, entire person, and whole person in a social setting. Thus, it integrates the medical and social domains and provides a comprehensive understanding of health [23]. The ICF has been utilized in defining research variables, locating literature in databases, describing patients' health conditions in guidelines and formal documents, and assisting in developing and selecting the proper assessment tools (PROMs) for patients through the rehabilitation pathway [24]. For example, the ICF has been deployed in the development of TOMs for physiotherapy, occupational therapy, and speech pathology disciplines [25]; it has also been implemented to select the most appropriate items for the assessment of ankylosing spondylitis, which cover most of the ICF core set and best represent the patients' health status [26]. The ICF has been implemented in clinical practice and research to categorize TOMs for body function and structure, activity, and participation [1, 2, 27]. Deploying the ICF has augmented neurorehabilitation strategies [28], simplified the common language of function and disability, encouraged innovative ways of measuring them [29], and provided more consistent results related to patients' health recovery than conventional PROMs [30].

2.6 The ICF categories and core set

The ICF is a common framework to understand and describe function and disability [31]. The first prospect is body function and structure, denoted as "b" and "s", respectively. It contains physiological and psychologic functions and anatomical characteristics. Activity denoted by "d" refers to a wide spectrum of purposeful planned actions performed by the individual within life situations, such as climbing stairs. Participation, also denoted by "d" is the activities that are crucial for economic and social life, such as holding a job. The environmental factors are the physical, social, and attitudinal factors individuals live and conduct their lives and are denoted by "e" [23, 31]. Personal factors are a particular background of an individual, such as gender, age, and education, but they are not yet coded within the ICF. The hierarchical classification of the ICF categories identifies four levels, represented by numerical codes, starting with the chapter number of one digit, followed by the second level, two digits, and then the third and fourth levels, each of one digit; the lower the level, the more incremental information. For example, b2 refers to sensory functions and pain (first level), b280 refers to the sensation of pain (second level), b2801 is the pain in the body part (third level), and b28013 is pain in the back (fourth level). The ICF categories are arranged in a stem-branch-leaf scheme, starting with the component letter with one, two, three, or four digits, corresponding to the code of the categories [24, 31]. The ICF qualifier is the state of the health level or the degree of severity of a problem of concern. It is coded as the first, second, third, or fourth number after the decimal point [24]. The ICF core set was developed based on a robust scientific methodology and provides a category list that is essential for specific medical conditions and contexts related to healthcare, which facilitates the creation of a patient's functional profile in a variety of situations, including clinical practice [31].

2.7 How the ICF has been deployed for the mapping of PROMs?

Given that the ICF is the universal consolidated language of defining function and health, HCPs and researchers have been deploying the ICF to map PROMS qualitatively using the linkage rules, quantitatively using the Rasch model, and a combined quantitative and qualitative mapping to transfer information from electronic records. Qualitative mapping can also be utilized to compare the content of measuring instruments [32]. The PROMs have been coded using the ICF core set; for example, the EQ-5D-5L Dimension can be coded by identifying its main domains: mobility (d4), self-care (d5), usual activities unspecified: remunerative employment (d850), pain/discomfort (b152), anxiety/depression (b152) [30]. The ICF qualifiers for this instrument have been implemented before and after rehabilitation intervention on a 0–4 scale outlining the level of impairment, limitation, or restriction, stated as (4) complete; (3) severe; (2) moderate; (1) mild; and (0) no problem [30].

2.8 Administering TOMs in telemedicine

Administration of TOMs in telemedicine should consider factors related to changes in the context and environments of testing, changes in the method of data collection, and the lack of HCP supervision. We should also consider telemedicine's objective to promote the health of individuals and communities.

2.9 Consider the psychometric properties

It is highly essential to deploy valid, reliable, and responsive TOMs, which contribute to the validity of results, the effectiveness of the intervention, and ultimately, the enhancement of the patients' and community's trust in healthcare service [33]. Validity refers to the extent to which an instrument measures what it is intended to measure [34], it entails the selection of an accurate, and appropriate assessment tool. For example, when treating a patient with diminished cardiovascular fitness, the six-minute walk test (6 MWT) is appropriate to assess aerobic capacity and endurance [35]. Criterion, concurrent, and predictive validity were also considered in clinical practice and research [1, 34]. Validity considers the population and the context of evaluation, suggesting that any changes in them would make changes in validity [1, 34]. For example, validity values of the six-MWD for geriatrics differ from those related to patients with stroke, COPD, or spinal cord injury (SCI), values of criterion and construct validity values also differ [35]. Reliability is the degree to which the TOM is free of random error, therefore, a test with high reliability produces consistent findings over several tries, and relative reliability identifies the inter-rater, intra-rater reliability, and internal consistency [1, 34]. Systematic errors can potentially influence reliable tests, leading to incorrect results. For example, errors due to fatigue, lack of attention, inaccuracy, or a lack of clear instructions and inaccurate interpretation [1, 34]. Responsiveness indicates response to change, which is the ability of the measure to identify change throughout the time of the construct to be examined [1, 33]. Thus, PROMs should be sensitive to detect changes induced by the healthcare intervention provided by TM. Limitations of responsiveness include the multi-trial scales, the PROMs that provide a categorical or limited number of response options, and PROMs with extended reporting periods are unlikely to detect responsiveness if they are implemented frequently over a short period [13].

2.10 The necessity for validation in the tele-contexts

Given that validity is defined concerning the context of measurement, including the study population and settings, it is crucial to consider the effects of utilizing different modes or procedures than the one used for validation of the PROMs [13]. In telemedicine, the application of TOMs raises many questions about the population, the PROMs, the technology, and the healthcare system [36]; besides, contextual factors, especially the site impact, the overall usage of the TM system [37]. The change in how data collection has been performed by the use of mHealh, web-based measures, sensors, cameras, movement trackers, or any combination of them, with possibility of miscalibration, misconduct, and potential measurement errors, including both random and systematic errors, draws questions about the PROMs applicability, validity, and reliability in remote settings and highlights the necessity for validation in tele-contexts [13, 18]. In total, the population, the measuring environment, the PROMs, and the context of evaluation along with the data collection methods should be re-evaluated in TM practice as they impose potential variations in validity and reliability values. On the contrary, electronic data collection facilitates the incorporation of data within health records, with increasing possibilities for integration in clinical practice workflow.

2.11 The complex barriers to administering PROMs in telemedicine

Barriers to integrating TOMs into telemedicine can be explained by considering the complex barriers of deploying both PROMs and TM systems in clinical practice. Barriers to deploying PROMs were attributed to personal, professional, as well as institutional factors, while the deployment of TM systems is challenged by the high cost of development, difficulties in implementing and utilizing high-tech solutions at personal and institutional levels, the low rates of technology acceptance, especially for the elderly, who claim that it is a disruption of their privacy and security, the low confidence in diagnostic accuracy despite of its adequacy, and the digital literacy, especially for elderly [8]. Specifically, barriers to implementing TOMs in telemedicine may include, but are not limited to, patient health literacy, HCPs' resistance to deploying PROMs in practice, insufficient understanding of the optimal way to utilize TOMs results in clinical practice [36], issues related to platform design, inexperience with PROMs devices, computer literacy, and lack of IT infrastructure for data collection [18, 20]. In total, the Implementation of PROMs in telemedicine is challenged by patients, HCPs, and healthcare system-related factors, along with the difficulties in deploying the TM system. Therefore, it is recommended to provide adequate training to HCPs, with consideration of their contexts, and enhance awareness about TOMs for patients and administrative leaders [19]; additionally, it is recommended to consider PROMs impeded in telemedicine for patients with chronic disorders who require numerous consecutive visits, where PRO is essential for follow-up and monitoring. Any new patient admission requires the awareness and training of patients, HCPs, and administrative leaders [36].

2.12 Telemedicine and TOMs; the proposed approaches to simplify the complex equation

To simplify the concept of integrating TOMs in telemedicine, we worked in an organized manner to map the reported TOMs in the developed TM systems for noncommunicable diseases (NCDs) over the last 5 years. We identified keywords and synonyms, and developed search strings. We then searched on three databases: EBSCO, WOS, and PubMed. The resulting studies were screened through two stages: for the title and abstract, and then for the whole document. Accordingly, we randomly selected the mapped RCTs to represent the developed TM systems for the NCDs, including musculoskeletal [38], cancer [39, 40], metabolic disorders including DM [37, 41], cardiovascular disorders [42, 43], and chronic pulmonary diseases [44, 45]. Mapping of these RCTs has resulted in the identification of the STEERING model to develop TM systems for effectively enhancing TOMs and the identification of the three-pronged approach to integrate TOMs into TM systems.

2.13 The STEERING model: Develop effective TM systems to enhance TOMs

An effective TM system that contributes to the enhancement of the TOMs is based on eight pillars: self-management, tracking, education, enhanced adherence strategies, reminders, identified usefulness, networking, and generalized vs. individualized features, as shown in **Figure 1**.

2.13.1 Self-management (SM)

Involves the transfer of knowledge and utilization of patients' self-regulation skills to control their chronic disease, manipulate risk factors, and engage in healthy behaviors [46, 47]. SM skills encompass identifying goals, self-monitoring, reflective thinking, self-evaluation, decision-making, execution of certain behaviors, coping skills, and control of physical, emotional, and cognitive responses to changes in health conditions [46, 48]. Telemedicine has been successfully implemented to promote SM behaviors of chronic diseases and has contributed to the enhancement of TOMs [49–51]. The implemented SM programs were multicomponent, deployed mostly for adults, and occasionally for children and caregivers, either in clinical or home environments by multidisciplinary HCPs. Additionally, SM programs provide support for disease and symptoms management, drug management, psychosocial concerns, lifestyle modifications, communication, social support, and career planning [51].

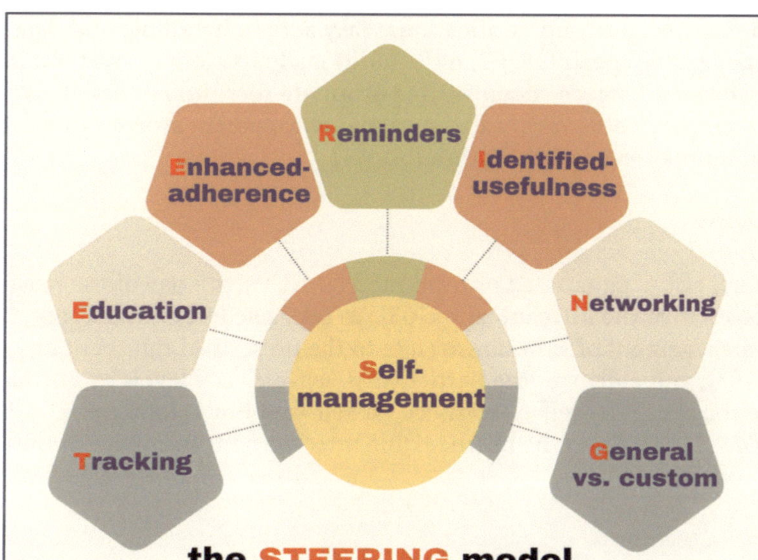

Figure 1.
The STEERING model: development of an effective TM system that has the potential to enhance TOMs; self-management is the gear.

2.13.2 Tracking

Refers to the information relating to itemized coding of procedures and costs associated with healthcare delivery, used as a means for tracking healthcare utilization, patterns of care, and treatment outcomes [52], it is an integral component of any TM system, that allows ongoing remote monitoring of changes in participant status of the body function and structure, activity, and participation through utilizing TOMs and other means [50, 53]. The literature highlighted the benefits of self-monitoring, implemented in TM, compared to traditional monitoring methods, and showed its contribution to enhancing SM and TOMs [54–56].

2.13.3 Education

Health education, in variable forms, is effective in enhancing knowledge and satisfaction and promoting readiness to engage in health behaviors [46, 57], and it has been implemented along with SM and contributed to enhancing its efficiency and effectiveness, along with improvements of TOMs [50, 57–60]. such as fasting blood glucose, blood pressure, and QOL in chronic kidney disease [61], anxiety, weight loss, physical activity, and the post-enrolment rate at hospitals in chronic care [50].

2.13.4 Enhanced adherence

Adherence is the extent to which the users follow the program as intended [62]. Despite the effectiveness of TM in augmenting patients and healthcare systems in chronic disease management, there is a high rate of attrition and dropout among patients with health conditions [62–64]. Nonadherence has threatened treatment effectiveness, led to an increased number of hospitalizations, and is considered a significant concern in developing the TM system [62]. Engagement strategies to enhance adherence involve but are not limited to, portability [18], the development of customized features, push-up notifications, easy access, handling, and data sharing, along with adjustable speed [18, 62, 64]. Additionally, patient characteristics, and meeting their specific needs, along with appropriate recruitment channels pose the potential to enhance adherence; adherence and engagement scores can be computed and assist in more effective application [62, 64].

2.13.5 Reminders

Reminders, either automated or prompted by HCPs, are one of the mastery experience procedures of the mHealth apps [65], as they encourage adherence, commitment, and management of time constraints to the prescribed interventions targeting SM [62, 65–67], and enhances the participants' self-efficacy levels by encouraging users to use the app, read self-care advice, or self-monitor symptoms [65]. Reminders can also be used to scale up the telemedicine interventions in cohort studies as a retention procedure [62].

2.13.6 Identified usefulness

This is one of the influential factors toward adherence to telemedicine. Typically, the belief factors, including perceived usefulness have been a part of the Technology Acceptance Model (TAM); a powerful tool implemented widely to measure the users' acceptance of technology-based interventions such as telemedicine [68]. It is essential to discuss with patients and caregivers the actual benefits of the TM system and to avoid overstatement, as the expectation-confirmation theory states that the patients would confirm such usefulness while using the tool. Meeting users' expectations through confirmation, has the potential to maximize their intention to use and enhance satisfaction, and therefore facilitate lifestyle improvements [69, 70].

2.13.7 Networking

Creating variable forms of networking, such as study communities [67], community clinical linkages [71], or peer-led SM programs [72] has enhanced users' engagement, facilitated the transfer of knowledge and experience among patients, peers, researchers, and HCPs, augmented reminders about self-care tasks, served as a useful tool to update participants about the progress, empowered participants to overcome barriers and share their experience, facilitates problem-solving, daily management, and behavioral modifications, provided the social and emotional support, and enhanced suers' linkages to clinical care, therefore, these benefits have the potential for motivation, self-efficacy, and SM and eventually improvement of TOMs and PM [67, 71, 72].

2.13.8 Generalized vs. customized features

The development of TM systems is initiated by targeting certain populations, identifying their needs, and developing general features to meet the population's needs [10]. However, researchers recommend personalization of some features to enhance functionalities of the TM systems such as tailored education, symptoms management advice [66, 73], and the closed loop feedback system which allows HCPs to react in time with individualized adjustment to patient care [74]. The self-development of goals, reminders, and positive feedback upon achieving these goals have shown effectiveness in enhancing personal acceptance and commitment, facilitating personalized care, empowering behavioral changes, and eventually, improving the TOMs [75]. Moreover, personalized reminders, feedback, and stories have enhanced adherence, engagement, and SM [53, 62, 65].

Based on the mentioned methodology, we analyzed randomly several TM systems that were developed for variable NCDs, the mapped system, shown in **Table 1**. has been built upon the "STEERING" model. Self-management, tracking, and education have been reported in 9/9 of the mapped systems, networking and generalized vs. individualized features have been reported in 8/9 of the mapped systems, enhanced adherence and reminders have been reported in 7/9 of the charted systems, the identified usefulness has been charted only in one system; we assume that such low value is attributed to the usual practice of including awareness of the interventions in the education module. Almost seven out of nine interventions have positively enhanced the TOMs either in the body function and structure, participation, or in the environmental factors' domain.

2.14 TOMs in the scope of telemedicine and the ICF core set

TM refers to the utilization of ICT to provide healthcare services while the patient is physically presented in a different environment, this obliges the inclusion of new OMs related to the tele-contexts and constructs. On the other hand, the ICF classifies

Study	Disease	TM system			Effectiveness	S	T	E	E	R	I	N	G
		Software	Hardware	Cloud									
Plow and Golding [38]	NMSK	√	—	√	(+) physical activity, physical function, self-regulation, self-efficacy	√	√	√	√	√	—	√	√
Maguire et al. [39]	Cancer	√	—	√	(+) HRQOL, self-efficacy, anxiety, & supportive care.	√	√	√	√	√	—	√	√
McManus et al. [42]	Hypertension	√	—	√	(+) control SBP, & cost-efficient	√	√	√	—	√	—	√	√
Yang et al. [41]	TY2DM	√	√	√	(+) glycaemic control, (+) total & HDL cholesterol	√	√	√	—	√	—	√	√
Agarwal et al. [37]	TY2DM	√	—	—	(−) in 1ry OMs (HbA1c)	√	√	√	√	—	√	—	√
Basch et al. [40]	Metastatic cancer	√	—	—	(+) 2ry OMs: physical function, symptom control, & HRQOL	√	√	√	√	√	—	√	—
Stamenova et al. [44]	COPD	√	√	√	(−) SM skills, knowledge, symptoms, healthcare use	√	√	√	√	√	—	√	√
Moor et al. [45]	Idiopathic pulmonary fibrosis	√	√	√	- (+) Psychology well-being, & Satisfaction. - allow medication adjustment. (−) HRQoL	√	√	√	√	√	—	√	√
Maddison et al. [43]	CVD	√	√	√	(−) 1ry OMs. (+) utilization & cost-efficient. - lead to less sedentary	√	√	√	√	—	—	√	√

Table 1.
The STEERING model for the development of an effective TM system to enhance the TOMs; (+) indicates improvement, (−) indicates no improvement.

human function and health based on body function and structure, activity, participation, and with consideration of environmental factors. Utilizing the ICF framework in clinical practice and research has brought several advantages as described previously, which triggered our attempt to use the ICF classification to map the OMs, including both TOMs and PMs, across the developed TM systems. We hope that the results of this attempt will help researchers and HCPs plan, administer, and interpret the interventions including TOMs within the context of telemedicine.

We employed the results of the search strategy described previously to analyze the randomly selected RCTs, accordingly, we identified the three-pronged approach to utilize the OMs across the developed TM systems as shown, in **Figure 2**. The first dimension is the procedure OMs, which refers to the pre-trial procedure that is implemented to initiate TM systems. The second is the TOMs, sorted based on the ICF's body function and structure, activity, and participation, and refers to the change in the health status of the participants. The tele-OMs refer to the measurements of constructs related to the tele-contexts and are equivalent to the environmental factors of the ICF. It is worth noting that the three-pronged approach identified in **Figure 2** and described in **Table 2** is not synonymous with functional profile, nor is a mapping of the OMs using the ICF categories; such work requires more detailed description along with more collaboration of multidisciplinary teams, which is beyond the concept of this chapter. Rather, the three-pronged approach is an attempt to facilitate the administration of the OMs into telemedicine based on the ICF domains.

2.14.1 Procedure OMs

Refers to the pre-trial procedures that are implemented by researchers and HCPs to initiate TM systems. This includes screening, randomization, allocation, and setting up the TM system for NCDs. For example, screening of patients with hypertension focused on baseline values of blood pressure > 140/90 mm Hg (b420), participants'

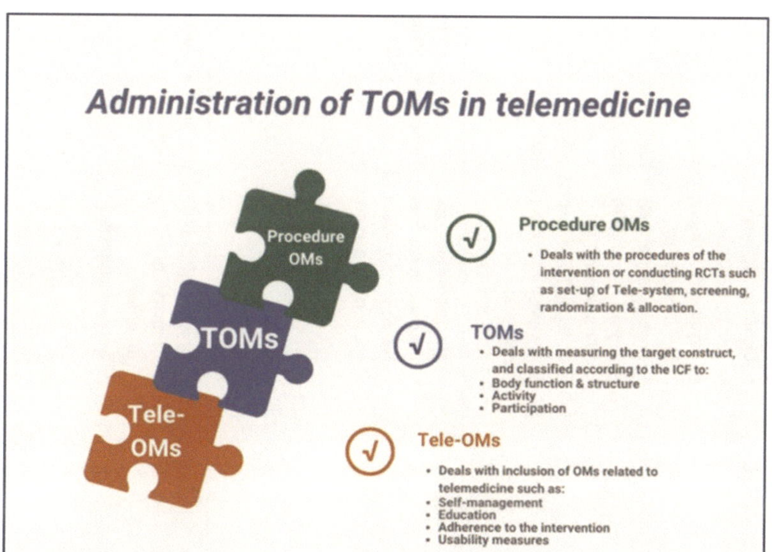

Figure 2.
Administration of OMs into telemedicine through the three-pronged approach: (1) Procedure OMs, (2) TOMs, and (3) tele-OMs.

Study	Disease	Procedure OMs	TOMs based on the ICF classification			Tele-OMs environmen
			Body function & structure OMs	Activity OMs	Participation OMs	
Plow and Golding [38]	NMSK	• Confirm diagnosis • Age 18–76 years, • Physician's consent to engage in PA program, • Engage in ≤90 min of PA • Engage in unhealthy eating < 10 on survey) • GHQ: < 17 on mental composite & <16 physical composite • Access to Internet	—	• PADS-revised • Adapted portions of Senior Fitness Test (6MWT, Bicep curls, 1 M chair stand)	• Exercise Confidence Survey • Social Support & Exercise Survey • The Goal Setting for Exercise Scale	• Attrition rate, • Adverse events, • % phone calls completed after the manual, • % entries in mHealth apps & paper diary • GAS
Maguire et al. [39]	Cancer	• No distant metastasis • No concurrent chemotherapy • Receiving 6 cycles of supported chemotherapy	• Body temperature • Neutropenic sepsis • MSAS	• FACT-G	• HRQoL-4D • SCNS • SF34 • STAI-R • WLQ • Planned-unplanned hospital admission	• DCTAQ • (CASE-Cancer) • Cost effectiveness of ASyMS • Clinical practice changes
McManus et al. [42]	Hypertension	• Baseline BP > 140/90 mm Hg • Participants willing to self-monitor • Access to internet	• Systolic BP • Side effects symptoms	• Healthy eating • PA • Weight	• EuroQoL-5D-5L • Cost of service • Salt & alcohol reduction	• Digital tool engagement • Motivate healthy behaviors • PEI • Drug adherence
Yang et al. [41]	TY2DM	• HP for >1 year, • Taking HP medics >3 months, • SBP or DBP =140/90 at screening	• HbA1c • SMBG, • FPG • Weight,	—	—	• DTSQs • MMAS-6

Study	Disease	Procedure OMs	TOMs based on the ICF classification			Tele-OMs environmen
			Body function & structure OMs	Activity OMs	Participation OMs	
			• WC, BMI • Lipid profile • -SBP, DBP,			
Agarwal et al. [37]	TY2DM	• >18, −receive care for TY2DM, -HbA1c =8.0% • Use, able or willing to use active email • Read English language. • Get phone loaded with Bluestar app +training • Medication & comorbidities	• HbA1c • SDSCA • Blood Glucose	• SDSCA (general & specific diet, exercise, foot care • No. of cigarettes)	• EuroQol-5D • EQ5D VAS (self-rated health on VAS)	• PAID, • uMARS-adapted • Utilization measures: • No. engagements/week • Use of each feature/week • Satisfaction
Basch et al. [40]	Metastatic cancer	• Adult +21 with advanced metastatic cancer • Receive outpatient systemic cancer treatment • Understand English, Spanish, Mandarin-Chinese • Info about device, Internet, and email use	• Fatigue, nausea, pain, vomiting, Dyspnea, insomnia, appetite loss, diarrhea, constipation)	Physical function	• EORTC • QLO-C30 • Date of Death form	• Symptom control • Patient satisfaction • PRO feedback • CRA & nrse perspective • Physicians response • Off-study chart abstrct form
Stamenova et al. [44]	COPD	• Clinical diagnosis of COPD, ≥18 years. English-speaking • With Wi-Fi internet @ home & community • Physical & cognitive ability to use technology	• Oxygen, • BP • Tmperatur • Weight • MRC • CAT	• SGRQ • ED presentations • hospital admissions & stays • no. of excrbtions	• BCKQ • Vendor recorded use data	• SM using • PIH Scale • No. of times thresholds exceeded. • Visits to family Drs • No. of call to outpatnt clinic • No of daths
Moor et al. [45]	Idiopathic Pulmonary fibrosis	• Adults (≥18 year), + diagnosis of IPF	• FEV1, -FVC • DLCOc • Dyspnea	• EQ-VAS (generic health status)	• EQ-5D-5L, • well-beng • HADS	• Satisfaction & • Adherence • Home monitoring VAS.

Study	Disease	Procedure OMs	TOMs based on the ICF classification			Tele-OMs environmen
			Body function & structure OMs	Activity OMs	Participation OMs	
		• About to start on antifibrotic ttt • Able to speak, read, or write Dutch	• Fatigue • Cough • Urge to cough • Stability IPF		• K-BILD • PESaM • GRC • Adjusts in medics & hsptalzton	• Patient experience
Maddison et al. [43]	CVD	• Min 6-month diagnosis of CHD. -adults (≥18). • Clinically stable CHD • English-speaking, • No limitations to max exercise test; completed =150 in/week moderate to vigorous PA	• O2-max • Glucose con • Fasted • Blood lipid • Height • Weight • BMI • BP • WC • HC	• Physical activity	• HRQoL. • Adverse events of health	• Exercise adherence • Exercise-related motivation (self-eficacy, intention, confidence, locus causality)

- EuroQol 5-Dimension Questionnaire
- HADS: Hospital Anxiety and Depression Scale
- DCTAQ: Daily Chemotherapy Toxicity Self-Assessment Questionnaire
- HbA1c: hemoglobinA1c
- FBG: fasting blood glucose
- SMBG: self-monitored blood glucose
- DTSQs: The Diabetes Treatment Satisfaction Questionnaire status version
- BP: blood pressure, SBP: systolic BP,
- HP: hypertension, DBP: diastolic BP
- MMAS-6: The 6-item Morisky Medication Adherence Scale
- QLQ-C30 version 3: Core Quality of Life
- EORTC: The European Organization for Research and Treatment of Cancer
- EORTC QLQ-BR45: Updated Breast Cancer Module
- MARS: Mobile App Rating Scale
- SCNS-SF34: supportive Care Needs Survey Short-Form
- STAI-R: State-Trait Anxiety Inventory-Revised
- CASE-CANCER: Communication and Attitudinal Self-Efficacy Scale for cancer
- WLQ: Work Limitations Questionnaire
- PADS-revised: Physical Activity and Disability Survey–revised
- CHD: Coronary Heart Disease
- K-BILD: King's Brief Interstitial Lung Disease health status questionnaire
- PESaM: Patient Experiences and Satisfaction with Medication questionnaire
- GRC: Global Rating of Change
- DLCOc: Diffusing Capacity Of The Lungs For Carbon Monoxide
- SGRQ: St. George's Respiratory Questionnaire
- BCKQ: Bristol COPD Knowledge Questionnaire
- WC: Waist Circumference,

Study	Disease	Procedure OMs	TOMs based on the ICF classification			Tele-OMs environmen
			Body function & structure OMs	Activity OMs	Participation OMs	
• PAID: problem areas in diabetes • GAS: goal attainment scaling • PEI: patient enablement instrument • MRC: medical research council • CAT: COPD assessment test • SDSCA: the summary of diabetes self-care activities measure • MSAS: Memorial Symptom Assessment Scale: global, psychological, and physical symptoms			• HC: Hip Circumference • PIH: Partners in Health • FACT-G: Functional Assessment of Cancer Therapy -General			

Table 2.
Examples of administering TOMs in clinical research/RCTs.

willingness to self-monitoring, and their access to the internet [42]. We tried to link these measures to their equivalent ICF categories; however, we could not locate an ICF equivalent to self-monitoring, instead, we located the closest category: self-care (d5), self-care unspecified (d599), or looking after one's health (d570). The same issue applies to access to the internet within the e category; we located the closest category, products and technology for communication (e125), and products and technology, unspecified (e199).

2.14.2 Treatment OMs

Refers to the measurement of the intended change in the health status of participants. Regardless of the classification of these measures by the original work, here we classified the TOMs according to the ICF; therefore, TOMs will be grouped by body function and structure, activity, and participation. In the mentioned study of measuring OMs related to hypertension [42], body function expressed in systolic blood pressure (b420), weight equivalent to the body weight maintenance function (b530), physical activity could be equivalent to mobility unspecified (d499), or walking (d450), and moving (d469), healthy eating could be equivalent to eating (d550), salt and alcohol reduction could be equivalent to Products or substances for personal consumption (e110). The EuroQoL-5D-5L was coded previously to its main domains: mobility (d4), self-care (d5), and usual activities unspecified: remunerative employment (d850), pain/discomfort (b152), anxiety/depression (b152) [30].

2.14.3 Tele-OMs

Refers to the measures used to implement the telemedicine interventions through the tele-context, this dimension encompasses the environmental factors' domain of the ICF as well as the performance measure of the healthcare service. This could include some instruments used to be implemented in routine clinical practice; however, administration of these instruments in tele-context requires revalidation and consideration of the new environment. For example, deploying self-management, self-monitoring, remote education, engagement, and adherence in tele-context would impose differences from the routine clinical practice. In the above-mentioned intervention, researchers implemented several instruments to measure patients' interaction with the tele-context [42] such as engagement with the digital tool which is closely equivalent to products and technology, unspecified (e199), motivate healthy behaviors is closely equivalent to support and relationships, unspecified (e399), drug adherence is closely equivalent to products or substances for personal consumption (e110), cost of service is closely equivalent to health services, systems and policies (e580), and the patient enablement instrument focuses on participant's ability to cope with life and illness, ability to keep health and help himself, and confident about health are equivalent to self-care unspecified (e599), along with understand illness which is equivalent to mental functions, unspecified (b199).

In concrete terms, the proposed approach to integrating OMs into telemedicine focuses on the deployment and distribution of these instruments over the pathway of conducting clinical interventions and research, starting from the preparatory phase until the final evaluation phase. Here we raise three major concerns: the first is that the distribution of the OMs is not always consistent with the ICF domain; for example, the EuroQoL-5D-5L was categorized under the ICF-participation domain while it constitutes body function, activity, and participation. The second concern is that we could not locate the exact ICF equivalent category for several measures, especially those related to tele-OMs, and we either identified an unspecified ICF category or kept that instrument without locating the equivalent category. This highlights the necessity for further work to identify concepts related to telemedicine in the ICF core set. Third, the procedure OMs, as described previously, has the potential to include measures from all ICF domains: body function, structure, activity, participation, and environmental factors. However, the personal factor is missing in the ICF despite its significance [76].

3. Conclusion

In conclusion, this chapter provides an overview of treatment outcomes, its measures, and reporting, focused on the value of integrating it into clinical practice and research, along with the barriers and facilitations of its implementation. The chapter also highlights the main issues of implementing TOMs in telemedicine, exemplified by the necessity of evaluating the TOMs in the tele-context for validity and reliability. We identified two measures to facilitate the administration of TOMs in telemedicine; the first is the STEERING model, which, we claim, would contribute to the development of an effective TM system that helps promote TOMs. The second is the three-pronged approach, which could facilitate the administration of TOMs through clinical intervention and research related to telemedicine.

This is groundwork that we hope to build upon in the future to provide more consolidated models and approaches that help HCPs and researchers implement TOMs in tele-contexts in clinical practice and research. Although we conducted a robust methodology in identifying the interventions eligible for analysis, we could only work with a small number of them to align the space of this chapter. We strongly recommend that future work include a large number of studies to further validate the STEERING model and the three-pronged approach. Finally, we highlighted the requirement to update the ICF core set to include telemedicine as an emerging discipline, however, few studies have been conducted on this aspect, and we urge researchers to focus on this area of research.

Conflict of interest

The author(s) declared no potential conflicts of interest with respect to the research, authorship, and/or publication of this chapter.

Author details

Suad J. Ghaben[1,2*] and Arimi Fitri Mat Ludin[3]

1 Department of Physiotherapy, Faculty of Applied Medical Science, Al-Azhar University, Gaza, Palestine

2 Physiotherapy Program and Center for Healthy Ageing and Wellness, Faculty of Health Sciences (H-CARE), Faculty of Health Sciences, Universiti Kebangsaan Malaysia, Jalan Raja Muda Abdul Aziz, Kuala Lumpur, Malaysia

3 Biomedical Science Program and Center for Healthy Ageing and Wellness (H-CARE), Faculty of Health Sciences, Universiti Kebangsaan Malaysia, Jalan Raja Muda Abdul Aziz, Kuala Lumpur, Malaysia

*Address all correspondence to: dr.suad.physio@gmail.com

References

[1] Stokes EK. Rehabilitation Outcome Measures. 1st ed. Churchill Livingstone; 2011. 190 p

[2] Hill K, Denisenko S, Miller K, Clements T, Batchelor F, Morgan P. Clinical Outcome Measurement in Adult Neurological Physiotherapy. 4th ed. Melbourne: Australian Physiotherapy Association, National Neurology Group; 2010. pp. 3-6

[3] Liu Y, Avant KC, Aungsuroch Y, Zhang X-Y, Jiang P. Patient outcomes in the field of nursing: A concept analysis. International Journal of Nursing Sciences. 2014;**1**(1):69-74

[4] Moyse K, Enderby P, Chadd K, Gadhok K, Bedwell M, Guest P. Outcome measurement in speech and language therapy: A digital journey. BMJ Health & Care Informatics. 2020;**27**(1):1-6

[5] Kaplan SL. Outcome Measurement and Management: First Steps for the Practicing Clinician. USA: Philadelphia: F.A.Davis; 2007

[6] Van Herck P, De Smedt D, Annemans L, Remmen R, Rosenthal MB, Sermeus W. Systematic review: Effects, design choices, and context of pay-for-performance in health care. BMC Health Services Research. 2010;**10**(1):1-13

[7] World Health Organization. Telemedicine Opportunities and Developments in Member States. Geneva: WHO; 2010. ISBN 978 92 4 156414 4

[8] Khemapech I, Sansrimahachai W, Toachoodee M. Telemedicine–meaning, challenges and opportunities. Siriraj Medical Journal. 2019;**71**(3):246-252

[9] Brienza DM, McCue M. Introduction to Telerehabilitation. London: Springer London; 2012. pp. 1-11

[10] Ghaben SJ, Mat Ludin AF, Mohamad Ali N, Beng Gan K, Singh DKA. A framework for design and usability testing of telerehabilitation system for adults with chronic diseases: A panoramic scoping review. Digital Health. 2023;**9**:20552076231191014

[11] Shem K, Irgens I, Alexander M. Chapter 2 - getting started: Mechanisms of telerehabilitation. In: Alexander M, editor. Telerehabilitation. New Delhi: Elsevier; 2022. pp. 5-20

[12] Yoshida Y, Patil SJ, Brownson RC, Boren SA, Kim M, Dobson R, et al. Using the RE-AIM framework to evaluate internal and external validity of mobile phone–based interventions in diabetes self-management education and support. Journal of the American Medical Informatics Association. 2020;**27**(6): 946-956

[13] Cella D, Hahn EA, Jensen SE, Butt Z, Nowinski CJ, Rothrock N, et al. Patient-reported outcomes in performance measurement. 2015

[14] Huemer M, Bösch F. Measuring what matters: Why and how to include patient reported outcomes in clinical care and research on inborn errors of metabolism. Journal of Inherited Metabolic Disease. 2023;**46**(5):796-805

[15] Van der Wees PJ, Nijhuis-Van Der Sanden MW, Ayanian JZ, Black N, Westert GP, Schneider EC. Integrating the use of patient-reported outcomes for both clinical practice and performance measurement: Views of experts from 3 countries. The Milbank Quarterly. 2014;**92**(4):754-775

[16] Nguyen H, Butow P, Dhillon H, Sundaresan P. A review of the barriers to using patient-reported outcomes (PROs) and patient-reported outcome measures (PROMs) in routine cancer care. Journal of Medical Radiation Sciences. 2021; **68**(2):186-195

[17] Sørensen NL, Hammeken LH, Thomsen JL, Ehlers LH. Implementing patient-reported outcomes in clinical decision-making within knee and hip osteoarthritis: An explorative review. BMC Musculoskeletal Disorders. 2019; **20**:1-8

[18] Golden AH, Gabriel MH, Russo J, Price M, Ruhmel S, Nilsson A, et al. Let's talk about it: An exploration of the comparative use of three different digital platforms to gather patient-reported outcome measures. Journal of Patient-Reported Outcomes. 2023;**7**(1):130

[19] Barth CA, Donovan-Hall M, Blake C, Akhtar NJ, Al-Barawi S, Kazibwe H, et al. "Otherwise ... he will be a beggar": A focus group study to understand the perspectives of physiotherapists about measuring rehabilitation outcomes and impact in low-resource and conflict-affected settings. Disability and Rehabilitation. 2023;**45**:1-12

[20] Spencer KL, Absolom KL, Allsop MJ, Relton SD, Pearce J, Liao K, et al. Fixing the leaky pipe: How to improve the uptake of patient-reported outcomes–based prognostic and predictive models in cancer clinical practice. JCO Clinical Cancer Informatics. 2023;7:e2300070

[21] Nguyen H, Butow P, Dhillon H, Morris L, Brown A, West K, et al. Using patient-reported outcomes (PROs) and patient-reported outcome measures (PROMs) in routine head and neck cancer care: What do health professionals perceive as barriers and facilitators? Journal of Medical Imaging and Radiation Oncology. 2020;**64**(5): 704-710

[22] Santana M-J, Ahmed S, Lorenzetti D, Jolley RJ, Manalili K, Zelinsky S, et al. Measuring patient-centred system performance: A scoping review of patient-centred care quality indicators. BMJ Open. 2019;**9**(1):1-10

[23] WHO. Towards a Common Language for Functioning, Disability and Health ICF. Geneva: WHO; 2002

[24] Heerkens Y, Hendriks E, Oostendorp R. Assessment instruments and the ICF in rehabilitation and physiotherapy. Medical Rehabilitation. 2006;**10**:11-20

[25] Perry A, Morris M, Unsworth C, Duckett S, Skeat J, Dodd K, et al. Therapy outcome measures for allied health practitioners in Australia: The AusTOMs. International Journal for Quality in Health Care. 2004;**16**(4): 285-291

[26] Kiltz U, Van Der Heijde D, Boonen A, Cieza A, Stucki G, Khan M, et al. Development of a health index in patients with ankylosing spondylitis (ASAS HI): Final result of a global initiative based on the ICF guided by ASAS. Annals of the Rheumatic Diseases. 2014. DOI: 10.1136/annrheumdis-2013-203967

[27] Grover P, Holt D. Outcome Measurement in Rehabilitation. 2017.

[28] Lexell J, Brogårdh C. The use of ICF in the neurorehabilitation process. NeuroRehabilitation. 2015;**36**(1):5-9

[29] Madden RH, Bundy A. The ICF has made a difference to functioning and disability measurement and statistics. Disability and Rehabilitation. 2019; **41**(12):1450-1462

[30] Calvo M, Subirats L, Ceccaroni L, Maroto JM, De Pablo C, Miralles F. Automatic assessment of socioeconomic impact on cardiac rehabilitation. International Journal of Environmental Research and Public Health. 2013;**10**(11): 5266-5283

[31] ICF Research Branch. ICF Core Sets in Clinical PRactice. ICF-Based Documentation Tool Göttingen. 2nd ed. Germany: Hogrefe; 2020. Available from: https://www.icf-core-sets.org/

[32] Kelvin L. ICF-based classification and measurement of functioning. European Journal of Physical and Rehabilitation Medicine. 2008;**44**: 315-328

[33] Mokkink LB, Prinsen CA, Bouter LM, de Vet HC, Terwee CB. The consensus-based standards for the selection of health measurement instruments (COSMIN) and how to select an outcome measurement instrument. Brazilian Journal of Physical Therapy. 2016;**20**:105-113

[34] Leslie G, Portney DG. Concepts of measurement validity. In: Pine J, editor. Foundations of Clinical Research: Applications to Evidence-Based Practice. 4th ed. Philadelphia, USA: F.A Davis; 2020. pp. 127-140

[35] Physiopedia. Six Minute Walk Test / 6 Minute Walk Test. Available from: https://www.physio-pedia.com/Six_Minute_Walk_Test_/_6_Minute_Walk_Test

[36] Schougaard LMV, Larsen LP, Jessen A, Sidenius P, Dorflinger L, de Thurah A, et al. AmbuFlex: Tele-patient-reported outcomes (telePRO) as the basis for follow-up in chronic and malignant diseases. Quality of Life Research. 2016;**25**:525-534

[37] Agarwal P, Mukerji G, Desveaux L, Ivers NM, Bhattacharyya O, Hensel JM, et al. Mobile app for improved self-management of type 2 diabetes: Multicenter pragmatic randomized controlled trial. JMIR mHealth and uHealth. 2019;**7**(1):e10321

[38] Plow M, Golding M. Using mHealth technology in a self-management intervention to promote physical activity among adults with chronic disabling conditions: Randomized controlled trial. JMIR mHealth and uHealth. 2017;**5**(12): e6394

[39] Maguire R, McCann L, Kotronoulas G, Kearney N, Ream E, Armes J, et al. Real time remote symptom monitoring during chemotherapy for cancer: European multicentre randomised controlled trial (eSMART). BMJ. 2021;**374**(8301):1-14

[40] Basch E, Schrag D, Henson S, Jansen J, Ginos B, Stover AM, et al. Effect of electronic symptom monitoring on patient-reported outcomes among patients with metastatic cancer: A randomized clinical trial. Journal of the American Medical Association. 2022; **327**(24):2413-2422

[41] Yang Y, Lee EY, Kim H-S, Lee S-H, Yoon K-H, Cho J-H. Effect of a mobile phone–based glucose-monitoring and feedback system for type 2 diabetes management in multiple primary care clinic settings: Cluster randomized controlled trial. JMIR mHealth and uHealth. 2020;**8**(2):e16266

[42] McManus RJ, Little P, Stuart B, Morton K, Raftery J, Kelly J, et al. Home and online management and evaluation of blood pressure (HOME BP) using a digital intervention in poorly controlled hypertension: Randomised controlled trial. BMJ. 2021;**372**(8276):1-13

[43] Maddison R, Rawstorn JC, Stewart RA, Benatar J, Whittaker R, Rolleston A, et al. Effects and costs of real-time cardiac telerehabilitation: Randomised controlled non-inferiority trial. Heart. 2019;**105**(2):122-129

[44] Stamenova V, Liang K, Yang R, Engel K, van Lieshout F, Lalingo E, et al. Technology-enabled self-management of chronic obstructive pulmonary disease with or without asynchronous remote monitoring: Randomized controlled trial. Journal of Medical Internet Research. 2020;**22**(7):e18598

[45] Moor CC, Mostard RL, Grutters JC, Bresser P, Aerts JG, Chavannes NH, et al. Home monitoring in patients with idiopathic pulmonary fibrosis. A randomized controlled trial. American Journal of Respiratory and Critical Care Medicine. 2020;**202**(3):393-401

[46] Ryan P, Sawin KJ. The individual and family self-management theory: Background and perspectives on context, process, and outcomes. Nursing Outlook. 2009;**57**(4):217-225 e6

[47] Hessler DM, Fisher L, Bowyer V, Dickinson LM, Jortberg BT, Kwan B, et al. Self-management support for chronic disease in primary care: Frequency of patient self-management problems and patient reported priorities, and alignment with ultimate behavior goal selection. BMC Family Practice. 2019;**20**:1-10

[48] Martz E. Promoting Self-Management of Chronic Health Conditions: Theories and Practice. New York, USA: Oxford University Press; 2017

[49] Wang H, Ho AF, Wiener RC, Sambamoorthi U. The association of mobile health applications with self-management behaviors among adults with chronic conditions in the United States. International Journal of Environmental Research and Public Health. 2021;**18**(19):10351

[50] Obro LF, Heiselberg K, Krogh PG, Handberg C, Ammentorp J, Pihl GT, et al. Combining mHealth and health-coaching for improving self-management in chronic care. A scoping review. Patient Education and Counseling. 2021;**104**(4):680-688

[51] Allegrante JP, Wells MT, Peterson JC. Interventions to support behavioral self-management of chronic diseases. Annual Review of Public Health. 2019;**40**:127-146

[52] Pubmed-Mesh. Administrative claims, healthcare. 2016. Available from: https://www.ncbi.nlm.nih.gov/mesh/2009747

[53] Cho Y, Zhang H, Harris MR, Gong Y, Smith EL, Jiang Y. Acceptance and use of home-based electronic symptom self-reporting systems in patients with cancer: Systematic review. Journal of Medical Internet Research. 2021;**23**(3):e24638

[54] Turner-McGrievy GM, Beets MW, Moore JB, Kaczynski AT, Barr-Anderson DJ, Tate DF. Comparison of traditional versus mobile app self-monitoring of physical activity and dietary intake among overweight adults participating in an mHealth weight loss program. Journal of the American Medical Informatics Association. 2013;**20**(3):513-518

[55] Greenwood DA, Young HM, Quinn CC. Telehealth remote monitoring systematic review: Structured self-monitoring of blood glucose and impact on A1C. Journal of Diabetes Science and Technology. 2014;**8**(2):378-389

[56] Ong T, Van Citters AD, Dowd C, Fullmer J, List R, Pai S-A, et al. Remote monitoring in telehealth care delivery across the US cystic fibrosis care network. Journal of Cystic Fibrosis. 2021; **20**:57-63

[57] Bashi N, Fatehi F, Fallah M, Walters D, Karunanithi M. Self-management education through mHealth: Review of strategies and structures. JMIR mHealth and uHealth. 2018;**6**(10):e10771

[58] Chatterjee S, Davies MJ, Heller S, Speight J, Snoek FJ, Khunti K. Diabetes structured self-management education programmes: A narrative review and current innovations. The Lancet Diabetes & Endocrinology. 2018;**6**(2): 130-142

[59] Howell D, Harth T, Brown J, Bennett C, Boyko S. Self-management education interventions for patients with cancer: A systematic review. Supportive Care in Cancer. 2017;**25**:1323-1355

[60] Jang I. A systematic review on mobile health applications' education program for patients taking oral anticoagulants. International Journal of Environmental Research and Public Health. 2021;**18**(17):8902

[61] Sarker MHR, Moriyama M, Rashid HU, Rahman MM, Chisti MJ, Das SK, et al. Chronic kidney disease awareness campaign and mobile health education to improve knowledge, quality of life, and motivation for a healthy lifestyle among patients with chronic kidney disease in Bangladesh: Randomized controlled trial. Journal of Medical Internet Research. 2022;**24**(8): e37314

[62] Jakob R, Harperink S, Rudolf AM, Fleisch E, Haug S, Mair JL, et al. Factors influencing adherence to mHealth apps for prevention or management of noncommunicable diseases: Systematic review. Journal of Medical Internet Research. 2022;**24**(5):e35371

[63] Meyerowitz-Katz G, Ravi S, Arnolda L, Feng X, Maberly G, Astell-Burt T. Rates of attrition and dropout in app-based interventions for chronic disease: Systematic review and meta-analysis. Journal of Medical Internet Research. 2020;**22**(9):e20283

[64] Winter N, Russell L, Ugalde A, White V, Livingston P. Engagement strategies to improve adherence and retention in web-based mindfulness programs: Systematic review. Journal of Medical Internet Research. 2022;**24**(1): e30026

[65] Shi N, Wong AK, Wong FK, Sha L. Mobile health application-based interventions to improve self-management of chemotherapy-related symptoms among people with breast cancer who are undergoing chemotherapy: A systematic review. The Oncologist. 2023;**28**(4):e175-ee82

[66] Mollard E, Michaud K. Self-management of rheumatoid arthritis: Mobile applications. Current Rheumatology Reports. 2021;**23**:1-8

[67] Druce KL, Dixon WG, McBeth J. Maximizing engagement in mobile health studies: Lessons learned and future directions. Rheumatic Disease Clinics. 2019;**45**(2):159-172

[68] Kim Y, Lee HS. Quality, perceived usefulness, user satisfaction, and intention to use: An empirical study of ubiquitous personal robot service. Asian Social Science. 2014;**10**(11):1

[69] Leung L, Chen C. E-health/m-health adoption and lifestyle improvements: Exploring the roles of technology

readiness, the expectation-confirmation model, and health-related information activities. Telecommunications Policy. 2019;**43**(6):563-575

[70] Wang J, Cao Y. Factors affecting users' continuance intention toward Mobile health: Integration of theory of consumption value and expectation confirmation. Open Access Library Journal. 2023;**10**(3):1-15

[71] Steinman L, Heang H, van Pelt M, Ide N, Cui H, Rao M, et al. Facilitators and barriers to chronic disease self-management and mobile health interventions for people living with diabetes and hypertension in Cambodia: Qualitative study. JMIR mHealth and uHealth. 2020;**8**(4):e13536

[72] Park PH, Wambui CK, Atieno S, Egger JR, Misoi L, Nyabundi JS, et al. Improving diabetes management and cardiovascular risk factors through peer-led self-management support groups in Western Kenya. Diabetes Care. 2015; **38**(8):e110-e1e1

[73] Azizoddin D, Adam R, Kessler D, Enzinger A, editors. Leveraging mobile health technology and multidisciplinary methodology to optimize self-management education for advanced cancer pain: development of stamp. The 54th Hawaii International Conference on System Sciences. 2021. Kauai, Hawaii, USA. USA: University of Hawai'i at Mānoa Hamilton Library; 2021

[74] Qudah B, Luetsch K. The influence of mobile health applications on patient-healthcare provider relationships: A systematic, narrative review. Patient Education and Counseling. 2019;**102**(6): 1080-1089

[75] Cooke M, Richards J, Tjondronegoro D, Raj Chakraborty P, Jauncey-Cooke J, Andresen E, et al. myPainPal: Co-creation of a mHealth app for the management of chronic pain in young people. Informatics for Health and Social Care. 2021;**46**(3):291-305

[76] Karhula M, Saukkonen S, Xiong E, Kinnunen A, Heiskanen T, Anttila H. ICF personal factors strengthen commitment to person-centered rehabilitation–A scoping review. Frontiers in Rehabilitation Sciences. 2021;**2**:1-11

Chapter 8

Teleophthalmology in Retinal Diseases

Kamal El-Badawi, Christine Goodchild, Hadassah Drukarch and Serena Salvatore

Abstract

Recent advancements in teleophthalmology have transformed retinal disease management, benefiting healthcare providers and patients. By enabling remote monitoring, teleophthalmology significantly reduces the need for in-person consultations. Easy-to-use devices like at-home Optical Coherence Tomography (OCT) systems empower patients to generate high-quality images crucial for tailored treatment. Artificial intelligence (AI) aids in quick, affordable screenings by analysing fundus photographs and OCT images. These innovations underscore teleophthalmology's pivotal role in streamlining patient care and optimising healthcare resources. Legal, ethical, and logistical considerations surrounding teleophthalmology, drawn from literature and experiences at Bristol Eye Hospital, are also discussed.

Keywords: teleophthalmology, retinal diseases, telemedicine, optical coherence tomography (OCT), artificial intelligence (AI)

1. Introduction

Teleophthalmology leverages electronic communication technologies to exchange medical information across various locations, enhancing patient eye health. This field encompasses multiple methods of eye care, including real-time virtual consultations with eye specialists and the store-and-forward model, where digital ocular images are acquired and sent to remote specialists for analysis, remote monitoring and care planning.

Several key factors drive the rapid growth of teleophthalmology in retinal diseases. Firstly, there's a significant increase in the worldwide incidence of conditions like age-related macular degeneration (AMD) and diabetic retinopathy (DR), with estimates suggesting AMD could impact nearly 300 million people by 2040 [1]. Secondly, a large portion of these individuals are elderly, often from low socioeconomic backgrounds and living in rural areas, highlighting the urgent need to make healthcare more accessible to these groups [2]. Thirdly, as the prevalence of these conditions rises, clinicians' production needs to catch up with the demand for patient care. This gap necessitates alternative methods to deliver care efficiently.

The diagnosis and monitoring of retinal disorders heavily depend on imaging technologies. Fundus photography and optical coherence tomography (OCT) now enable capturing high-quality retinal images. Teleophthalmology allows for analysing these images outside traditional clinic settings, providing a solution for people who face barriers to accessing care, such as financial limitations, travel restrictions, or logistical issues. This method ensures broader access to specialised retina care, eliminating the need for extensive travel. However, several other critical factors need to be considered.

2. Technological foundations of teleophthalmology

2.1 Key technologies enabling teleophthalmology

The evolution of imaging devices and data transmission has significantly enhanced the efficiency and outreach of teleophthalmology. From its early days in the 1970s, utilising telephones and televisions, initially perceived as "cumbersome" with technical challenges, teleophthalmology has significantly progressed [3].

2.1.1 Digital communication tools

Teleophthalmology communication involves data acquisition, transfer, and reception by retina professionals (**Figure 1**). Advances in these three fundamental areas enable the success of teleophthalmology services.

Effective and efficient communication is vital to the success of teleophthalmology programs, especially in clinics that manage a large volume of patients and need to transmit high-quality images quickly. The introduction of 5th generation (5G)

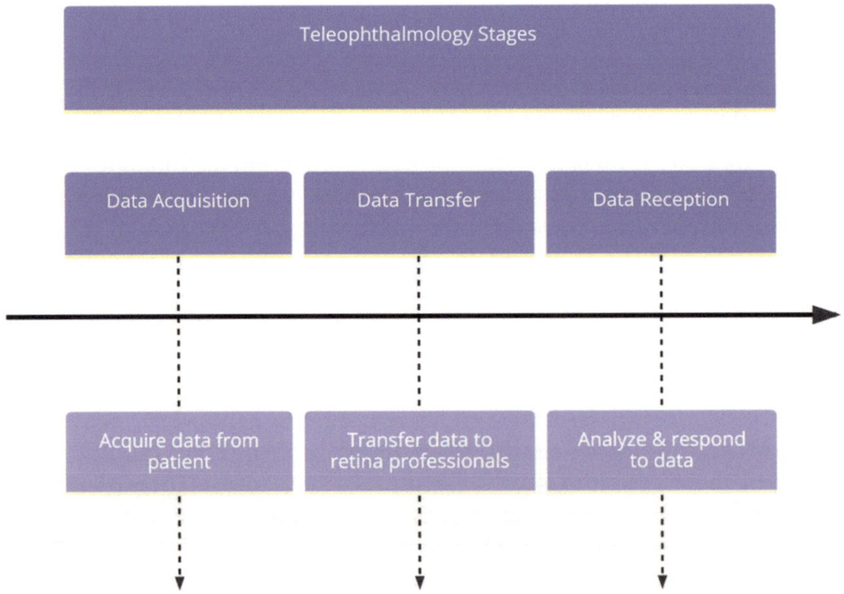

Figure 1.
Flow diagram showing the various stages of teleophthalmology.

wireless communication technologies has led to significant advancements in this area. 5G offers low latency, increased capacity, and quicker data transmission compared to the older 4G technology, making it ideal for supporting the demands of modern telemedicine. However, while 5G performs exceptionally well in urban settings where base stations can be placed approximately 250 meters apart, its effectiveness diminishes in rural areas, where different data transmission methods may be necessary. In addition to quickly transferring high-resolution images, 5G technology facilitates multimedia streaming. This capability enhances teleophthalmology by supporting remote consultations and allowing for real-time examinations using a slit lamp.

2.1.2 Retinal imaging and diagnostics advances

The first recorded photograph of the human retina was taken in 1886. The landscape changed dramatically with the introduction of scanning laser ophthalmoscopy (SLO) in 1981 and OCT in 1991 [4]. These innovations heralded a new era in eye care, characterised by rapid advancements and a shift from gradual improvements to a fast-paced evolution in diagnostic capabilities.

This shift was not just about the technology itself but also how it transformed our understanding and treatment of eye conditions. With these new tools, doctors gained a more nuanced view of the retina, enabling them to diagnose and treat eye diseases with unprecedented precision.

2.1.3 Fundus photography

Traditionally, mydriatic drops were indispensable for accurate retinal fundus imaging, but the advent of non-mydriatic cameras eliminated the need for such drops, sparing patients from temporary vision impairment. Utilising non-mydriatic cameras in fundus visualisation, particularly in diabetic eye screening programmes, has demonstrated notable benefits [5]. The application of this imaging modality is also associated with the advantages of remote monitoring, a crucial element in facilitating teleophthalmology [6].

2.1.4 Scanning laser ophthalmoscopy

SLO generates images through low-powered laser light penetrating the retina in a confocal raster technique. The resulting images of the retina and optic nerve head surpass the quality of standard fundus photography, with notable benefits observed, especially in patients with cataracts [7].

Based on SLO, the Optos or optomap® ultra-widefield (UWF™) (Optos Plc) imaging system captures ultrawide retinal images covering up to 82% of the retina [8]. This system incorporates non-invasive fundus autofluorescence (FAF) retinal images and invasive retinal images like fundus fluorescein angiography and indocyanine green (ICG) angiography.

2.1.5 Optical coherence tomography

OCT is a non-invasive imaging method providing high-resolution cross-sectional retinal images that unveil the retinal internal microstructure. It offers a detailed view of the retina's intricate structure, aiding in anatomical assessment, identifying disease-related abnormalities, and monitoring disease progression. OCT, combined with clinical findings and other imaging modalities, exhibits high sensitivities and specificities in diagnosing retinal pathologies [9].

OCT angiography has also emerged as a non-invasive technique for imaging the retina and choroid microvasculature. The first clinical studies using this innovative technology were published in 2014 [10]. Barriers to accessibility, such as physical accessibility, limited funding, and scarce resources, have sparked interest in remote monitoring OCT devices, showing promising potential.

3. Integration of artificial intelligence and robotics for teleophthalmology in retinal diseases

3.1 Artificial intelligence (AI)

In the evolving landscape of ophthalmology, integrating AI and deep learning (DL) technologies has opened new frontiers in diagnosing and treating retinal diseases. Initially, the medical community was sceptical about AI's diagnostic capabilities compared to the seasoned eye of trained clinicians. Yet, through rigorous trials and research, AI has demonstrated significant promise in enhancing retinal diagnosis accuracy and efficiency. A notable milestone was the Iowa Detection Program in 2013, which marked a breakthrough in diagnosing DR through retinal imaging [11].

Subsequent studies, such as the work by Abramoff et al. in 2016, further cemented AI's role by showcasing DL's high sensitivity and specificity in detecting DR through colour fundus photography [12]. This advancement underscored the potential of AI in ophthalmology and highlighted its capability to prevent blindness through early and accurate detection.

DL has since become the method of choice for developing algorithms that significantly improve the analysis of retinal images. However, despite these advancements, challenges still need to be addressed, including research gaps and the need for improved diagnostic accuracy by integrating AI with traditional imaging methods [13]. Moreover, deploying AI in retinal diagnosis faces practical challenges in rural settings, where poor image quality can hamper diagnostic performance.

3.2 Robotics

Parallel to the advancements in AI, robotic devices have been making remarkable progress in ophthalmology [14]. The primary focus of robotics in ophthalmology has been on complex and intricate procedures such as retinal interventions and cataract procedures [15]. Robotic systems, equipped with advanced imaging technologies and microsurgical instruments, enable surgeons to perform highly precise manoeuvres with enhanced dexterity and control. This level of precision is particularly crucial in procedures involving delicate eye structures. Cybersurgery, the concept of remote surgical intervention, has yet to be established in ophthalmology, as the issue of transmitting tactile information across low latency networks (ideally <200 ms) using haptic feedback systems must be solved [16]. Robot-assisted technology is being studied in intravitreal injections for patients with retinal pathologies with greater efficiency [17]. Despite the technological strides, patient receptiveness to robotic interventions, particularly in procedures like intravitreal injections, varies, with several factors influencing their willingness to embrace such innovations [18].

4. Teleophthalmology in retinal diseases: case studies

4.1 The case of diabetic retinopathy

Teleophthalmology is the backbone of multiple nationally and regionally implemented retinal screening initiatives, such as screening for DR in the United Kingdom (UK), Singapore, and India. DR screening initiatives are designed to achieve early identification and treatment of patients with potentially vision-threatening diseases, thereby mitigating the risk of sight loss.

4.1.1 United Kingdom

In the UK, the overarching body responsible for coordinating DR screening programs is the National Screening Committee. England, Wales, Scotland and Northern Ireland each have their local committee overseeing the screening efforts. Each program may have minor variations in its approach, but they share a standard core structure.

The process begins with mydriatic colour fundus photographs, which are then analysed by specialist graders, ranging from non-clinical technicians and optometrists to nurses, all trained in DR screening and supported by a supervising medical retina specialist. Outcomes are communicated to relevant services, leading to referrals for further investigations if necessary. Individuals with no identifiable retinopathy are informed via their general practitioners (GPs). Following the screening, patients may undergo additional diagnostic workup, accelerated surveillance, or continue on the current surveillance program [19]. Each local service is responsible for monitoring and enhancing its screening programme, and quality control regulations ensure high-quality care nationwide. Annual reports compile data on factors such as the number of patients invited to screening, the uptake of screening invites, referrals made, and outcomes [20].

The patient uptake of the DR screening programme is slowly increasing, with 78.3% national uptake in 2021/22. This shows increasing confidence in this new form of healthcare delivery; however, the rates are still lower than expected [21]. Multiple studies have identified patient and non-patient-related barriers, including competing priorities, screening anxiety, poor glycaemic control, misinformation, incorrect address, unavailability of clinical notes and forgetting appointments [22].

To bridge this gap, there are ongoing projects to improve patient education, address barriers, and enhance service outreach. Initiatives include optimising care for low-risk people, such as changing screening intervals from 1 to 2 years, depending on the outcome of consecutive screen results [23]. The national health service (NHS) diabetic eye screening program has carried out work to assess the use of AI systems in grading DR photographs, which has identified programs such as Retmarker and EyeArt as having acceptable sensitivity for referable retinopathy, false-positive rates, compared to human graders, and was cost-effective [24].

Telescreening for DR in the remote setting allows for retinal image grading, treatment decisions, and surveillance, with or without the assistance of AI, overcoming limitations associated with the availability of retinal graders on a global scale [25]. Other countries that have employed telehealth in DR screening include a few noteworthy instances, which are detailed below.

4.1.2 Singapore

In Singapore, 17% of individuals with DR exhibit sight-threatening DR (STDR) [26]. The Singapore Integrated DR Program, the national telemedicine DR screening initiative launched in 2010, screens nearly 200,000 diabetic patients annually using colour fundus photographs. These images are captured at 18 sites, transmitted through networks, and analysed by trained graders. Outcomes are communicated to clinics, with 90% receiving results within an hour of grading and 100% on the same day. The potential cost savings of this telemedicine program in Singapore are estimated to be 21.6 million dollars annually. Ongoing efforts are underway to integrate AI and DL into their DR systems [27].

4.1.3 India

In India, 3.6% of individuals with DR have STDR [28]. Due to the absence of recent studies on DR prevalence in India, obtaining up-to-date statistics for guiding screening and treatment programs takes a lot of work. Rural populations in India face limitations in accessing screening centres, prompting a shift towards the preferred remote monitoring and screening method. Despite challenges, many individuals in these areas have network connections and mobile phones. Smartphone-based imaging devices, such as the Remidio Fundus on Phone (FOP) camera, have demonstrated comparable capabilities to produce colour fundus photographs accurately compared to standard mydriatic fundus cameras [29]. In 2017, 16,226 individuals with diabetes underwent screening using the Remidio FOP camera, with 7% referred for further diagnostic workup and offered treatment [29].

4.1.4 China

China is actively working to develop effective strategies for detecting and managing DR. A study conducted by Nanchang First Hospital used the remote medical platform "Eye Grader" to store and transfer photos taken and uploaded by trained technicians and analysed in a grading centre. In 2022, when compared to ophthalmologist grading, GPs demonstrated a sensitivity of 93.99%, a specificity of 88.97%, and an overall accuracy of 92.86%. Suspected cases identified by GPs were subsequently referred for further diagnostic workup [30]. The high accuracy of this program shows the immense potential of teleophthalmology. However, it relies on the advanced telecommunication capabilities present in China.

4.1.5 Kenya

A prospective regional telemedicine screening program was conducted by nursing staff in Nairobi, Kenya, with local ophthalmologists reviewing the images. Implementation challenges included insufficient numbers and uneven distribution of ophthalmologists, low literacy levels among the population, limited medical insurance coverage, transportation and communication difficulties, and medication shortages. Despite these obstacles, patients expressed satisfaction with the program, particularly appreciating the information provided and the convenience of clinic attendance. However, accessibility emerged as the primary limiting factor, raising concerns about feasibility. Without sustainable and accessible means of attendance, specific populations may not receive adequate care [31].

4.1.6 Iran

A study analysed the implementation of the Iranian Retinopathy Teleophthalmology Screening (IRTOS) program. This secure web-based program used the local language and was adopted for patient use. Trained GPs interpreted colour fundus photographs, with subsequent referral and review by the specialist. DR recognition by GPs had a sensitivity and a specificity of 82.8% and 86.2% , respectively. Follow-up was an essential aspect of this program, which found that a text message-based communication update improved adherence to management plans, including urgent follow-up [32].

4.2 The case of retinopathy of prematurity

Retinopathy of Prematurity (ROP) is preventable and may lead to visual impairment or blindness if not promptly identified and treated. Preterm infants, especially those with low gestational age and birth weight, are at the highest risk. Approximately 60% of infants weighing less than 1500 g develop ROP. While most cases of ROP do not progress beyond mild stages that do not require treatment, 4% of screened infants require treatment [33]. Screening methods include binocular indirect ophthalmoscopy (BIO) and wide-field digital retinal imaging (WFDRI) [34].

BIO, the gold standard for ROP screening, requires an in-person examination by an experienced ophthalmologist. Telescreening programmes for ROP rely on WFDRI, which a trained individual can take. Images obtained through telescreening can be remotely analysed by human graders or AI, with studies in China providing evidence of its benefits [35]. Remote analysis of images addresses the decreasing availability of BIO screeners due to liability claims and poor reimbursement [36]. During the COVID-19 pandemic, telescreening for ROP proved effective, safe, and feasible compared to in-clinic screening and analysis [37]. Children identified through telescreening were then brought in for further evaluation using BIO.

Teleophthalmology in ROP has demonstrated long-term time and cost-effectiveness [38]. Its objective documentation ensures transferability, facilitates second opinions, supports education, and contributes to research work [39]. An example of a successful screening programme is seen in the San Francisco Bay Area. Dr. Moshfeghi developed the ROP screening programme, the Stanford University Network for Diagnosis of Retinopathy of Prematurity. Established in 2005 to address a shortage of graders and ROP specialists, the program served two local Neonatal Intensive Care Units (NICUs) and expanded to six NICUs. Utilising telescreening, trained nurses captured wide-angle retinal photographs, which were securely transferred via email or courier for remote interpretation by an ROP specialist at the Stanford University Byers Eye Institute reading centre. Outcomes were confirmed, and families were promptly informed of the results, with outpatient ophthalmology follow-up or BIO offered within 24 hours. Results were also compared to the gold standard of BIO assessment by a paediatric ophthalmologist within 1 week of discharge from the hospital. The telemedicine approach for detecting ROP requiring treatment demonstrated a sensitivity of 100%, specificity of 99.8%, a positive predictive value of 93.8%, and a negative predictive value of 100%, establishing it as a valuable tool in ROP screening [40].

4.3 The case of choroidal naevi

Integrating teleophthalmology into the management of choroidal naevi presents a promising advancement in patient care. Research by Lamis Al Harby et al. on a virtual clinic pathway for choroidal naevi management, the NAEVUS study, demonstrated an 83.1% agreement in management decisions between virtual and traditional face-to-face consultations, highlighting the safety and efficiency of telehealth services [41]. However, the study noted an increased rate of over-referrals in virtual pathways, suggesting the need for optimisations in cost-effectiveness. Similarly, Kelsey Roelofs and Ezekiel Weis found that teleophthalmology offers a highly reliable method for detecting naevus growth, with a remarkable sensitivity and specificity of 100 and 99%, respectively, compared to in-person evaluations [42]. Together, these findings underscore the potential of teleophthalmology and teleoncology in enhancing access to care, reducing the need for physical visits, and efficiently managing choroidal naevi with high accuracy and safety.

5. Teleophthalmology at University Hospitals of Bristol and Weston's (UHBW): our experience

In 2017, Bristol Eye Hospital, part of the University Hospitals of Bristol and Weston, introduced teleophthalmology. The advent of the COVID-19 pandemic significantly increased its usage due to heightened demand. To manage this surge and ensure social distancing, BEH expanded its services to a separate site in February 2021, establishing virtual clinics outside its primary location. Initially, these clinics operated from the Nightingale Hospital, a facility adapted for the COVID-19 response, serving patients with retina and glaucoma issues through virtual healthcare.

The diagnostic hub for these services has since relocated twice, now finding its current home in The Galleries shopping centre, located in the heart of Bristol city centre. The diagnostic hub is equipped with appropriate equipment for measuring and capturing patients' ocular findings, including Early Treatment Diabetic Retinopathy Screening (ETDRS) visual acuity (VA) charts, intraocular pressure check with iCare rebound tonometer, Humphrey visual fields machines for glaucoma patients and retinal imaging using spectral domain OCT (Triton, Topcon Corp) and Optos or optomap® ultra-widefield (UWF™) (Optos Plc).

The diagnostic hub operates with the support of nurses, technicians, and imaging staff responsible for recording patient data and capturing medical images. All collected information is digitally uploaded to an electronic patient record and imaging system for future analysis. These teleophthalmology services are asynchronous, meaning data and images are not assessed in real-time. Initially, a trained optometrist specialising in medical retina examines the data and images. If issues are detected, the case is escalated, and the patient is scheduled for a teleconsultation with a consultant ophthalmologist. During this consultation, conducted over the phone, the ophthalmologist discusses the results of the virtual examination and explores treatment options with the patient. Based on this discussion, patients may be directly scheduled for additional diagnostic tests, further review, or treatment, either in-person or virtual.

This healthcare model has significantly increased the unit's capacity to see patients promptly. Despite relocating twice in the last 3 years, the diagnostic hub has scheduled appointments for over 20,000 patients within the medical retina service [43]. In its initial year, 2021, the hub managed 4611 patient appointments, which grew to 6958 in 2022 and 8569 in 2023. An internal review of the data revealed that 70% of the patients treated at the virtual hub were dealing with diabetic eye conditions, such as non-proliferative DR and diabetic macular oedema, which had progressed beyond the criteria for the diabetic retina screening program. This includes moderate nonproliferative DR, characterised by signs like blot haemorrhages and intraretinal microvascular abnormalities; proliferative DR, marked by the growth of new blood vessels; and diabetic maculopathy. Other conditions treated included AMD, central serous chorioretinopathy, retinal vein occlusion, choroidal naevus, and retinal dystrophies. Of those assessed at the diagnostic hub, only 15% required a follow-up teleconsultation with a consultant ophthalmologist, and fewer than 1% needed an in-person appointment. The hub's innovative approach earned it the "Innovation and Improvement" award at the Recognising Success 2023 event. Looking ahead, the plan is to leverage this virtual diagnostic hub and telemedicine further to maintain a patient-centred approach, ensuring that patients receive care from the appropriate provider at the right time and in the most suitable location.

Additionally, with the upcoming integration of shared care imaging systems between primary care opticians and tertiary centres, the role of telehealth at BEH, especially for retinal diseases, is set to expand even more.

6. Teleophthalmology and remote monitoring

The COVID-19 pandemic has highlighted the importance and potential of using digital technologies, such as smartphones and tablets, for remote monitoring [44]. While home monitoring for VA is well-developed, with many applications available, using OCT for home monitoring is rare [45]. An example of innovation in this area is the Notal Vision Home OCT device, which can capture high-quality OCT images. This device is crucial in identifying fluid accumulation in the retina, a critical indicator for retinal diseases that significantly influence treatment decisions [46]. The AI analysis of these home-based OCT scans has been shown to match the accuracy of human graders in 96% of cases, particularly in monitoring neovascular AMD, showcasing the potential of at-home monitoring systems [47].

However, the cost of these self-monitoring devices remains a significant barrier to their widespread adoption [48]. Despite this, they offer a valuable solution for improving access to care, especially for older individuals who may face difficulties with mobility and travel. Sight-threatening conditions like AMD and diabetic macular oedema depend heavily on regular OCT imaging for early detection, initiation of treatment, and ongoing monitoring. This requirement can place a substantial burden on patients, caregivers, and healthcare resources [49]. Implementing remote monitoring for these patients appears promising in reducing the frequency of visits not requiring treatment and facilitating personalised treatment plans [50]. Efforts are ongoing among researchers and companies to enhance the technology's affordability for broader use. For instance, Siloton Ltd. has developed a photonic chip named Akepa for OCT devices, which is small, durable, cost-effective, and suitable for mass production, aiming to make portable OCT machines more affordable [51].

Mobile applications (apps) have seen practical success in AMD patient monitoring [52]. Apps like Alleye and Okkohealth provide clinicians with timely alerts [53]. A particular study highlighted the effectiveness of the Alleye app, which uses threshold-based alerts for VA to signal worsening conditions reliably. These alerts can hasten the consideration for anti-vascular endothelial growth factor (anti-VEGF) treatments, underlining the critical role of thorough monitoring in preventing disease progression [50].

7. Teleophthalmology in patients' consultation and education

7.1 Virtual consultations: methods and best practices

As technology advances, there is a growing push for healthcare services that are both accessible and efficient. Healthcare professionals are advised to consider the appropriateness of virtual consultations for each patient individually. This decision should consider the patient's preferences, the specific health issue, and whether the necessary resources for a virtual consultation are available.

Video consultations have proven to be particularly timesaving for routine monitoring and check-ups, especially in the field of medical retina. This efficiency, however, hinges on several factors, including the patient's ability to use digital tools, their technical expertise, and their capacity to solve technical problems. Setting up a digital environment for a consultation, navigating the internet, and effectively using technology requires skills that not everyone possesses. As a result, older adults and those not tech-savvy may need help accessing the healthcare services they need in the UK [54].

In the UK, the General Medical Council (GMC), which oversees doctors, has recognised the increasing importance of telemedicine by updating its professional standards [55]. It offers detailed guidance for clinicians on when and how to conduct remote consultations, emphasising the importance of patient consent and ensuring continuity of care, particularly in primary healthcare settings. The GMC's guidelines on good medical practice and the Royal College of General Practitioners' recommendations published at the onset of the COVID-19 pandemic address these critical issues [56]. They also stress the significance of both verbal and nonverbal communication during video consultations. Once patients have agreed, a guide helps both clinicians and patients prepare for video consultation appointments or follow-ups [57].

In 2021–2022, ophthalmology had the highest clinic attendance rate across all specialties in the UK, leading to the adoption of telemedicine to improve referral processes. Moorfield's Eye Hospital's implementation of a virtual clinic for medical retina, as outlined by the Royal College of Ophthalmologists, UK, was analysed and found to be effective and safe, meeting high clinical standards [58].

With telemedicine becoming more common in ophthalmology, training in telemedicine is increasingly recognised as essential for expanding service delivery to various patient groups. However, while the UK has yet to formally incorporate telemedicine training for its trainees, ophthalmology residency programs in the United States (US) have successfully integrated such initiatives. This training covers remote patient history collection, ophthalmic examinations, logistical setup, and documentation practices. Notably, it has boosted clinicians' confidence in performing telemedicine consultations [59].

7.2 Effective virtual consultations

Effective verbal and non-verbal communication plays a crucial role in the success of remote healthcare delivery. This is especially true for patients with visual impairments, such as those treated in the medical retina speciality, where clear verbal communication and resolving connectivity issues are vital for effective telemedicine [60].

The successful incorporation of telemedicine into daily clinical operations requires the cooperative efforts of doctors, technicians, and allied health staff [61]. Teleophthalmology encounters several obstacles to effective communication, including vague goals for consultations, poor internet connectivity, and challenges in verbal and non-verbal interactions during video consultations. Tackling these issues calls for government and healthcare organisations to invest in better internet infrastructure. Setting up dedicated communication hubs with reliable internet could serve as a viable remedy, echoing the setup of internet cafes.

Enhancing video consultation communication involves positioning the positioning the patient close to the webcam to improve visual interaction and stressing the importance of verbalising emotions to compensate for the absence of in-person cues. Issues like technical difficulties and unfamiliarity with the telemedicine platform can cause confusion and delays. Providing easy-to-follow troubleshooting guides and ensuring access to technical support through expert tech support teams or training administrative personnel can alleviate these concerns [61].

For conditions like retinal diseases, which often result in varying degrees of visual impairment, the significance of verbal communication is even more pronounced. Hosting seminars and workshops to improve communication with visually impaired patients can bolster healthcare professionals' effectiveness in remote consultations. By systematically addressing communication hurdles, telemedicine can become a more reliable and efficient means of providing healthcare remotely.

7.3 Patient education through telemedicine platforms

Patient education through telemedicine platforms has emerged as a crucial element in modern healthcare delivery, facilitating effective communication and information dissemination between healthcare providers and patients. This approach provides patients access to valuable information, fostering a collaborative approach to managing retinal disorders and promoting better outcomes through shared knowledge and understanding.

Lifestyle adaptations are crucial in managing ophthalmology pathologies, including diseases like DR and AMD [62]. A study in the American Journal of Lifestyle Medicine explored the use of telemedicine and various multimedia formats to improve patient engagement, which is vital in enhancing health outcomes [63]. Despite limited research on health outcomes and patient education using telemedicine, a growing body of evidence highlights the benefits of digital health technologies in improving lifestyle medicine. Tools such as wearable monitoring devices and smartphone applications could be utilised in conjunction with video consultations to educate patients about the reality of their condition and how lifestyle changes can improve their overall well-being.

8. Clinical outcomes, patients' satisfaction and cost-effectiveness of telemedicine in retinal diseases

8.1 Clinical outcomes between traditional and telemedicine approaches

Studies on telemedicine are essential for understanding its effectiveness in remote healthcare delivery, focusing on important metrics such as treatment eligibility, missed diagnosis rates, and clinic attendance. Significant research in this field includes work on DR and ROP [64].

The Tribal Vision Project in the US revealed that telemedicine screenings increased the likelihood of patients getting screened for DR without any noticeable difference in DR progression compared to traditional screenings [65]. In the UK, telemedicine has significantly lowered DR rates, changing the leading cause of blindness in the working-age population as of 2021 [66]. Lorenz et al. found that telemedicine using WFDRI over 6 years effectively reduced vision loss secondary to ROP [67].

Further, telemedicine has been shown to decrease unnecessary specialist referrals, saving substantial resources [68]. A study at Moorfields Eye Hospital demonstrated that telemedicine could reduce wait times for routine clinic referrals without compromising patient safety, highlighting the efficiency of virtual clinics over traditional face-to-face ones [69].

However, the success of telemedicine heavily relies on the availability of trained diagnosticians, pointing to a workforce shortage [70]. These findings suggest that healthcare providers and policymakers could benefit from integrating traditional and telemedicine practices more effectively, although more research is needed for direct clinical outcome comparisons [71]. Mobile health apps for monitoring chronic conditions like AMD and DR have also emerged as supportive tools, enabling patient engagement and providing a cost-effective monitoring solution. Despite the potential benefits, the clinical effectiveness of these apps varies, with limitations in follow-up duration and the need for real-world studies restricting their adjunctive use in telemedicine-based care.

8.2 Clinician satisfaction

During the COVID-19 pandemic, the adoption of teleophthalmology saw mixed satisfaction levels among clinicians, influenced by their subspecialty and the volume of video consultations. Retina specialists reported the highest satisfaction, although challenges such as inadequate equipment and technical issues were common concerns [72].

8.3 Patient satisfaction and adherence in telemedicine

Evaluating patient satisfaction and treatment adherence has become vital in determining the effectiveness and viability of telemedicine in ophthalmology, especially following the COVID-19 pandemic. There's been a noticeable trend toward patients preferring telephone consultations over traditional in-person visits [73]. By incorporating various tools such as multimodal imaging, video consultations, and home monitoring devices, healthcare providers can strengthen their clinical decision-making processes, thereby earning patient trust and boosting satisfaction levels.

Telemedicine has proven effective in breaking down geographical barriers and reducing travel inconvenience for patients, leading to higher satisfaction levels. Surveys have indicated that patient satisfaction with telemedicine services in eye care falls between 80 and 99% [74]. A specific study from Saudi Arabia highlighted that the primary cause of patient dissatisfaction was concerns about the timeliness of being assessed by an ophthalmologist following a screening test that suggested a need for referral [75]. Addressing this concern requires a well-structured referral system supported by efficient IT infrastructure to maintain high-quality patient care. Furthermore, introducing AI tools like chatbots can significantly enhance the patient experience. Chatbots can provide essential information on eye health, explain common eye procedures and treatments, and guide patients through pre-and post-operative care. This innovative approach in telemedicine encourages patients to play an active role in managing their eye health, thereby improving their adherence to treatment plans [76].

8.4 Cost-effectiveness and resource utilisation

The optimisation of cost-effectiveness and resource utilisation in teleophthalmology has become a focal point in healthcare systems striving to deliver efficient and high-quality care. In rural settings, establishing teleophthalmology centres emerges as a cost-effective solution, as the early diagnosis of undiagnosed pathologies can alleviate the substantial burden on patient care. This approach prevents additional travel, treatment, and post-operative monitoring costs [77]. Conversely, in densely populated areas with extensive DR programs, handheld portable non-mydriatic fundus cameras are viable and cost-effective alternatives [6]. However, it is essential to note that such technology may not be readily available in regions with lower economic status.

In the US, costs of assessment in the retinal diagnosis of DR were cheaper using telemedicine-based digital retinal imaging compared to conventional fundus examination [78]. The research found that telemedicine interventions led to notable cost savings by reducing the number of in-person visits and associated travel expenses for patients. Moreover, the study highlighted the efficient utilisation of healthcare resources, demonstrating that telemedicine allowed for a more streamlined allocation of specialist time and expertise [79].

An article examined resource utilisation in teleophthalmology clinics for medical retina conditions. The findings indicated that the virtual model allowed for more efficient scheduling and reduced waiting times, optimising the utilisation of clinical and administrative resources. This study underscores the cost-effectiveness and resource-efficient nature of telemedicine in medical retina within the UK, providing valuable insights for healthcare policymakers and practitioners seeking to implement and enhance teleophthalmology services [80].

To harness the full potential of telemedicine on a larger scale, increased government funding for screening programmes is essential. These programs aim to identify patients with early-stage DR and AMD [78]. Telemedicine is pivotal in facilitating early detection and timely intervention, ultimately preventing complications and reducing the overall economic burden associated with advanced sight-threatening eye disease and sight loss.

9. Legal, ethical, and regulatory considerations around telemedicine in medical retina

As with any transformative technology, teleophthalmology operates within a web of legal frameworks, ethical norms, and regulatory considerations that must be navigated with diligence. Considering the scope of this chapter, this section will discuss some of the critical considerations in this regard.

9.1 Legal considerations

9.1.1 Information security and data privacy considerations

At the forefront of legal considerations is the adherence to information security and data privacy standards to ensure that telemedicine infrastructures provide an environment for safe and effective care delivery. Telemedicine services encompass transferring patient health information via text, sound, images, and other data formats to aid in disease prevention, diagnosis and management. Where teleophthalmology is integrated in medical retina, this information generally includes detailed retinal images, patient-specific VA data, intraocular pressure readings, OCT scans, and patient-reported outcomes. Additionally, it may involve the transmission of electronic health records, medication history and laboratory test results pertinent to the patient's ocular health. From a data privacy perspective, such information is highly sensitive, revealing detailed personal health details, potential genetic predispositions, specific medical conditions, and personal identifiers. Introducing AI, big data, and advanced analytics tools into healthcare has further heightened this sensitivity. These technologies can aggregate and analyse vast amounts of data from diverse sources, uncovering previously inaccessible insights [81, 82]. This capacity amplifies the potential for personalised medicine and raises significant privacy concerns as it could inadvertently reveal even more intimate and detailed aspects of an individual's health status and predispositions [83–86]. As a consequence, the processing of such information requires robust technical and organisational governance measures to ensure that its use is restricted to authorised personnel only and for the intended medical purposes. Such measures should align with legal standards, such as the Health Insurance Portability and Accountability Act (HIPAA) in the United States, the General Data Protection Regulation (GDPR) in the European Union, and other relevant regional and international frameworks.

The GDPR constitutes the poster child of data privacy law, influencing data privacy regulation across the globe [87, 88]. It lays down rules for data subjects' protection and the free movement of data within the EU. The GDPR is a principles-based regulation that sets out six fundamental principles for processing personal data: lawfulness, fairness and transparency, purpose limitation, data minimisation, accuracy, storage limitation, and integrity and confidentiality. In line with its lawfulness requirement, the GDPR furthermore outlines several grounds for lawful processing[1], including consent and tasks carried out in the public interest, and it lays down the rights data subjects can rely on while balancing these against the obligation posed on organisations processing personal data.

As a first note, in the context of telemedicine delivery, healthcare providers should implement high standards of transparency, ensuring that patients are aware of the processing of their data where they are subjected to medical procedures involving telemedicine devices and applications. In practice, this involves clear communication about the types of data collected, the purposes for which it is used, the entities with whom it is shared, and the measures taken to protect patient privacy and data security. There are various ways in which this transparency can be achieved, including privacy notices and patient education initiatives. Patients should be informed about their rights regarding their data, including access, correction, and deletion rights, as well as how to exercise these rights. Additionally, healthcare providers must ensure that patients understand how their data contributes to their care, the benefits and risks of telemedicine, and any options to opt out or restrict certain uses of their data. With the advent of new regulations around AI, these obligations will be strengthened significantly, requiring healthcare providers to be transparent about their use of AI and, where the use of AI is not prohibited, to put measures in place to mitigate potential risks of such use.

Furthermore, the digital nature of telemedicine raises significant information security concerns. Protection against these threats to secure telemedicine platforms is complex and requires a multi-disciplinary, multi-stakeholder approach [89]. To protect sensitive patient information from unauthorised access and security threats, healthcare providers must implement robust technical and organisational information security measures. These include conducting regular risk assessments, enforcing robust data encryption methods, performing continuous security audits, and keeping software and protocols up to date. Regarding these requirements, the GDPR also

[1] *See* article 6(1) of the GDPR.

emphasises accountability, ensuring that entities processing personal data are responsible for and able to demonstrate compliance with these principles.

Beyond the above-described foundational framework for data privacy protection, the GDPR contains several further provisions specifically about healthcare and health data, which—according to the GDPR—should be defined as "personal data related to the physical or mental health of a natural person, including the provision of health care services, which reveal information about his or her health status"[2]. In other words, health data encompasses information about an individual's past, current, or future physical or mental health status. This includes data collected during registration for, or the provision of, health care services, unique identifiers for health purposes, test results from body parts or biological samples, and information about diseases, disabilities, disease risk, medical history, treatments, or physiological or biomedical state of the data subject obtained from healthcare professionals, hospitals, medical devices, or a medical device or an in vitro diagnostic test.

As a point of departure, the GDPR prohibits processing specific types of sensitive personal data, including health and genetic data. As such, health data enjoys enhanced protection as a 'special category of personal data' under the GDPR. However, this prohibition has several exceptions, some of which relate specifically to health data processing. Though conditioned by very high substantive and procedural requirements and subject to a certain level of discretion by Member States, where the data subject has given her 'explicit consent', the processing is, in principle, allowed[3]. In addition, the processing of health data is permitted when necessary to protect the vital interests of the data subject or another person who is unable or legally incapable of giving consent[4]. Under strict conditions, the GDPR also allows for the processing of health data where this is considered to be necessary for reasons of substantial public interest or other specific purposes, including preventive or occupational medicine, medical diagnosis, the provision of health or social care or treatment or the management of health or social care systems and services".

Moreover, where sufficient safeguards are put in place, the GDPR permits the processing of health data for public health reasons, such as protecting against serious cross-border threats to health, without requiring the data subject's consent[5]. The relevance of these grounds for processing health data became particularly clear in recent years during the fight against the COVID-19 pandemic. Depending on the case and context, the processing of health data in light of telemedicine may be based on a variety of grounds for lawfulness.

Finally, the GDPR mandates a Data Protection Impact Assessment (DPIA) for high-risk processing activities, mapping potential risks and devising a strategy for mitigation[6]. For instance, a DPIA is required when processing special categories of personal data on a large scale, among which health-related data. Consequently, the performance of a DPIA is typically necessary for handling health data, except when the data processing involves patients' personal information managed directly by an individual doctor or another healthcare professional. Additionally, the GDPR mandates a DPIA in the case of automated decision-making or the systematic and extensive evaluation of personal aspects relating to a data subject based on automated

---

[2] *See* article 4(15) of the GDPR.

[3] *See* article 9(2)(a) of the GDPR.

[4] *See* article 9(2)(c) of the GDPR.

[5] *See* articles 9(2)(i) and 35 of the GDPR.

[6] *See* article 35 of the GDPR.

processing, including profiling—which may include health data—, and based on which decisions are made that may affect them. Though the latter may be less relevant considering the current state-of-the-art telemedicine applications, its relevance may increase as we encounter advanced levels of autonomy.

9.1.2 Other considerations

Beyond data privacy considerations, a legal analysis of telemedicine integration in retinal disorders also requires considerations of various other aspects, including safety and liability. Traditionally, the concept of safety has been narrowly construed to refer primarily to hazards with direct physical effects on individuals, such as mechanical or chemical dangers. With the incorporation of advanced technologies into our direct surroundings, however, this perspective has shifted. Integrating digital technologies—both hardware and software—into the workflows across many different domains, including healthcare delivery, has led to heightened interconnectivity and an evolving landscape of human-robot interactions. This expansion challenges the traditional, limited view of safety, suggesting a need to broaden its definition to encompass a wider range of risks and implications in the era of advanced technology [90]. Beyond the physical dimension of safety, this also includes temporal, societal, cyber and social interaction dimensions [90]. This shift in perspective on the scope and meaning of safety is particularly relevant in the field of medical retina, where telemedicine introduces new dynamics in patient care. For instance, there are concerns about the accuracy and reliability of diagnostic algorithms, the security of patient data in transit, and the potential for delayed treatment due to technological failures or miscommunications. In this context, legal considerations must include the reliability and accuracy of telemedicine technologies, the responsibility for decisions made based on telemedicine consultations, and the protocols for data security and patient confidentiality.

Introducing advanced technologies into healthcare delivery, while beneficial, is not a straightforward process and presents new risks that are not associated with traditional medical procedures and instruments. Although there are numerous obvious advantages to continuously innovating in healthcare delivery, such as integrating telemedicine, its practical implementation reveals several shortcomings that could lead to harm in ways that might not be easily rectifiable or monitored by humans [91]. Liability issues arise when errors occur, whether due to technological malfunctions, misinterpretations of data by healthcare providers, or system security breaches. The virtual nature of patient interaction in telemedicine brings unique challenges in the attribution of liability and malpractice. In the complex healthcare technology ecosystem, where there is a significant interplay between humans and machines and a diverse array of stakeholders, pinpointing liability for specific harms becomes exceedingly difficult. This is especially true for risks that emerge from the combination of, and interactions among, components controlled by various entities, as opposed to issues arising from a single entity's incompetence [92]. These factors pose a challenge to the innovation management, especially as the division of autonomy in technology-enabled healthcare delivery is shifting rapidly. Early examples of this can be found in robot-assisted surgery (RAS), where increasing levels of autonomy complicate the scene [93]. The same can be said for healthcare delivery through telehealth devices and applications, where liability attribution for the risks arising from the interplay between stakeholders remains unclear, and legal frameworks to address this issue comprehensively are currently lacking.

9.2 Ethical considerations

Teleophthalmology must align with the medical ethics requirements of maintaining high standards of patient care, ensuring patients' overall well-being, and respecting their fundamental human rights [94]. Beyond complying with the four key pillars of medical ethics—autonomy, justice, beneficence, and non-maleficence—, this also includes considering privacy and confidentiality, accessibility to care, disclosure of medical errors, and expectations around informed consent.

Regarding the latter, informed consent has gained renewed significance in the digital age, where patients are increasingly pushed toward 'participation', requiring them to 'consume' information and produce data–also referred to as 'prosumption' [95]. In traditional healthcare settings, obtaining informed consent involves detailed discussions between patients and healthcare providers [96]. However, the digital landscape introduces unique challenges. In this context, transparent communication becomes paramount as patients interact with healthcare professionals virtually, necessitating a clear understanding of telemedicine's implications, risks, and benefits in care delivery [97]. In the subspecialty of medical retinal care, informed consent in the digital age is crucial. Teleophthalmology requires explicit consent from patients to ensure they comprehend the virtual nature of consultations and the potential eye health implications of telehealth devices and applications. With advancements in imaging and remote monitoring devices, patients must be informed about the data collection methods deployed and the impact of their use on the care they receive. This also safeguards patient autonomy, establishing a stronger trust foundation between patient and provider.

Furthermore, the principle of justice in the context of telemedicine underscores the importance of equitable access to healthcare services. Telemedicine has the potential to bridge gaps in healthcare delivery, especially for patients in remote or underserved areas. Ethically, it is vital to address disparities in access to telemedicine services, ensuring that all patients, regardless of their geographical location or socioeconomic status, have equal opportunities to benefit from advancements in medical retina care. Closely tied to this is the ethical obligation to ensure the well-being of patients and avoid harm. In telemedicine, this translates to maintaining high standards of care, ensuring that the services provided are in the patient's best interest and do not expose them to unnecessary risks. This includes the competent use of technology, adherence to clinical guidelines, and continuous monitoring of patient outcomes. Finally, in line with the ethical principle of transparency, any medical error or adverse events that occur in telemedicine must be disclosed to the patient promptly and honestly. This includes clearly explaining the error, its implications, and the steps taken to rectify the situation or prevent future occurrences.

9.3 Regulatory considerations

Finally, regulatory considerations are equally crucial, as integrating telemedicine into the practice of medical retina is not only a technological evolution but also a regulatory challenge. Beyond the complexity of compliance with evolving regulatory frameworks, telemedicine, like all healthcare services, falls under the purview of various regulatory bodies, further complicating the scene. Navigating the regulatory landscape and understanding how to translate regulatory obligations into actionable measures is essential for the responsible and sustainable implementation of telemedicine in this specialised field. To achieve this, healthcare providers must adopt a proactive approach to staying abreast of evolving regulations, ensuring compliance with existing standards, and communicating lacunas to the relevant regulatory authorities in line with their chosen innovation strategy [98]. Moreover, in shaping these efforts, the role of trust and confidence in influencing consumer acceptance of innovation cannot be undermined [99]. Where consumers do not merely benefit from innovation but also become strongly intertwined in the innovation process itself, acceptance does not solely depend on whether their needs and value expectations are met in an economic sense but also on trust and alignment with core values and rights. This also applies to digital healthcare innovation, where the successful rollout of new technologies and technology-driven processes relies on usability and desirability, as well as trust and concerns related to handling personal data [100–102]. Healthcare providers must acknowledge that telemedicine's successful rollout in medical retina relies heavily on patient trust and confidence. Consequently, they should be transparent about their regulatory compliance efforts, as this transparency directly impacts patient trust and acceptance of telemedicine services.

10. Challenges and limitations of teleophthalmology

10.1 Digital limitations and challenges

The rapid growth of teleophthalmology is met with numerous technical challenges and limitations. Research indicates that bandwidth limitations are a notable obstacle, especially in remote or underprivileged areas lacking robust internet infrastructure [103]. Even with the rollout of 5G technology, significant areas within teleophthalmology still need enhancement, such as the widespread availability of advanced ophthalmic imaging technologies necessary for remote diagnosis and monitoring. This highlights the importance of developing solutions specifically designed to address the limitations of resources [27].

Data security and privacy concerns emerge due to the dependence on digital devices and platforms. Additionally, the varying levels of technological literacy among patients and healthcare providers can make integrating teleophthalmology into existing healthcare frameworks challenging.

These technical issues become particularly critical in diagnosing and managing retinal diseases, where high-resolution imaging is crucial for accurate assessment and ongoing monitoring. Continuous improvements in imaging technology, data transmission efficiency, and the user-friendliness of interfaces are required to overcome these technical barriers. Such enhancements must ensure that teleophthalmology meets the strict clinical precision and reliability standards. Government investment and clinical governance oversight are indispensable to support the development of these technologies.

10.2 Accessibility and disparity issues and strategies for overcoming them

Teleophthalmology highlights the existing health inequalities, with stark differences in healthcare access between developed and developing countries. These barriers are evident at the individual, health system, and societal levels.

At the health system level, disparities are seen in online health portals for telemedicine consultations. These platforms are less frequently used by older adults, racial and ethnic minorities, those with low health literacy, and individuals from lower socioeconomic backgrounds [104]. The effectiveness of telemedicine also depends on clinicians' familiarity with and education on virtual clinic operations, presenting a significant barrier to its adoption. In response, American organisations are prioritising the training of medical students in telemedicine to equip them with the skills needed to conduct virtual clinics [105].

On an individual level, telemedicine services are primarily designed for non-disabled users, neglecting those with sensory impairments, low technological proficiency, or cognitive challenges [106]. This results in difficulties for patients with poor digital literacy in online services, thereby affecting the quality of care they receive [107].

Initiatives to improve access to telemedicine are in progress, focusing on technical training and support programs that have been shown to increase the use of health portals among vulnerable groups. Other potential solutions include offering free or low-cost internet services, providing more straightforward technology options like 2G or 3G for data transmission, and ensuring that software complies with legal and accessibility standards [108].

The COVID-19 pandemic further exposed the disparities in teleophthalmic care, with ethnic and racial minorities, older adults, and non-English speakers being less likely to utilise teleophthalmic services. Addressing these disparities requires more effort [109]. Successfully overcoming these barriers could significantly enhance telemedicine's role in reducing disease burdens, especially in paediatric populations [110].

11. Future directions and innovations

11.1 5G technology

5G networks play a pivotal role in teleophthalmology by facilitating the rapid transmission of high-quality retinal images and relevant data essential for accurate diagnoses. Future applications of 5G could revolutionise remote treatments, such as telephotocoagulation, allowing for the collection, planning, and implementation of treatment across vast distances, potentially on an intercontinental scale [111]. However, the high costs associated with 5G technology pose challenges. Alternative solutions like Wi-Fi hotspots have proven effective in certain communities to bypass internet access issues [112]. As the development of 6G begins, it is anticipated to enhance connectivity and accessibility further, benefiting both rural and urban areas [27].

11.2 Big data, internet of things (IoT), and AI

Big data analytics are crucial in understanding extensive datasets to reveal patterns and insights not visible with traditional analysis methods [113]. The Fight Retinal Blindness database exemplifies this, tracking retinal disease outcomes and influencing clinical practices globally. DL systems, using big data, such as Singapore's SELENA+ program, have made significant strides in disease pattern recognition using extensive image datasets [114].

IoT refers to the network of interconnected devices that exchange data autonomously. When combined with AI, IoT devices can monitor health outcomes efficiently, requiring clinicians only for final decision-making. This synergy has proven effective in retinal disease screening and diagnosis, offering accuracy that often surpasses human experts [115].

AI and machine learning (ML) are set to transform retinal disease diagnosis and screening, streamlining the process while ensuring the invaluable oversight of ophthalmologists [116]. The World Health Organisation stresses the importance of evaluating AI and ML tools based on several factors, including equity and resource utilisation [117]. Computer-aided diagnosis (CADx) systems, empowered by AI and ML, are facilitating the rise of teleophthalmology, especially in remote clinic setups, broadening access to care [118].

Convolutional Neural Networks (CNNs), a subset of DL, are revolutionising image recognition capabilities, including in retinal pathology diagnosis [119]. Recent advancements also highlight the application of AI in analysing OCT images, offering the potential for precise disease stage identification and treatment customisation [120]. Such technology promises real-time disease detection capabilities comparable to retina specialists in community settings [112].

Despite the potential of AI in ophthalmology, ethical considerations and the need to account for social, economic, and lifestyle factors in diagnosis and treatment planning remain crucial. AI systems might not fully grasp these aspects, potentially harming patients [121].

11.3 Collaborative efforts and global initiatives in teleophthalmology care

Global initiatives are crucial in enhancing tele-retinal healthcare, with the World Health Organization (WHO) World Report on Vision highlighting the need to incorporate eye health into universal health coverage [122]. The Lancet Global Health recognises the effectiveness of AI in screening programs for DR and ROP in both high-income and low- to middle-income countries.

International collaborations, such as those with the UK, are vital for enhancing teleophthalmology programs in developing countries. The UK's diabetic eye screening programme is a model for such initiatives and is being piloted in the Philippines. Despite ideal conditions for screening in the Philippines, challenges such as a lack of trained staff and appropriate equipment highlight the need for global support [123].

A recent publication calls on retinal specialists in affluent countries to help improve outcomes for those at risk of retinal diseases. Key objectives include improving detection and diagnostic processes for early treatment, reducing treatment burden on patients and healthcare systems, enhancing monitoring and management of retinal conditions, and improving care coordination throughout the patient's healthcare journey [124].

12. Conclusion

The landscape of teleophthalmology in retinal diseases represents a transformative advancement in healthcare delivery, primarily propelled by significant technological advancements. This cutting-edge methodology has proven invaluable, offering the ability to remotely perform diagnoses, monitor progress, and administer treatments for various retinal conditions. Specifically, establishing the virtual diagnostic hub at the BEH exemplified substantial enhancements in patient care efficiency well before the global emergence of COVID-19, which catalysed the broader international integration of virtual healthcare services.

Looking forward, it is imperative for future teleophthalmology initiatives to be meticulously designed to cater to the nuanced needs of diverse patient demographics. This includes focusing on ethnic minorities, individuals challenged by limited health and digital literacy, and those from lower socioeconomic backgrounds. These efforts are essential to ensure equitable access to and benefits from telehealth technologies across all population segments.

Despite its considerable potential to revolutionise care provision for patients with retinal diseases, teleophthalmology faces challenges. The integration of high-speed internet networks, AI, and big data analytics has significantly enhanced the efficiency and accuracy of remote care delivery. Nonetheless, the escalating incidence of DR, juxtaposed with relatively stagnant growth in the number of healthcare practitioners, underscores the indispensable role of AI and ML technologies in facilitating prompt detection, efficient communication, and effective management of populations at risk.

The evolution and expansion of teleophthalmology, particularly in the screening and management of retinal pathologies, depend heavily on sustained financial investment, formal recognition, and implementation by governments, as well as active collaboration on a global scale. Overcoming the hurdles of resource constraints, fostering international cooperation, and adapting to rapidly advancing technological landscapes are imperative actions to propel teleophthalmology forward. Nonetheless, these advancements hinge on the awareness, initiative, and concerted efforts of a broad spectrum of stakeholders, including clinicians, researchers, allied healthcare professionals, and, critically, policymakers. The latter group holds significant sway in enacting impactful changes and ensuring the sustainable growth of teleophthalmology. The collective engagement and forward-thinking policies are not merely advantageous but essential for realising the full potential of teleophthalmology in improving patient outcomes and expanding access to specialised retinal care.

Author details

Kamal El-Badawi[1], Christine Goodchild[2,3], Hadassah Drukarch[4] and Serena Salvatore[2*]

1 East Kent Hospitals University NHS Foundation Trust, Margate, UK

2 University Hospitals of Bristol and Weston NHS Foundation Trust, Bristol, UK

3 Royal Victoria Eye and Ear Hospital, Dublin, Ireland

4 Responsible AI Institute, United States

*Address all correspondence to: serena.salvatore@uhbw.nhs.uk

References

[1] Vyawahare H, Shinde P. Age-related macular degeneration: epidemiology, pathophysiology, diagnosis, and treatment. Cureus. 2022;**14**(9):e29583

[2] Burton MJ, Ramke J, Marques AP, Bourne RRA, Congdon N, Jones I, et al. The lancet global health commission on global eye health: Vision beyond 2020. The Lancet Global Health. 2021;**9**(4):e489-e551

[3] Glazer E, Marshall C, Cunningham N. Remote pediatric consultation in the inner city: Television or telephone? American Journal of Public Health. 1978;**68**(11):1133-1135

[4] Mohankumar AGB. Scanning Laser Ophthalmoscope. Treasure Island, FL: StatPearls Publishing; 2023

[5] Harper CA, Livingston PM, Wood C, Jin C, Lee SJ, Keeffe JE, et al. Screening for diabetic retinopathy using a non-mydriatic retinal camera in rural Victoria. Australian and New Zealand Journal of Ophthalmology. 1998;**26**(2):117-121

[6] Jin K, Lu H, Su Z, Cheng C, Ye J, Qian D. Telemedicine screening of retinal diseases with a handheld portable non-mydriatic fundus camera. BMC Ophthalmology. 2017;**17**(1):89

[7] Terasaki H, Sonoda S, Tomita M, Sakamoto T. Recent advances and clinical application of color scanning laser ophthalmoscope. Journal of Clinical Medicine. 2021;**10**(4):718

[8] Patel SN, Shi A, Wibbelsman TD, Klufas MA. Ultra-widefield retinal imaging: An update on recent advances. Therapeutic Advances in Ophthalmology. 2020;**12**:1-12

[9] Hadziahmetovic M, Nicholas P, Jindal S, Mettu PS, Cousins SW. Evaluation of a remote diagnosis imaging model vs dilated eye examination in referable macular degeneration. JAMA Ophthalmology. 2019;**137**(7):802-808

[10] Tsokolas G, Tsaousis KT, Diakonis VF, Matsou A, Tyradellis S. Optical coherence tomography angiography in neurodegenerative diseases: A review. Eye Brain. 2020;**12**:73-87

[11] Abràmoff MD, Folk JC, Han DP, Walker JD, Williams DF, Russell SR, et al. Automated analysis of retinal images for detection of referable diabetic retinopathy. JAMA Ophthalmology. 2013;**131**(3):351-357

[12] Abràmoff MD, Lou Y, Erginay A, Clarida W, Amelon R, Folk JC, et al. Improved automated detection of diabetic retinopathy on a publicly available dataset through integration of deep learning. Investigative Ophthalmology & Visual Science. 2016;**57**(13):5200-5206

[13] Hao S, Liu C, Li N, Wu Y, Li D, Gao Q, et al. Clinical evaluation of AI-assisted screening for diabetic retinopathy in rural areas of Midwest China. PLoS One. 2022;**17**(10):e0275983

[14] Alafaleq M. Robotics and cybersurgery in ophthalmology: A current perspective. Journal of Robotic Surgery. 2023;**17**(4):1159-1170

[15] Pandey SK, Sharma V. Robotics and ophthalmology: Are we there yet? Indian Journal of Ophthalmology. 2019;**67**(7):988-994

[16] Wu CT, Lin TY, Lin CJ, Hwang DK. The future application of artificial

intelligence and telemedicine in the retina: A perspective. Taiwan Journal of Ophthalmology. 2023;**13**(2):133-141

[17] Ullrich F, Michels S, Lehmann D, Pieters RS, Becker M, Nelson BJ. Assistive device for efficient intravitreal injections. Ophthalmic Surgery, Lasers and Imaging Retina. 2016;**47**(8):752-762

[18] Aw KL, Suepiantham S, Rodriguez A, Bruce A, Borooah S, Cackett P. Patients' perception of robot-driven technology in the management of retinal diseases. Ophthalmology and Therapy. 2023;**12**(5):2529-2536

[19] NHS. What is diabetic eye screening? United Kingdom. 2022. Available from: https://www.nhs.uk/conditions/diabetic-eye-screening/ [Accessed: January 24, 2024]

[20] NHS. Diabetic eye screening: 2021 to 2022 data. 2023. Available from: https://www.gov.uk/government/publications/diabetic-eye-screening-2021-to-2022-data

[21] Public Health England. NHS Public Health Functions Agreement 2014-15: Public Health Functions to be Exercised by NHS England Service. London, England: Strategy Unit Department of Health; 2013

[22] Strutton R, Du Chemin A, Stratton IM, Forster AS. System-level and patient-level explanations for non-attendance at diabetic retinopathy screening in Sutton and Merton (London, UK): A qualitative analysis of a service evaluation. BMJ Open. 2016;**6**(5):e010952

[23] Stratton IM, Aldington SJ, Taylor DJ, Adler AI, Scanlon PH. A simple risk stratification for time to development of sight-threatening diabetic retinopathy. Diabetes Care. 2013;**36**(3):580-585

[24] Diabetes UK. State of the Nation. London, England; 2013. Available from: https://diabetes-resources-production.s3-eu-west-1.amazonaws.com/diabetes-storage/migration/pdf/0160b-state-nation-2013-england-1213.pdf

[25] Nguyen HV, Tan GS, Tapp RJ, Mital S, Ting DS, Wong HT, et al. Cost-effectiveness of a National Telemedicine Diabetic Retinopathy Screening Program in Singapore. Ophthalmology. 2016;**123**(12):2571-2580

[26] Khoo DH, Tan KT, Yeo KT, Chew W, Yong V, Tan YT. Diabetic retinopathy—results of a two year screening programme in two medical units in Singapore. Annals of the Academy of Medicine, Singapore. 1990;**19**(4):484-488

[27] Li J-PO, Liu H, Ting DSJ, Jeon S, Chan RVP, Kim JE, et al. Digital technology, tele-medicine and artificial intelligence in ophthalmology: A global perspective. Progress in Retinal and Eye Research. 2021;**82**:100900

[28] Vashist P, Senjam SS, Gupta V, Manna S, Gupta N, Shamanna BR, et al. Prevalence of diabetic retinopahty in India: Results from the National Survey 2015-19. Indian Journal of Ophthalmology. 2021;**69**(11):3087-3094

[29] Rajalakshmi R, Behera UC, Bhattacharjee H, Das T, Gilbert C, Murthy GVS, et al. SPEED Study group. Spectrum of eye disorders in diabetes (SPEED) in India. Report # 2. Diabetic retinopathy and risk factors for sight threatening diabetic retinopathy in people with type 2 diabetes in India. Indian Journal of Ophthalmology. Feb 2020;**68**(Suppl 1):S21-S26

[30] Li L, Jin Y, Wang JH, Wang SS, Yuan FX. Potency of teleophthalmology as a detection tool for diabetic retinopathy. Scientific Reports. 2023;**13**(1):19620

[31] Kurji K, Kiage D, Rudnisky CJ, Damji KF. Improving diabetic retinopathy screening in Africa: patient satisfaction with teleophthalmology versus ophthalmologist-based screening. Middle East African Journal of Ophthalmology. 2013;**20**(1):56-60

[32] Safi S, Ahmadieh H, Katibeh M, Yaseri M, Nikkhah H, Karimi S, et al. Modeling a telemedicine screening program for diabetic retinopathy in iran and implementing a pilot project in Tehran Suburb. Journal of Ophthalmology. 2019;**2019**:2073679

[33] Adams GG, Bunce C, Xing W, Butler L, Long V, Reddy A, et al. Treatment trends for retinopathy of prematurity in the UK: Active surveillance study of infants at risk. BMJ Open. 2017;7(3):e013366

[34] Wilkinson AR, Adams GGW, Fleck BW, Nieto-Hernandez R, Adams G, Anderson J, et al. UK screening and treatment of retinopathy of prematurity updated 2022 guidelines. Early Human Development. 2023;**177-178**:105715

[35] Greenwald MF, Danford ID, Shahrawat M, Ostmo S, Brown J, Kalpathy-Cramer J, et al. Evaluation of artificial intelligence-based telemedicine screening for retinopathy of prematurity. Journal of American Association for Pediatric Ophthalmology and Strabismus. 2020;**24**(3):160-162

[36] Day S, Menke AM, Abbott RL. Retinopathy of prematurity malpractice claims: the ophthalmic mutual insurance company experience. Archives of Ophthalmology. 2009;**127**(6):794-798

[37] Guo Z, Ma N, Wu Y, Yuan H, Luo W, Zeng L, et al. The safety and feasibility of the screening for retinopathy of prematurity assisted by telemedicine network during COVID-19 pandemic in Wuhan, China. BMC Ophthalmology. 2021;**21**(1):258

[38] Brady CJ, D'Amico S, Campbell JP. Telemedicine for retinopathy of prematurity. Telemedicine Journal and E-Health. 2020;**26**(4):556-564

[39] Chiang MF, Melia M, Buffenn AN, Lambert SR, Recchia FM, Simpson JL, et al. Detection of clinically significant retinopathy of prematurity using wide-angle digital retinal photography: A report by the American Academy of Ophthalmology. Ophthalmology. 2012;**119**(6):1272-1280

[40] Fijalkowski N, Zheng LL, Henderson MT, Wang SK, Wallenstein MB, Leng T, et al. Stanford University network for diagnosis of retinopathy of prematurity (SUNDROP): Five years of screening with telemedicine. Ophthalmic Surgery, Lasers & Imaging Retina. 2014;**45**(2):106-113

[41] Harby LA, Ali Z, Rajai A, Roberts SA, Peto T, Leung I, et al. Prospective validation of a virtual clinic pathway in the management of choroidal naevi: The NAEVUS study report no. 1: Safety assessment. British Journal of Ophthalmology. 2022;**106**(1):128-134

[42] Roelofs K, Weis E. Tele-oncology: A validation study of choroidal and Iris Nevi. Ocular Oncology and Pathology. 2019;**5**(4):298-302

[43] UHBW. Bristol Eye Hospital Assessment Service moves to The Galleries, Broadmead. Bristol, UK: UHBW; 2023. Available from: https://www.uhbw.nhs.uk/p/march-2023/bristol-eye-hospital-assessment-service-moves-to-the-galleries-broadmead/print

[44] Golinelli D, Boetto E, Carullo G, Nuzzolese AG, Landini MP, Fantini MP.

Adoption of digital technologies in health care during the COVID-19 pandemic: Systematic review of early scientific literature. Journal of Medical Internet Research. 2020;**22**(11):e22280

[45] Nagino K, Sung J, Midorikawa-Inomata A, Eguchi A, Fujimoto K, Okumura Y, et al. Clinical utility of smartphone applications in ophthalmology: A systematic review. Ophthalmology Science. 2024;**4**(1):100342

[46] Kim JE, Tomkins-Netzer O, Elman MJ, Lally DR, Goldstein M, Goldenberg D, et al. Evaluation of a self-imaging SD-OCT system designed for remote home monitoring. BMC Ophthalmology. 2022;**22**(1):261

[47] Liu Y, Holekamp NM, Heier JS. Prospective, longitudinal study: Daily self-imaging with home OCT for neovascular age-related macular degeneration. Ophthalmology Retina. 2022;**6**(7):575-585

[48] Land MR, Patel PA, Bui T, Jiao C, Ali A, Ibnamasud S, et al. Examining the role of telemedicine in diabetic retinopathy. Journal of Clinical Medicine. 2023;**12**(10):3537

[49] Schmidt-Erfurth U, Garcia-Arumi J, Bandello F, Berg K, Chakravarthy U, Gerendas BS, et al. Guidelines for the management of diabetic macular Edema by the European Society of retina specialists (EURETINA). Ophthalmologica. 2017;**237**(4):185-222

[50] Balaskas K, Drawnel F, Khanani AM, Knox PC, Mavromaras G, Wang YZ. Home vision monitoring in patients with maculopathy: Current and future options for digital technologies. Eye (London, England). 2023;**37**(15):3108-3120

[51] SetSquared. Siloton: Photonics technology to prevent sight loss 2023. Available from: https://setsquared-bristol.co.uk/news/siloton-photonics-technology-to-prevent-sight-loss/

[52] Faes L, Bachmann LM, Sim DA. Home monitoring as a useful extension of modern tele-ophthalmology. Eye. 2020;**34**(11):1950-1953

[53] Okkohealth. Every patient needs on-time treatment. 2024. Available from: https://okkohealth.com/en-gb/

[54] Schutz S, Walthall H, Snowball J, Vagner R, Fernandez N, Bartram E, et al. Patient and clinician experiences of remote consultation during the SARS-CoV-2 pandemic: A service evaluation. Digital Health. 2022;**8**:1-21

[55] GMC. Remote consultations. Available from: https://www.gmc-uk.org/professional-standards/ethical-hub/remote-consultations#:~:text=You%20must%20seek%20informed%20consent,and%20audio%20recordings%20of%20patients

[56] GMC. Good medical practice 2019. Available from: https://www.gmc-uk.org/professional-standards/professional-standards-for-doctors/good-medical-practice

[57] Donaghy E, Atherton H, Hammersley V, McNeilly H, Bikker A, Robbins L, et al. Acceptability, benefits, and challenges of video consulting: A qualitative study in primary care. British Journal of General Practice. 2019;**69**(686):e586-ee94

[58] Kern C, Kortuem K, Hamilton R, Fasolo S, Cai Y, Balaskas K, et al. Clinical outcomes of a hospital-based teleophthalmology service: What happens to patients in a virtual clinic? Ophthalmology Retina. 2019;**3**(5):422-428

[59] Aziz K, Sherif NA, Meshkin RS, Lorch AC, Armstrong GW. Telemedicine

curriculum in an ophthalmology residency program. Journal of Academic Ophthalmology. 2017;**14**(1):e93-e102

[60] Wherton J, Shaw S, Papoutsi C, Seuren L, Greenhalgh T. Guidance on the introduction and use of video consultations during COVID-19: Important lessons from qualitative research. BMJ Leader. 2020;**4**(3):120-123

[61] Zanaboni P, Knarvik U, Wootton R. Adoption of routine telemedicine in Norway: The current picture. Global Health Action. 2014;**7**:22801

[62] Serre K, Sasongko MB. Modifiable lifestyle and environmental risk factors affecting the retinal microcirculation. Microcirculation. 2012;**19**(1):29-36

[63] Kuwabara A, Su S, Krauss J. Utilizing digital health technologies for patient education in lifestyle medicine. American Journal of Lifestyle Medicine. 2020;**14**(2):137-142

[64] Labiris G, Panagiotopoulou EK, Kozobolis VP. A systematic review of teleophthalmological studies in Europe. International Journal of Ophthalmology. 2018;**11**(2):314-325

[65] Mansberger SL, Sheppler C, Barker G, Gardiner SK, Demirel S, Wooten K, et al. Long-term comparative effectiveness of telemedicine in providing diabetic retinopathy screening examinations: A randomized clinical trial. JAMA Ophthalmology. 2015;**133**(5):518-525

[66] Liew G, Michaelides M, Bunce C. A comparison of the causes of blindness certifications in England and Wales in working age adults (16-64 years), 1999-2000 with 2009-2010. BMJ Open. 2014;**4**(2):e004015

[67] Lorenz B, Spasovska K, Elflein H, Schneider N. Wide-field digital imaging based telemedicine for screening for acute retinopathy of prematurity (ROP). Six-year results of a multicentre field study. Graefe's Archive for Clinical and Experimental Ophthalmology. 2009;**247**(9):1251-1262

[68] Kern C, Fu DJ, Kortuem K, Huemer J, Barker D, Davis A, et al. Implementation of a cloud-based referral platform in ophthalmology: Making telemedicine services a reality in eye care. British Journal of Ophthalmology. 2020;**104**(3):312-317

[69] Faes L, Fu DJ, Huemer J, Kern C, Wagner SK, Fasolo S, et al. A virtual-clinic pathway for patients referred from a national diabetes eye screening programme reduces service demands whilst maintaining quality of care. Eye. 2021;**35**(8):2260-2269

[70] Society M. Workforce Census illustrates severe shortage of eye doctors. 2023. Available from: https://www.macularsociety.org/about/media/news/2023/march/workforce-census-illustrates-severe-shortage-of-eye-doctors/

[71] Hanumunthadu D, Adan K, Tinkler K, Balaskas K, Hamilton R, Nicholson L, et al. Outcomes following implementation of a high-volume medical retina virtual clinic utilising a diagnostic hub during COVID-19. Eye. 2022;**36**(3):627-633

[72] Al Owaifeer AM, Al-Swailem SA, Al Dehailan AM, Al Naim A, Al Molhim MF, Khandekar RB. Physician satisfaction with virtual ophthalmology clinics during the COVID-19 pandemic: A tertiary eye care center experience. Cureus. 2022;**14**(4):e23837

[73] Shahid SM, Anguita R, daCruz L. Telemedicine for postoperative consultations following vitrectomy for retinal detachment repair during

the COVID-19 crisis: A patient satisfaction survey. Canadian Journal of Ophthalmology. 2021;**56**(2):e46-ee8

[74] Kumari Rani P, Raman R, Manikandan M, Mahajan S, Paul PG, Sharma T. Patient satisfaction with tele-ophthalmology versus ophthalmologist-based screening in diabetic retinopathy. Journal of Telemedicine and Telecare. 2006;**12**(3):159-160

[75] Alhumud A, Al Adel F, Alwazae M, Althaqib G, Almutairi A. Patient satisfaction toward a tele-retinal screening program in endocrinology clinics at a tertiary hospital in Riyadh, Saudi Arabia. Cureus. 2020;**12**(5):e7986

[76] Ittarat M, Cheungpasitporn W, Chansangpetch S. Personalized care in eye health: Exploring opportunities, challenges, and the road ahead for chatbots. Journal of Personalized Medicine. 2023;**13**(12):1679

[77] Shih KC, Wong JKW, Lian JX, Lam CLK, Lai JSM. Diagnostic accuracy of tele-ophthalmology versus face-to-face consultation: Abridged secondary publication. Hong Kong Medical Journal. 2023;**29**(Suppl. 1(1)):18-21

[78] Dolar-Szczasny J, Barańska A, Rejdak R. Evaluating the efficacy of teleophthalmology in delivering ophthalmic care to underserved populations: A literature review. Journal of Clinical Medicine. 2023;**12**(9):3161

[79] Li Z, Wu C, Olayiwola JN, Hilaire DS, Huang JJ. Telemedicine-based digital retinal imaging vs standard ophthalmologic evaluation for the assessment of diabetic retinopathy. Connecticut Medicine. 2012;**76**(2):85-90

[80] Than J, Sim PY, Muttuvelu D, Ferraz D, Koh V, Kang S, et al. Teleophthalmology and retina: A review of current tools, pathways and services. International Journal of Retina and Vitreous. 2023;**9**(1):76

[81] Raghupathi W. Data mining in healthcare. In: Healthcare Informatics: Improving Efficiency through Technology, Analytics, and Management. Boca Raton, Florida, United States: CRC Press, Taylor & Francis Group; 2016

[82] Singhal S, Kayyali B, Levin R, Greenberg Z. The next wave of healthcare innovation: The evolution of ecosystems. United States: McKinsey & Company; 2020

[83] Alexandru A, Alexandru C, Coardos D, Tudora E. Healthcare, big data and cloud computing. WSEAS Transactions on Computer Research. 2016;**4**:123-131

[84] Olaronke I, Oluwaseun O. Big data in healthcare: Prospects, challenges and resolutions. Future Technologies Conference (FTC). 2016;**2016**:1152-1157

[85] Asadi Someh I, Breidbach CF, Davern M, Shanks G. Ethical implications of big data analytics. In: Research-in-Progress Papers, 24. İstanbul, Turkey: Twenty-Fourth European Conference on Information Systems (ECIS); 2016

[86] Zillner S, Neururer S. Big Data in the Health Sector. In: Cavanillas JM, Curry E, Wahlster W, editors. New Horizons for a Data-Driven Economy: A Roadmap for Usage and Exploitation of Big Data in Europe. Cham: Springer International Publishing; 2016. pp. 179-194

[87] Gunst S, De Ville F. The Brussels Effect: How the GDPR Conquered Silicon Valley. Alphen aan Den Rijn, The Netherlands: European Foreign Affairs Review. 2021. pp. 437-458

[88] Rustad ML, Koenig TH. Towards a global data privacy standard. Florida Law Review. 2019;**71**(2):365

[89] Jalali MS, Landman A, Gordon WJ. Telemedicine, privacy, and information security in the age of COVID-19. Journal of the American Medical Informatics Association. 2021;**28**(3):671-672

[90] Martinetti A, Chemweno P, Nizamis K, Fosch VE. Redefining safety in light of human-robot interaction: A critical review of current standards and regulations. Frontiers in Chemical Engineering. 2021;**3**:666237

[91] Amodei D, Olah C, Steinhardt J, Christiano P, Schulman J, Mané D. Concrete Problems in AI Safety. 2016. arXiv preprint arXiv: 1606.06565

[92] Fosch-Villaronga E, Millard C. Cloud robotics law and regulation: Challenges in the governance of complex and dynamic cyber–physical ecosystems. Robotics and Autonomous Systems. 2019;**119**:77-91

[93] Fosch-Villaronga E, Khanna P, Drukarch H, Custers B. The role of humans in surgery automation. International Journal of Social Robotics. 2023;**15**(3):563-580

[94] Al-Atrache Y, Manfredi R, Brooks K, Wilson N. Chapter 22 - Medical Ethics, the Law, and Cultural Competency. In: Shesser R, Pourmand A, Keim A, editors. The Emergency Department Technician Handbook. New Delhi: Elsevier; 2024. pp. 229-235

[95] Bartlett A, Prainsack B. Personalized Medicine: Empowered Patients in the 21st Century? New York: New York University Press. 2017. 288 pp. Sociology of Health & Illness. 2019;41(7):1465-6

[96] Shah PTI, Turrin D, et al. Informed Consent [Internet]. Florida, United States: StatPearls Publishing; 2023 Available from: https://www.ncbi.nlm.nih.gov/books/NBK430827/

[97] Agrawal V, Agrawal S, Bomanwar A, Dubey T, Jaiswal A. Exploring the risks, benefits, advances, and challenges in internet integration in medicine with the advent of 5g technology: A comprehensive review. Cureus. 2023;**15**(11):e48767

[98] Fosch-Villaronga E, Heldeweg M. "Regulation, I presume?" said the robot – Towards an iterative regulatory process for robot governance. Computer Law & Security Review. 2018;**34**(6):1258-1277

[99] Rogers EM. Diffusion of Innovations. 4th ed. New York, United States: Free Press; 2010

[100] Jirotka M, Procter ROB, Hartswood M, Slack R, Simpson A, Coopmans C, et al. Collaboration and trust in healthcare innovation: The eDiaMoND case study. Computer Supported Cooperative Work (CSCW). 2005;**14**(4):369-398

[101] Kelly CJ, Young AJ. Promoting innovation in healthcare. Future Healthcare Journal. 2017;**4**(2):121-125

[102] Allain S. Healthcare Innovation for All: Trust and Equity Must be a Priority. 2022. Available from: https://jnjinnovation.com/news/blog-post/healthcare-innovation-for-all-trust-and-equity-must-be-a-priority

[103] Haimi M. The tragic paradoxical effect of telemedicine on healthcare disparities- a time for redemption: A narrative review. BMC Medical Informatics and Decision Making. 2023;**23**(1):95

[104] Grossman LV, Masterson Creber RM, Benda NC, Wright D, Vawdrey DK, Ancker JS. Interventions to increase patient portal use in vulnerable populations: A systematic review. Journal of the American Medical Informatics Association. 2019;**26**(8-9):855-870

[105] Pourmand A, Ghassemi M, Sumon K, Amini SB, Hood C, Sikka N. Lack of telemedicine training in academic medicine: Are we preparing the next generation? Telemedicine Journal and E-Health. 2021;**27**(1):62-67

[106] HRSA. Improving access to telehealth. 2023. Available from: https://telehealth.hhs.gov/providers/health-equity-in-telehealth/improving-access-to-telehealth

[107] Melhem SJ, Nabhani-Gebara S, Kayyali R. Digital trends, digital literacy, and E-health engagement predictors of breast and colorectal cancer survivors: A population-based cross-sectional survey. International Journal of Environmental Research and Public Health. 2023;**20**(2):1472

[108] NPSF. RCA2: Improving Root Cause Analyses and Actions to Prevent Harm. Boston, Massachusetts, United States: NPSF; 2015

[109] Dia M, Davoudi S, Sanayei N, Martin DC, Albrecht MM, Ness S, et al. Demographic and socioeconomic disparities in the hybrid ophthalmology telemedicine model. Journal of Telemedicine and Telecare. 2023. DOI: 10.1177/1357633X231211353

[110] Hennein L, Jastrzembski B, Shah AS. Use of telemedicine in pediatric ophthalmology in the underserved population. Seminars in Ophthalmology. 2023;**38**(2):116-123

[111] Kozak I, Payne JF, Schatz P, Al-Kahtani E, Winkler M. Teleophthalmology image-based navigated retinal laser therapy for diabetic macular edema: A concept of retinal telephotocoagulation. Graefe's Archive for Clinical and Experimental Ophthalmology. 2017;**255**(8):1509-1513

[112] Ruamviboonsuk P, Tiwari R, Sayres R, Nganthavee V, Hemarat K, Kongprayoon A, et al. Real-time diabetic retinopathy screening by deep learning in a multisite national screening programme: A prospective interventional cohort study. The Lancet Digital Health. 2022;**4**(4):e235-ee44

[113] Wu W-T, Li Y-J, Feng A-Z, Li L, Huang T, Xu A-D, et al. Data mining in clinical big data: The frequently used databases, steps, and methodological models. Military Medical Research. 2021;**8**(1):44

[114] Grzybowski A, Singhanetr P, Nanegrungsunk O, Ruamviboonsuk P. Artificial Intelligence for diabetic retinopathy screening using color retinal photographs: From development to deployment. Ophthalmology and Therapy. 2023;**12**(3):1419-1437

[115] Kelly JT, Campbell KL, Gong E, Scuffham P. The internet of things: Impact and implications for health care delivery. Journal of Medical Internet Research. 2020;**22**(11):e20135

[116] WHO. Recommendations on digital interventions for health system strengthening. Geneva, Switzerland: WHO; 2019. Available from: https://www.who.int/publications/i/item/9789241550505

[117] Holekamp NM. Moving from clinic to home: What the future holds for ophthalmic telemedicine. American Journal of Ophthalmology. 2018;**187**:xxviii-xxxv

[118] Ting DSW, Lin H, Ruamviboonsuk P, Wong TY, Sim DA. Artificial intelligence, the internet of things, and virtual clinics: Ophthalmology at the digital translation forefront. The Lancet Digital Health. 2020;**2**(1):e8-e9

[119] Ho E, Wang E, Youn S, Sivajohan A, Lane K, Chun J, et al. Deep ensemble learning for retinal image classification. Translational Vision Science & Technology. 2022;**11**(10):39

[120] Leandro I, Lorenzo B, Aleksandar M, Dario M, Rosa G, Agostino A, et al. OCT-based deep-learning models for the identification of retinal key signs. Scientific Reports. 2023;**13**(1):14628

[121] Abdullah YI, Schuman JS, Shabsigh R, Caplan A, Al-Aswad LA. Ethics of artificial intelligence in medicine and ophthalmology. The Asia-Pacific Journal of Ophthalmology. 2021;**10**(3):289-298

[122] WHO. The World Report on Vision. Geneva, Switzerland: WHO; 2019. Available from: https://www.iapb.org/learn/resources/the-world-report-on-vision/

[123] Belfast QU. The UK-Philippines Remote Retinal Evaluation Collaboration in Health: Diabetic Retinopathy (REACH-DR). Swindon, United Kingdom: UK Research and Innovation; 2022

[124] Loewenstein A, Berger A, Daly A, Creuzot-Garcher C, Gale R, Ricci F, et al. Save our Sight (SOS): A collective call-to-action for enhanced retinal care across health systems in high income countries. Eye. 2023;**37**(16):3351-3359

Chapter 9

Telemedicine in Dermatology

Mónica P. Novoa-Candia, Valeria Vela-Lopez and Mariana Orduz-Robledo

Abstract

Telemedicine is known as the practice of diagnosing and treating patients by medical professionals from a distant location. In dermatology, telemedicine offers a transformative approach to healthcare services, particularly in remote or rural areas. Telemedicine allows patients to access medical care conveniently, ensuring both doctor and patient's safety. Multiple advantages of telemedicine have been described, including lowering the necessity for expensive hospital trips and enabling remote consultations. Dermatology is a specialized field that is not universally accessible in all regions as ideally required. Therefore, telemedicine serves as a useful tool to facilitate access to evaluations for various dermatological conditions. However, despite its benefits, telemedicine in dermatology also encounters certain obstacles. In this chapter, we explore the dynamic and impact of telemedicine, specifically in the field of dermatology.

Keywords: telemedicine, dermatology, virtual healthcare, remote consultations, remote diagnosis

1. Introduction

Telemedicine, known as the practice of diagnosing and treating patients from a distant or rural location, has become increasingly important within modern healthcare practices. This approach has shown notable benefits, including improved healthcare access, enhanced quality of care, increased patient satisfaction, and decreased administrative expenses and costs. In dermatology, we talk about "Teledermatology," and it has emerged as a vital tool in healthcare services, particularly in rural areas or during times when in-person consultations are challenging, such as COVID-19. This innovative approach utilizes telecommunications technology to facilitate remote diagnosis, treatment, and management of various dermatological conditions. In this chapter, we aim to explore the current landscape of telemedicine in dermatology, discussing its applications, benefits, challenges, and future directions.

2. What is telemedicine?

Telemedicine involves health services supported by telecommunication and electronic technologies [1]. It is defined by the World Health Organization (WHO) as "the delivery of healthcare services, where distance is a critical factor, by all healthcare professionals using information and communication technologies for the exchange of valid information for diagnosis, treatment, and prevention of disease and injuries, research and evaluation, and for the continuing education of health care providers, all in the interests of advancing the health of individuals and their communities" [2].

The evolution of telemedicine spans many years, starting from the creation of the telegram, which served as a communication medium in its time, followed by the emergence of radio and telephone, both of which played significant roles in medical telecommunications. This journey includes the visionary concept of Hugo Gernsback, a renowned science fiction writer, who foresaw the potential of radio in providing remote medical care, as depicted in his work "The Radio Doctor – Maybe" [3, 4]. Additionally, figures like Gerson Cohen contributed to this evolution with innovations such as teleradiology, as described in his publication detailing a three-year experience of transmitting radiographs using commercial telephone lines between a clinic in Atlantic City and a county hospital in Philadelphia [5, 6].

Described in 1999 as "the use of telecommunications and computer technology to offer medical information and services remotely" [7], telemedicine has been studied over the years and is recognized as a method of delivering healthcare services via the Internet, typically utilizing the video conferencing technology [8].

From 2000 to the present day, there has been a rapid evolution in technology, including hardware such as smartphones, tablets, and telemedicine devices, as well as software like mobile applications, and improved connectivity through cellular and broadband networks. This technological progress has led to the development of various telemedicine devices, making remote care more accessible. The widespread adoption of smartphones has enabled consumers to access healthcare services conveniently through portable devices [1, 4, 9].

Furthermore, telemedicine's applications extend to various other areas, such as virtual medical appointments, remote chronic disease management, and telepharmacy services.

2.1 Teledermatology

Teledermatology utilizes telecommunications and information technologies to diagnose, monitor, treat, prevent, conduct research, and provide education remotely [3], involves remote consultation and treatment of patients with skin diseases by healthcare providers, and has become more acknowledged as a vital aspect of healthcare provision.

The majority of teledermatology research has been conducted particularly during the COVID-19 pandemic [10, 11]. Since then, numerous reviews and studies have been developed on this topic. In one such study conducted by Kennedy J. et al., it was revealed that 96.9% of the 591 dermatologists surveyed provided virtual consultations in 2020 [12].

There are four primary teledermatology practice models [13, 14]:

- Consultation: refers to the process where the referring physician seeks advice or guidance from the dermatologist concerning the patient's skin condition.

- Triage: where doctor can determine the priority of management and referrals.

- Direct care: doctor directly interacts with patients, either through video conferences or by patients sharing images of their skin lesions.

- Follow-up: where doctor can monitor the progress of the skin condition and how it responds to treatment over time.

Telemedicine, evolving within the field of dermatology, includes three primary applications: synchronous, asynchronous, and hybrid platforms [15, 16].

- Synchronous: utilizes real-time audio/video conferencing for direct interactions between patients and dermatologists and was the predominant approach during the pandemic [17]. This method provides a more personalized interaction similar to in-person consultations, enabling dermatologists to promptly gather information about patient symptoms and medical history [13].

- Asynchronous: involves patients forwarding clinical history and images directly to dermatologists through intermediary referring providers. It does not involve live teleconferencing and is often used for triaging, consultations, or follow-ups. A key advantage of this model is its flexibility for both dermatologists and patients, eliminating the need to schedule a specific time for communication, especially useful across different time zones [3, 13].

- Hybrid models: incorporate both approaches, enabling direct synchronous interactions for gathering patient history and providing education, while also facilitating the asynchronous transmission of high-quality images to ensure precise evaluation. It helps to solve problems with both methods by giving dermatologists a quick chat with the patient or doctor and also a clear picture of the skin problem [11, 13].

Each approach has its own characteristics and advantages, addressing the specific needs of both patients and dermatologists (**Table 1**).

The main features evaluated in teledermatology are accessibility, accuracy, cost-effectiveness, informed consent, and data security [13]. Accessibility is vital, facilitating patients to receive diagnosis and monitoring at home, while reducing exposure risks [18, 19]. Accuracy is comparable to face-to-face consultations, with studies demonstrating high diagnostic precision as we will talk about later [20]. Teledermatology proves cost-effective by reducing inpatient visits, transportation expenses, and lost productivity, particularly during the pandemic [21, 22]. Informed consent is essential, requiring patients to understand teledermatology features and data security policies, although debates persist on the method of obtaining consent [23, 24]. Data security measures, including pseudo anonymization and encryption, are crucial to safeguard patient privacy [13].

The accessibility and convenience offered by telemedicine have revolutionized the delivery of dermatological care, breaking down geographical barriers and improving patient access to specialists. Patients can now receive timely consultations and follow-ups without the need for travel, reducing both costs and logistical challenges associated with traditional healthcare delivery.

2.1.1 Teledermatology in specific diseases

Existing evidence confirms the diagnostic precision of teledermatology and its effectiveness in treating conditions, such as acne, atopic dermatitis, psoriasis, hair disorders, and even skin cancer [15].

Type	Advantages	Disadvantages
Synchronous	• Real-time communication between the doctor and the patient. • Experience more similar to face-to-face consultation. • There is no separation in time.	• Needs prior arrangement to agree to an appointment-convenient time. • Requires high-speed internet access – connectivity issues • The quality of videos may not match that of static images
Asynchronous	• The patient has the option to capture a static image of the skin disease. • Gives flexibility to the doctor and patients. • It does not require appointments or specific times. • Enables doctor to examine the image at a later time without disrupting their workflow.	• There is no real-time communication; so, the doctor may be unable to resolve any unclear details in the patient's medical history. • Delays in communication.
Hybrid	• Offering to the doctor a time-efficient consultation with the patient. • Can offer high-quality image of the dermatological disease.	• It can become expensive when multiple platforms are needed.

Table 1.
Advantages and disadvantages of each type of teledermatology.

In the context of acne, teledermatology has been extensively studied, especially using synchronous and asynchronous telemedicine [15, 25]. During the pandemic, teledermatology in acne management played a significant role, with a majority of visits conducted remotely. Studies have indicated a strong correlation between in-person and digital diagnosis of acne severity, demonstrating positive clinical outcomes with teledermatology. Prescription of isotretinoin via teleconsultations yielded mild adverse effects, with outcomes comparable to in-person visits [26, 27].

Another area of focus in teledermatology is atopic dermatitis (AD), showing promising results in the management of AD, with high diagnostic concordance rates and positive clinical outcomes observed across various studies [10, 15, 28]. Research indicates that both asynchronous and synchronous teledermatology approaches are effective in diagnosing and monitoring AD, with equivalent improvements in disease severity and patient-reported outcomes compared to in-person visits [29, 30]. Additionally, teledermatology has been recommended by leading medical organizations for its utility in therapeutic education, severity monitoring, and facilitating patient communication in AD management.

Moreover, telemedicine has been recognized as a valuable alternative for psoriasis follow-ups, particularly synchronous and asynchronous teledermatology [31, 32]. Studies have shown that teledermatology yields similar or superior efficacy in improving Psoriasis Area Severity Index (PASI) and Dermatology Life Quality Index (DLQI) scores compared to traditional in-person consultations [33]. Additionally, teledermatology has been associated with greater improvements in patient-physician relationships and treatment compliance [34]. Overall, teledermatology serves as a beneficial tool for monitoring systemic therapies, enhancing treatment adherence and improving clinical outcomes in psoriasis.

Despite the extensive exploration of teledermatology in managing various dermatological conditions such as those named before, a few studies have explored telemedicine's role in alopecia. A systematic review was conducted [35], analyzing 11 studies comprising 9622 patients, the majority of whom suffered from androgenetic alopecia (AGA), with telemedicine showing high diagnostic accuracy and positive outcomes. Notably, tele-trichology evaluation, coupled with telemedicine, aids in diagnosis and treatment initiation, particularly for alopecia areata (AA) and patients with AA undergoing specific treatments with Janus kinase (JAK) inhibitors [35]. Although teledermatology offers accessible care, its utilization for alopecia remains relatively low compared to other conditions.

In summary, teledermatology has demonstrated its effectiveness in diagnosing and managing a wide range of dermatological conditions. The utilization of synchronous and asynchronous telemedicine during the pandemic has highlighted its importance in providing remote care, with positive clinical outcomes observed across various studies.

2.2 Benefits and challenges of teledermatology

As mentioned before, teledermatology has positively transformed dermatology consultations by providing patients worldwide with increased access to specialized healthcare services. This form of consultation not only benefits patients in rural areas but also reduces waiting times for appointments with specialists such as a dermatologist [36]. It is well known that, for rural patients, it is expensive to assist for consultation in urban areas where most of the dermatologists are placed, so teledermatology could help reduce transportation, alimentation, and accommodation costs for these patients and their families. On the contrary, it would prevent patients or their families from wasting time traveling to medical appointments, which sometimes lead to them being absent from work, sometimes worsening their economic condition [37]. There is evidence to confirm where it was found that, by increasing telemedicine services, the coverage of patients who, due to mobility problems or lack of money, could not access in-person appointments expanded, which led insurance companies to include telemedicine in their plans [38].

It has been demonstrated that when using teledermatology, you could not only decrease time to diagnosis and treatment but also make patient follow-up timely and safe [37]. When holding medical meetings where difficult cases are evaluated, we could have dermatologists from different parts of the world to participate in important decisions, especially when it comes to diagnoses and treatments that would benefit patients. Barbieri JS et al. concluded in their study that teledermatology is a potential triage tool to classify cases into nonurgent versus emergent cases requiring immediate in-person consultation [39].

Regarding the barriers to teledermatology, they are still present in both developing and developed countries. Among them is the limitation of having equipment in good condition, with internet networks that cover all national territories and specifically speaking of dermatology, it would be having good image quality to properly evaluate each patient, especially when evaluating pigmented lesions [36]. Clemens Scott Kruse et al. made a systematic review where they evaluated barriers to adopting telemedicine worldwide, and they found about 33 barriers that they grouped in: organizational barriers, patient-related barriers, and staff and program barriers [40]. Also, it is important for countries to stablish some regulations and public policies to

Advantages	Disadvantages
• Faster and cost-effective • Increases patient access to specialized health services such as dermatology • Useful for patient triage • High patient and physician satisfaction • High diagnostic accuracy • Collaboration with other colleagues • Eliminates geographical barriers, facilitating access for patients to dermatologists worldwide • Tool to help educate patients and health workers • Minimize traveling of patients	• Requires good access to internet and good equipped technology • Not a full-body examination, so it can lead to miss incidental lesions • Cannot palpate lesions • Reimbursement is poor • Poor quality images sent by patients • Dermoscopy cannot be used • Fraud and abuse • Cases of misdiagnosis • Confidentiality • Patient privacy • Lack of regulations and public policies for telemedicine

Table 2.
Advantages and disadvantages of teledermatology.

ensure medicolegal responsibilities and privacy issues when making consultations via telemedicine to increase the safety of the patient and the treating doctor.

Regarding the privacy and security of doctors as well as patients, it is important that medical consultations are carried out via applications that are encrypted and that they are applications that are only used as a medical communication tool, thus avoiding access to information to third parties, which would allow both doctors and patients to have peace of mind when making consultations via telemedicine [40].

Additionally, countries and medical insurance companies should make regulations to ensure the privacy of both doctors and patients during medical consultations. This includes prohibiting the use of patient images, videos, and personal information for purposes other than the consultation itself. It must implement secure equipment for data transmission, which should undergo continuous evaluation and include encrypted systems with restricted access to information. In the article by P. J. Gómez Arias et al., fair measures for telemedicine use in Spain are described. Changes to the codes of ethics were made to facilitate appropriate telemedicine practices. Patients are required to sign informed consent allowing virtual evaluation [41].

Finally, we summarize in **Table 2** the advantages and disadvantages of teledermatology.

2.3 Future trends in teledermatology

Recent developments in telemedicine technology leverage artificial intelligence (AI) to enhance physicians' efficiency [1]. AI refers to a machine's ability to independently solve problems, while machine learning (ML) employs algorithms to derive desired output data by identifying patterns and relationships within input data. Data can be provided to algorithms in two main ways: supervised learning, where both input and output data are labeled, and unsupervised learning, which involves training algorithms with unlabeled data. In dermatology, supervised learning is predominantly used due to its image-centric nature, where recognizing structures within images is predominant [42].

Studies comparing dermatologists to machine-learning algorithms showed computer algorithms were superior to clinicians in diagnostic accuracy for pigmented skin lesion [43]. Phillips et al. conducted a study on a deep learning algorithm for identifying melanoma. Their results showed that the AI achieved better recognition of melanoma compared to dermatologists and significantly outperformed primary care physicians [44]. These new advances will make it possible to help dermatologists with the monitoring and diagnosis of tumors such as melanoma.

As is known, skin lesions can vary depending on the skin phototype and can sometimes confuse the dermatologist when making diagnoses, but, with the help of artificial intelligence this could be minimized since in the study carried out by Groh, Matthew et al. where they concluded that well-designed physician-machine partnerships can enrich the diagnostic precision of physicians [45]. Moreover, mobile applications are also improving telemedicine, and in a study made in Colombia by Juan Pablo Sáenz et al., the authors concluded that the adoption of a teledermatology approach utilizing mobile applications and a domain-specific ontology-driven knowledge base aims to offer prompt support to healthcare professionals such as a general practitioner who answers dermatological consultations in rural areas where dermatologists are not available [9].

For instance, Mohammed Saleh Al-Dhubaibi et al. detail a case of cutaneous larva migrans in a 35-year-old female patient who presented with a serpiginous skin lesion on her left ankle, where clinical suspicion led to the diagnosis and albendazole treatment was prescribed, all of these using the "AskUrDr-For-Doctors" online medical application (**Figure 1**) [46].

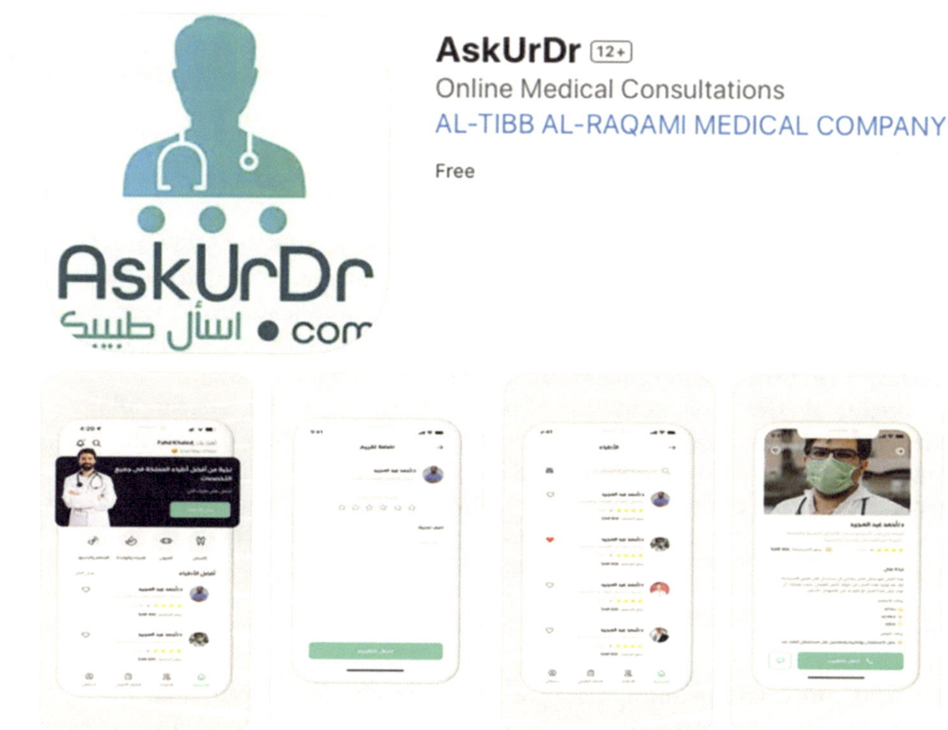

Figure 1.
Screenshot of the mobile application "AskUrDr-For-Doctors" only available in the country of application development.

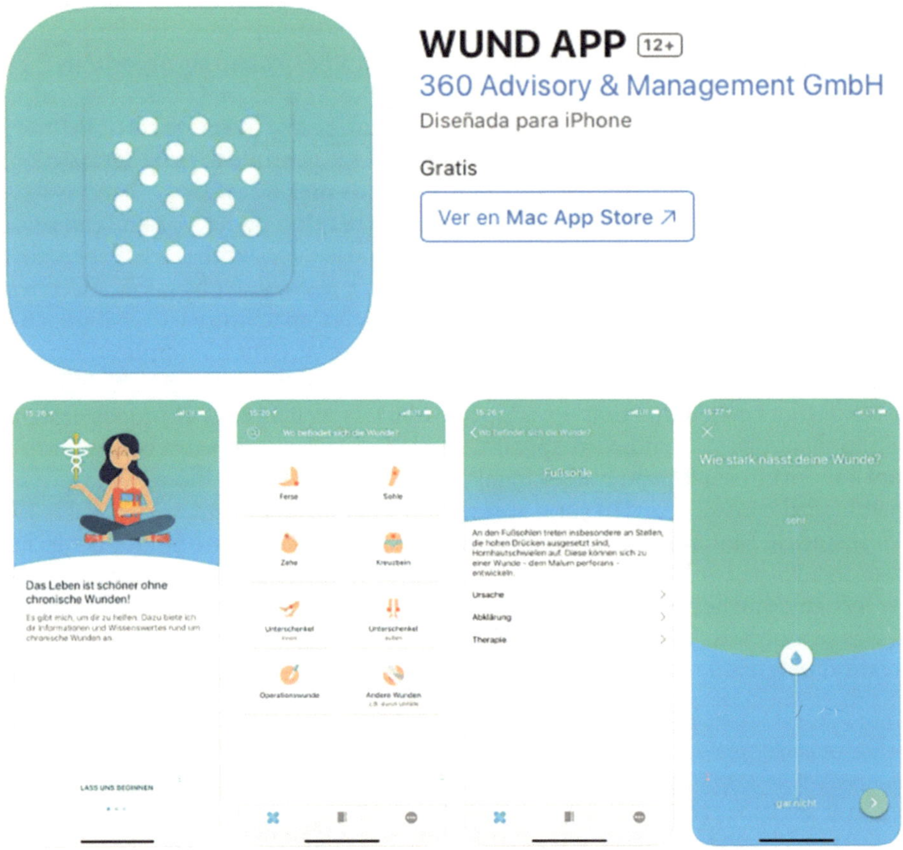

Figure 2.
Screenshot of the mobile application.

Another study on teledermatology and applications, conducted by Tassilo Degel et al., systematically evaluated mobile applications available in German or English for patients with chronic wounds. Out of 118 identified applications, 10 were patient-oriented. Following exclusion criteria, three applications underwent evaluation, with WUND APP (**Figure 2**) emerging as the top-rated option [47].

In conclusion, the implementation of new applications with teledermatology together with AI could screen large numbers of patients, sending those with distressing lesions to a dermatologist on time and discharging those with benign lesions earlier, decongesting the health system and thus giving priority to those who truly need a priority assessment with specialists like dermatologist [42].

3. Conclusions

Telemedicine is an expanding field that utilizes technology to facilitate the provision of healthcare services remotely to a wide variety of individuals in various locations. Within this domain, teledermatology stands out as a valuable tool for diagnosing and managing a wide spectrum of dermatological conditions. Furthermore, teledermatology serves as a potential triage mechanism, distinguishing between nonurgent cases and emergent cases necessitating immediate in-person consultation. Moreover, teledermatology holds promise in reducing costs for patients and their families while also overcoming geographical barriers, thereby enhancing patient access to dermatologists worldwide. Integrating teledermatology with artificial intelligence (AI) could further speed up the process by screening large volumes of patients and promptly referring those with concerning lesions to dermatologists for rapid assessment. In summary, teledermatology represents a powerful resource with the potential to revolutionize the delivery of dermatological services, making care more accessible, efficient, and impactful for a broader population.

Conflict of interest

The authors declare no conflict of interest.

Author details

Mónica P. Novoa-Candia[1*], Valeria Vela-Lopez[2] and Mariana Orduz-Robledo[3]

1 Pediatric Dermatology Department, Hospital Infantil de San José, Fundación Universitaria de Ciencias de la Salud (F.U.C.S), Bogotá, Colombia

2 Dermatology Resident, Fundación Universitaria de Ciencias de la Salud (F.U.C.S), Bogotá, Colombia

3 Dermatology Resident, Universidad del Bosque, Bogotá, Colombia

*Address all correspondence to: mopanoca@hotmail.com

References

[1] Haleem A, Javaid M, Singh RP, Suman R. Telemedicine for healthcare: Capabilities, features, barriers, and applications. Sensors International. 2021;**2**:100117

[2] Ryu S. Telemedicine: Opportunities and developments in member states: Report on the second global survey on eHealth 2009 (Global Observatory for eHealth Series, Volume 2). Healthcare Information Research. 2012;**18**(2):153

[3] Pasquali P, Sonthalia S, Moreno-Ramirez D, Sharma P, Agrawal M, Gupta S, et al. Teledermatology and its current perspective. Indian Dermatology Online Journal. 2020;**11**(1):12

[4] Jagarapu J, Savani RC. A brief history of telemedicine and the evolution of teleneonatology. Seminars in Perinatology. 2021;**45**(5):151416

[5] Gershon-Cohen J. Telognosis. Journal of the American Medical Association. 1952;**148**(9):731

[6] Думанский ЮВ, Владзимирский АВ, Лобас ВМ, Ливенс Ф, Dumanskyy YV, Vladzymyrskyy AV, et al. Атлас истории телемедицины Curatio Sine Distantia! АТЛАС ИСТОРИИ ТЕЛЕМЕДИЦИНЫ Atlas of the Telemedicine History. Donetsk, Ukraine: Донецк Donetsk Издательство «Ноулидж» Publishing House «Knowledge»; 2013

[7] Telemedicine: An overview. Health Devices. Mar 1999;**28**(3):88-103. PMID: 10212772

[8] Wang X, Zhang Z, Zhao J, Shi Y. Impact of telemedicine on healthcare service system considering patients' choice. Discrete Dynamics in Nature and Society. 2019;**2019**:1-16

[9] Sáenz JP, Novoa MP, Correal D, Eapen BR. On using a mobile application to support teledermatology: A case study in an underprivileged area in Colombia. International Journal of Telemedicine and Applications. 2018;**2018**:1-8

[10] Verma L, Turk T, Dennett L, Dytoc M. Teledermatology in atopic dermatitis: A systematic review. Journal of Cutaneous Medicine and Surgery. Mar-Apr 2024;**28**(2):153-157. DOI: 10.1177/12034754231223694. Epub 2024 Jan 11. PMID: 38205736; PMCID: PMC11015705

[11] Coates SJ, Kvedar J, Granstein RD. Teledermatology: From historical perspective to emerging techniques of the modern era. Journal of the American Academy of Dermatology. 2015;**72**(4):563-574

[12] Kennedy J, Arey S, Hopkins Z, Tejasvi T, Farah R, Secrest AM, et al. Dermatologist perceptions of teledermatology implementation and future use after COVID-19. JAMA Dermatology. 2021;**157**(5):595

[13] Ibrahim AE, Magdy M, Khalaf EM, Mostafa A, Arafa A. Teledermatology in the time of COVID-19. International Journal of Clinical Practice. Dec 2021;**75**(12):1-9, e15000. DOI: 10.1111/ijcp.15000. Epub 2021 Nov 4. PMID: 34714575; PMCID: PMC8646275

[14] Armstrong AW, Kwong MW, Ledo L, Nesbitt TS, Shewry SL. Practice models and challenges in teledermatology: A study of collective experiences from teledermatologists. PLoS One. 2011;**6**(12):e28687

[15] Hwang JK, del Toro NP, Han G, Oh DH, Tejasvi T, Lipner SR. Review of

teledermatology: Lessons learned from the COVID-19 pandemic. American Journal of Clinical Dermatology. 2024;**25**(1):5-14

[16] Lee JJ, English JC. Teledermatology: A review and update. American Journal of Clinical Dermatology. 2018;**19**(2):253-260

[17] Wang RH, Barbieri JS, Kovarik CL, Lipoff JB. Synchronous and asynchronous teledermatology: A narrative review of strengths and limitations. Journal of Telemedicine and Telecare. 2022;**28**(7):533-538

[18] Lee KJ, Finnane A, Soyer HP. Recent trends in teledermatology and teledermoscopy. Dermatology Practice Concept. 2018;**8**(3):214-223

[19] Markun S, Scherz N, Rosemann T, Tandjung R, Braun RP. Mobile teledermatology for skin cancer screening. Medicine. 2017;**96**(10):e6278

[20] Nami N, Massone C, Rubegni P, Cevenini G, Fimiani M, Hofmann-Wellenhof R. Concordance and time estimation of store-and-forward mobile teledermatology compared to classical face-to-face consultation. Acta Dermato Venereologica. 2015;**95**(1):35-39

[21] Livingstone J, Solomon J. An assessment of the cost-effectiveness, safety of referral and patient satisfaction of a general practice teledermatology service. London Journal of Prime Care (Abingdon). 2015;7(2):31-35

[22] Datta SK, Warshaw EM, Edison KE, Kapur K, Thottapurathu L, Moritz TE, et al. Cost and utility analysis of a store-and-forward teledermatology referral system. JAMA Dermatology. 2015;**151**(12):1323

[23] Nittari G, Khuman R, Baldoni S, Pallotta G, Battineni G, Sirignano A, et al. Telemedicine practice: Review of the current ethical and legal challenges. Telemedicine and e-Health. 2020;**26**(12):1427-1437

[24] Moghbeli F, Langarizadeh M, Ali A. Application of ethics for providing telemedicine services and information technology. Medical Archives. 2017;**71**(5):351

[25] Falotico JM, Gu L, Lipner SR. Not just pimple popping: The utility of hybrid telemedicine models beyond acne management amidst the ongoing COVID—19 pandemic. Journal of Cosmetic Dermatology. 2022;**21**(10):4105-4106

[26] Moreno-Ramírez D, Duarte-Ferreras MA, Ojeda-Vila T, García-Morales I, Conejo-Mir MD, Fernández-Orland A, et al. Telemedicine management of systemic therapy with isotretinoin of patients with moderate-to-severe acne during the COVID-19 pandemic: A longitudinal prospective feasibility study. Journal of the American Academy of Dermatology. 2022;**87**(5):1186-1189

[27] Onyekweli T, Agarwal A, Jaklitsch E, James A, Choudhary S, Ferris LK, et al. Teledermatology isotretinoin management for moderate-to-severe acne reveals similar outcomes to in-person management: A retrospective study. JAAD International. 2023;**11**:126-128

[28] Giavina-Bianchi M, Giavina-Bianchi P, Santos AP, Rizzo LV, Cordioli E. Accuracy and efficiency of telemedicine in atopic dermatitis. JAAD International. 2020;**1**(2):175-181

[29] Armstrong AW, Johnson MA, Lin S, Maverakis E, Fazel N, Liu FT.

Patient-centered, direct-access online care for management of atopic dermatitis. JAMA Dermatology. 2015;**151**(2):154

[30] Chiricozzi A, Talamonti M, De Simone C, Galluzzo M, Gori N, Fabbrocini G, et al. Management of patients with atopic dermatitis undergoing systemic therapy during COVID-19 pandemic in Italy: Data from the DA-COVID-19 registry. Allergy. 2021;**76**(6):1813-1824

[31] Koller S, Hofmann-Wellenhof R, Hayn D, Weger W, Kastner P, Schreier G, et al. Teledermatological monitoring of psoriasis patients on biologic therapy. Acta Dermato Venereologica. 2011;**91**(6):680-685

[32] Pelet del Toro N, Yahia R, Feldman SR, Van Voorhees A, Green L, Schwartzman S, et al. National psoriasis foundation telemedicine task force guidance for management of psoriatic disease via telemedicine. JAAD International. 2023;**12**:32-36

[33] Dahy A, El-Qushayri AE, Mahmoud AR, Al-Kelany TA, Salman S. Telemedicine approach for psoriasis management, time for application? A systematic review of published studies. Dermatologic Therapy. Nov 2020;**33**(6):1-6, e13908. DOI: 10.1111/dth.13908. Epub 2020 Jul 13. PMID: 32592525

[34] Armstrong AW, Chambers CJ, Maverakis E, Cheng MY, Dunnick CA, Chren MM, et al. Effectiveness of online vs in-person care for adults with psoriasis. JAMA Network Open. 2018;**1**(6):e183062

[35] Maskan Bermudez N, Perez S, Nguyen B, Tosti A. Teledermatology in alopecia: A systematic review. JAAD International. 2024;**14**:64-68

[36] McKoy K, Halpern S, Mutyambizi K. International teledermatology review. Current Dermatology Report. 2021;**10**(3):55-66

[37] Mocharnuk J, Lockard T, Georgesen C, English JC. Inpatient teledermatology: A review. Current Dermatology Report. 2022;**11**(2):52-59

[38] Greiwe J. Telemedicine lessons learned during the COVID-19 pandemic. Current Allergy and Asthma Reports. 2022;**22**(1):1-5

[39] Barbieri JS, Nelson CA, James WD, Margolis DJ, Littman-Quinn R, Kovarik CL, et al. The reliability of teledermatology to triage inpatient dermatology consultations. JAMA Dermatology. 2014;**150**(4):419

[40] Scott Kruse C, Karem P, Shifflett K, Vegi L, Ravi K, Brooks M. Evaluating barriers to adopting telemedicine worldwide: A systematic review. Journal of Telemedicine and Telecare. 2018;**24**(1):4-12

[41] Gómez Arias PJ, Abad Arenas E, Arias Blanco MC, Redondo Sánchez J, Galán Gutiérrez M, Vélez García-Nieto AJ. Aspectos medicolegales de la práctica de la teledermatología en España. Actas Dermo-Sifiliográficas. 2021;**112**(2):127-133

[42] Hartmann T, Passauer J, Hartmann J, Schmidberger L, Kneilling M, Volc S. Basic principles of artificial intelligence in dermatology explained using melanoma. JDDG: Journal der Deutschen Dermatologischen Gesellschaft. 2024;**22**(3):339-347

[43] Tschandl P, Codella N, Akay BN, Argenziano G, Braun RP, Cabo H, et al. Comparison of the accuracy of human readers versus machine-learning algorithms for

pigmented skin lesion classification: An open, web-based, international, diagnostic study. The Lancet Oncology. 2019;**20**(7):938-947

[44] Phillips M, Greenhalgh J, Marsden H, Palamaras I. Detection of malignant melanoma using artificial intelligence: An observational study of diagnostic accuracy. Dermatology Practical Concept. 2019;**2019**:e2020011

[45] Groh M, Badri O, Daneshjou R, Koochek A, Harris C, Soenksen LR, et al. Deep learning-aided decision support for diagnosis of skin disease across skin tones. Nature Medicine. 2024;**30**(2):573-583

[46] Al-Dhubaibi MS, Mohammed GF, Bahaj SS, AbdElneam AI. Cutaneous larva migrans: A case report diagnosed using teledermatology. Clinical Case Report. 26 Jun 2023;**11**(6):1-3, e7619. DOI: 10.1002/ccr3.7619. PMID: 37384230; PMCID: PMC10293577

[47] Dege T, Glatzel B, Borst V, Grän F, Goller S, Glatzel C, et al. Patient-Centered chronic wound care Mobile apps: Systematic identification, analysis, and assessment. JMIR mHealth and uHealth. 2024;**12**:e51592-e51592

Chapter 10

The Use of Innovative Digital Mobile Health Technology for Community Eye Care in Poor Resource Settings

Alozie Emeonye, Florence Nkwogu, Joseph Okeibunor and Sunny Ibeneme

Abstract

The practice of ophthalmology depends largely on ophthalmoscopy and photographic documentation of examination findings from patients. These images are used for patient education, monitoring, storage, expert reviews and treatment. In Africa, due to poor management and poor resources in some health systems, there is a dearth of infrastructure and equipment like fundus cameras. In such resource-poor settings, eye care personnel manage patients with available resources, or improvise with low-cost measures. Smartphone fundoscopy is one of such improvisations. This study describes a novel adapter for smartphone fundoscopy, used in conjunction with a tripod. It was built on existing research on smartphone fundoscopy. Fundus images were captured with a smartphone and a +20D lens, both coupled by an improvised adapter; the Chizaram-Condensing Lens Adapter for Smartphones (C-CLAS) on a tripod. This system works as an indirect ophthalmoscope. Videos of the fundus were recorded, and high-quality still-images were taken from segments of the videos. A total of 54 patients were used in the study, aged between 8 and 74 years. The C-CLAS captured high-quality fundus images from 39 patients (72%), in a variety of normal and pathological conditions. The use of a tripod rendered the procedure hands-free, introducing another dimension to smartphone fundoscopy.

Keywords: adapter, C-CLAS, condensing lens, fundoscopy, smartphone, tripod

1. Introduction

Fundus image capture is an integral part of ophthalmic practice where they serve the purposes of learning, documentation, patient management and education [1]. The gold standard of retinal image acquisition is the fundus camera, which is an expensive, bulky, stationary table-top equipment that is mostly used in the eye clinic setting [2]. In some parts of Africa, including Nigeria, due to poor health systems, some health institutions lack the capacity and resources necessary for basic health service delivery [3]. This has spurred discussions in several quarters on how to harness innovative technologies to bridge the digital divide and make services efficient, accessible, and affordable [4, 5].

Africa is currently the second most populous continent in the world, with an estimated population of 1 billion; and is predicted to rise to 4 billion by the end of the century [6]. This population growth comes with an exponential rise in the penetration of innovative technologies. Internet penetration, including the use of mHealth technologies for health is on the increase among African economies [6, 7]. mHealth is the application of mobile phone technologies for facilitating health service delivery [7]. The evolution of smartphones with novel designs, and functionalities is revolutionizing the field of digital eye health, especially among poor-resource settings where expensive equipment like fundus cameras are not affordable. In such settings, the simplest and cheapest approach is using a smartphone and an indirect condensing lens for patients with dilated pupils [8–12]. This chapter aims to contribute to the ongoing discussions on smartphone fundoscopy, with a particular focus on the unique features of the hardware (adapter) used, and its applications among impoverished contexts. It describes the Chizaram-Condensing Lens Adapter for Smartphones (C-CLAS), used in conjunction with a tripod-stand for retinal imaging; and also highlights key findings, challenges, ongoing progress and future directions in-view of adopting, implementing and scaling the adapter.

2. The C-CLAS study

2.1 Methodology

This study was conducted in the eye clinic of the Federal Teaching Hospital Owerri (FTHO), located in the capital of Imo State, Nigeria. FTHO is a tertiary-level healthcare center for training interns, resident doctors, and for research. Thus, this study was part of the requirements for postgraduate medical training in Nigeria and was focused on the application of mHealth technologies in the advancement of retinal imaging in this facility. All patients used in this study signed a written consent for their eyes to be imaged, and for their pictures to be used. Ethical clearance was obtained from the Ethics Committee of FTHO, Nigeria. This study targeted to sample 10% of the total fundoscopy procedures done each day at the FTH, Owerri across different age ranges, gender and pathologies. A total of 54 randomly selected patients aged 8–74 years, without significant media opacities who attended the eye clinic were used for this study. The project team assumed this to be a good representation of the cases in the eye clinic, and suitable for this study. We chose this facility because of large population of patients in need of retinal examination.

The C-CLAS adapter was designed and fabricated using locally-sourced polyvinylchloride PVC materials used in household plumbing. This material is lightweight, malleable, and was cut and molded to the design of the adapter using heat. An Infinix X650B- Hot 8 smartphone was used in this study. However, the adapter can also be used with other smartphone brands, making it versatile and customizable. The tripod-stand was purchased separately from an online retail store, and subsequently modified by adding a clamp for the adapter. The adapter was designed in two parts: A smartphone holder that clamps the smartphone in place, with a window for the camera and flashlight of the smartphone, and a tubular arm of fixed length (15 centimeters) with a lens mount at its end. The +20D Volk condensing lens has about 40°′ field of view, and an angular magnification of 3. The tubular arm length of 15 centimeters was chosen for reasons of weight balancing, and to enable the auto-focus of the smartphone camera easily acquire clear images. The fixed nature of the tubular arm meant the working distance between the lens and smartphone cannot be altered; and this worked well with different patients, irrespective of different ocular axial lengths and refractive errors due to the autofocus capability of the smartphone's camera.

The tubular arm was attached to the smartphone holder such that the window was aligned with the +20D lens on the lens mount; the unit functioning as a coaxial system, similar to an indirect ophthalmoscope. The picture of the C-CLAS is shown in **Figure 1**. The condensing lens mount was designed with a slight undersized fit to make it clamp the +20D lens firmly. An adhesive strap was added as an extra measure to secure the lens and prevent it from accidentally falling-off the mount. The device is hand-held (with one hand); but can also be coupled to a tripod. The use of a tripod reinforced the stability, and uniquely enabled the adapter to be used hands-free. In addition, the stability conferred by the tripod-stand also enabled the auto-focus feature of the smartphone to easily acquire a sharp focus of the fundus, thereby improving image quality. The tripod can be used with the legs shortened or extended (**Figure 2A** and **B**). The adapter can be used with the patient in standing, sitting or supine positions. A Ray tracing of the optics of the C-CLAS is shown in **Figure 3**.

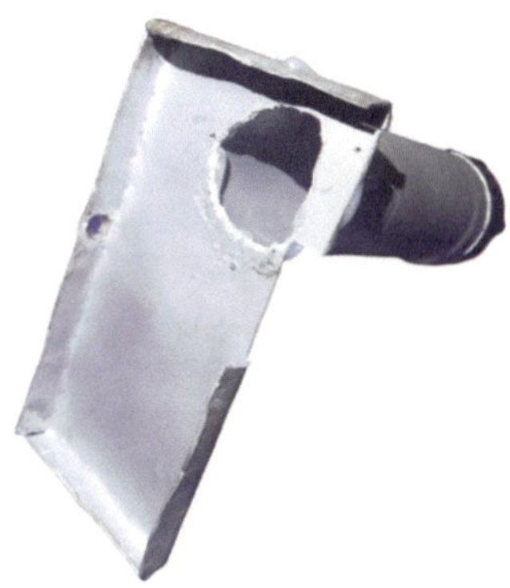

Figure 1.
The C-CLAS adapter.

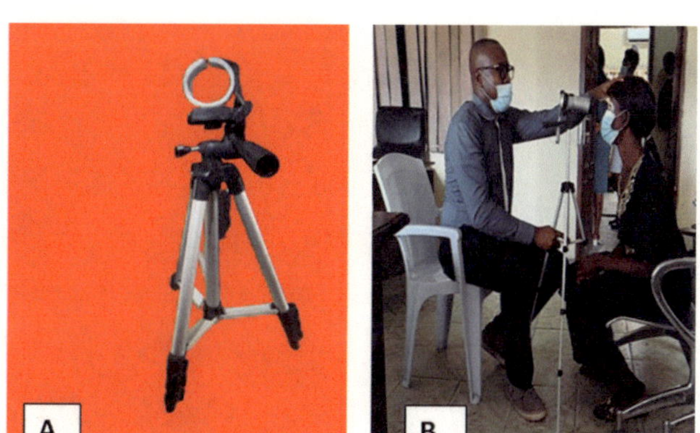

Figure 2.
Tripod shortened (A) and extended (B).

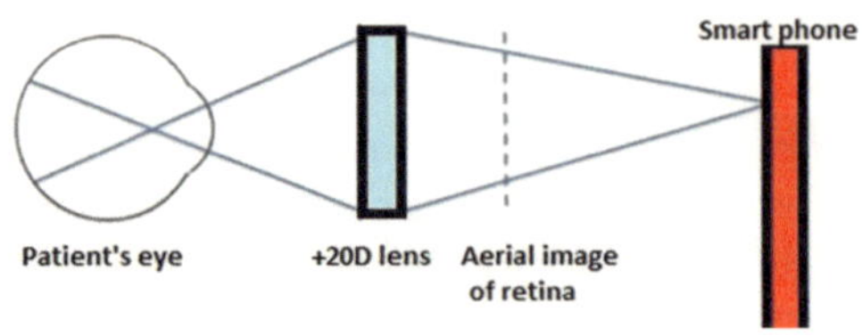

Figure 3.
Optics of the C-CLAS; based on the optics of indirect ophthalmoscopy.

It is important to note that good pupillary dilation prior to filming, and patient cooperation were necessary for easier imaging of the fundus. A minimum pupil aperture of 4 mm was required for imaging. The examination room was dimly lit, and the C-CLAS was placed about 5 centimeters in front of the eye, with the native video recorder and flashlight of the Infinix X650B turned on. The working distance between the lens and the eye was adjusted until an image of the area of interest in the retina filled the field of view (**Figure 4**). The auto-focus feature of the smartphone's 13-megapixel triple rear camera and quad flashlight adjusts for clarity automatically. A pre-recording zoom setting of 1.5 to 2× was found to be ideal for image capture, and video recording of the desired area of the fundus was commenced. Before filming, the smartphone's screen was cast on a large screen television or monitor, for a larger image and for teaching purposes. Live screen casting while filming also promoted social distancing among the team members, in-line with COVID-19 infection prevention protocols. A closer view of the C-CLAS is shown in **Figure 5**.

Some patients were intolerant to the intensity of the smartphone's flashlight, which was not dimmable. To address this, a double-layer of yellow adhesive paper-tape was placed over the smartphone's flashlight. This significantly reduced the intensity of the flashlight to a tolerable and comfortable level, while still retaining good image quality. However, the adapter can still be easily modified to incorporate either polarizing filters, or neutral density filters to reduce the light intensity. Once the areas of interest were filmed, the video gallery of the smartphone was accessed. The video is played and paused at the desired image, and screenshots were taken. No additional application was needed. Editing was not necessary as the pictures were good enough

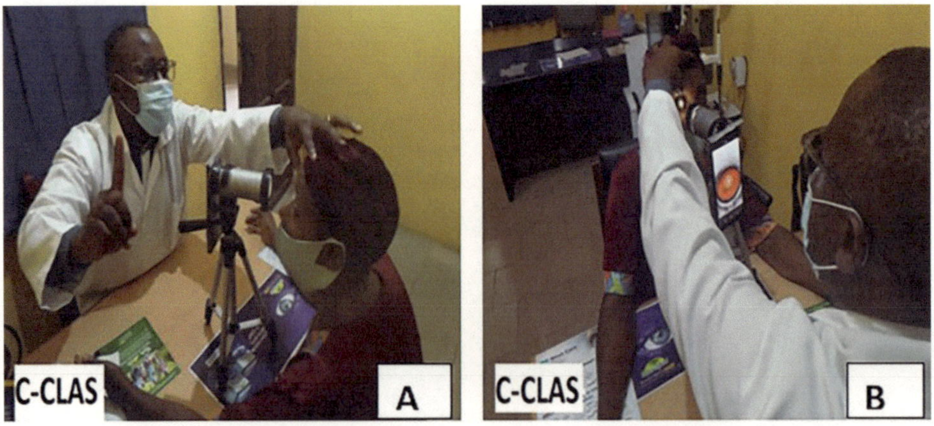

Figure 4.
Hands-free fundus recording with the C-CLAS. A: view from patient's side; B: view from doctor's side.

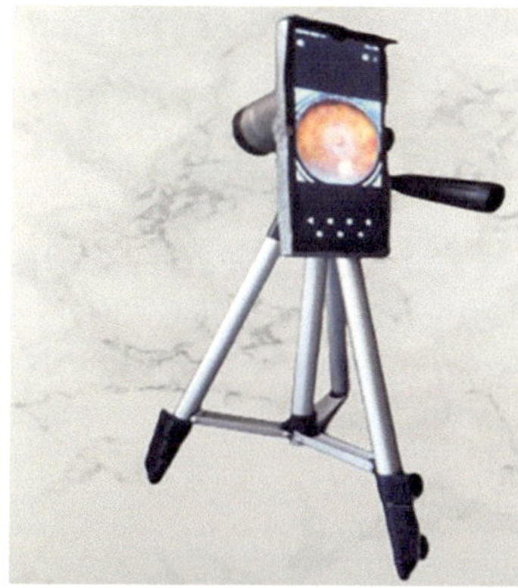

Figure 5.
A closer view of the C-CLAS system.

for interpretation. Lastly, the high-quality images from the patients were ready to be archived in the medical record or used for telemedicine purposes as necessary.

2.2 Results

The C-CLAS was initially validated with randomly selected cohorts and supervised by the Head of Department of the Ophthalmology, FTH Owerri, Nigeria. After validation, the prototype was tested to see how it performed before the commencement of this study. Of the 54 patients used in this study, 39 were co-operative, while 15 were uncooperative (mainly children).

It was observed that the C-CLAS was able to record good quality videos from which quality images were gotten in a variety of normal fundus (**Figure 6A–C**), and pathologic fundus (**Figure 7A–K**) among 39 cooperative patients. Of the 39 cooperative patients 24 patients (44%) had different pathologies, while 15 patients (28%) had normal findings (**Table 1**). It was also observed that the C-CLAS was able to uniquely record hands-free, when coupled to the tripod-stand among cooperative patients.

Another key finding of this study was that the researchers were able to self-acquire images of their own retina without needing assistance from anyone, by simple

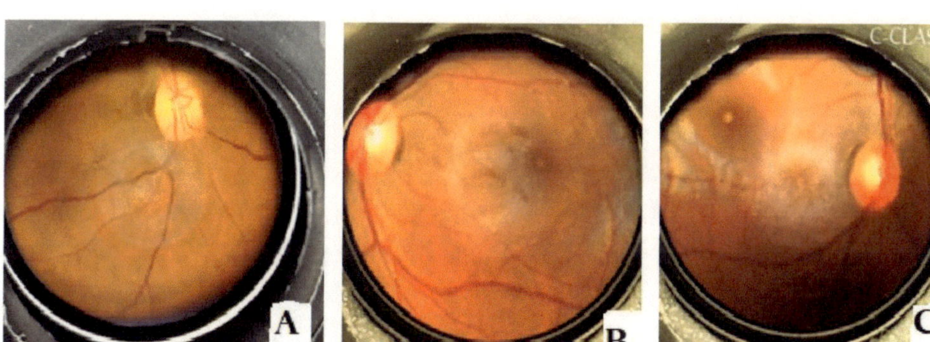

Figure 6.
(A-C) Normal findings.

positioning in front of the adapter, and putting a mirror on the opposite site. The mirror aided and guided the process.

2.3 Discussion

The use of the video camera and flashlight of a smartphone, manually and meticulously-aligned with a condensing lens (usually a +20D lens), has made it possible to capture fundus images at no or low-cost. Recently, this technique of using smartphones in conjunction with a +20D indirect ophthalmoscopy condensing lenses has

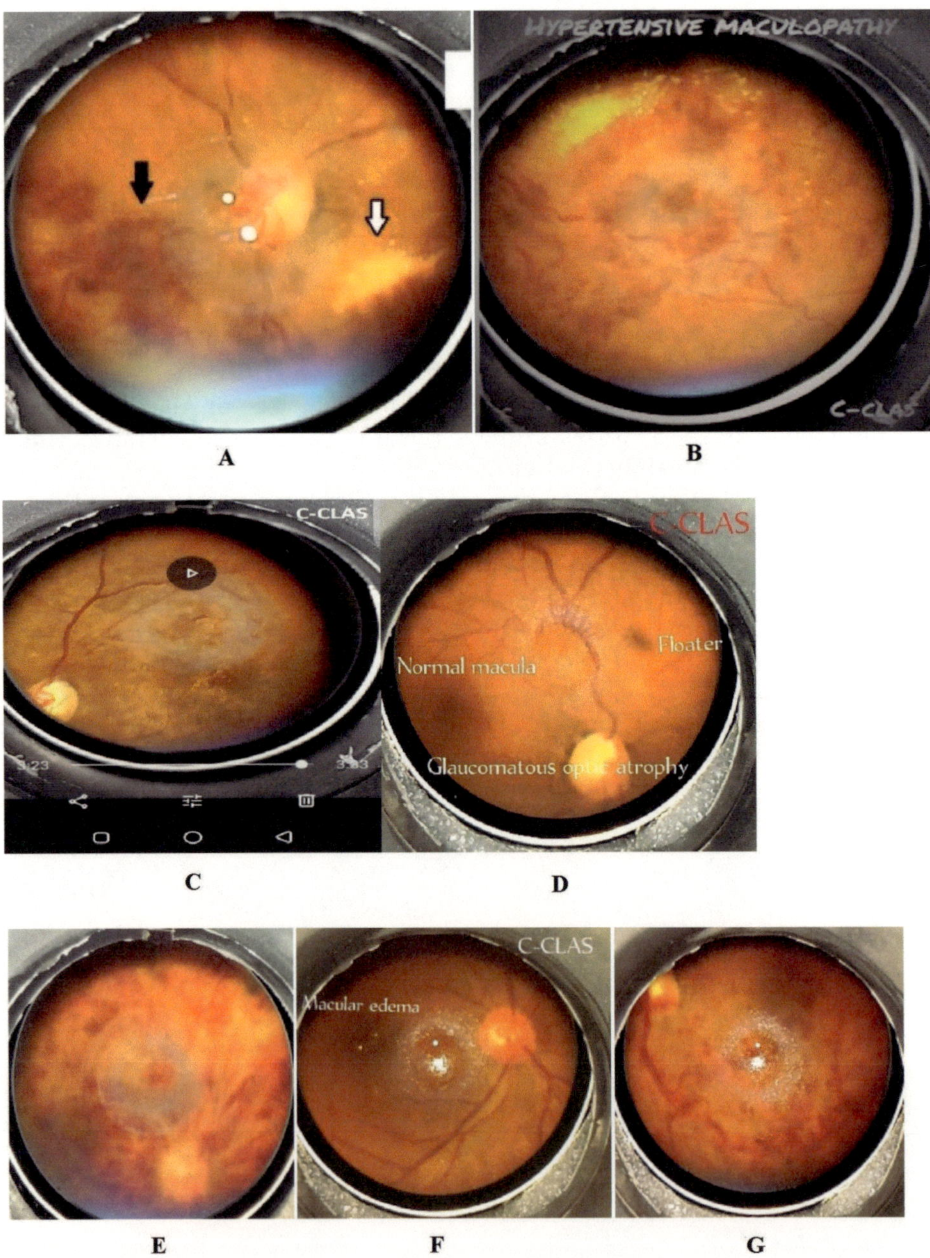

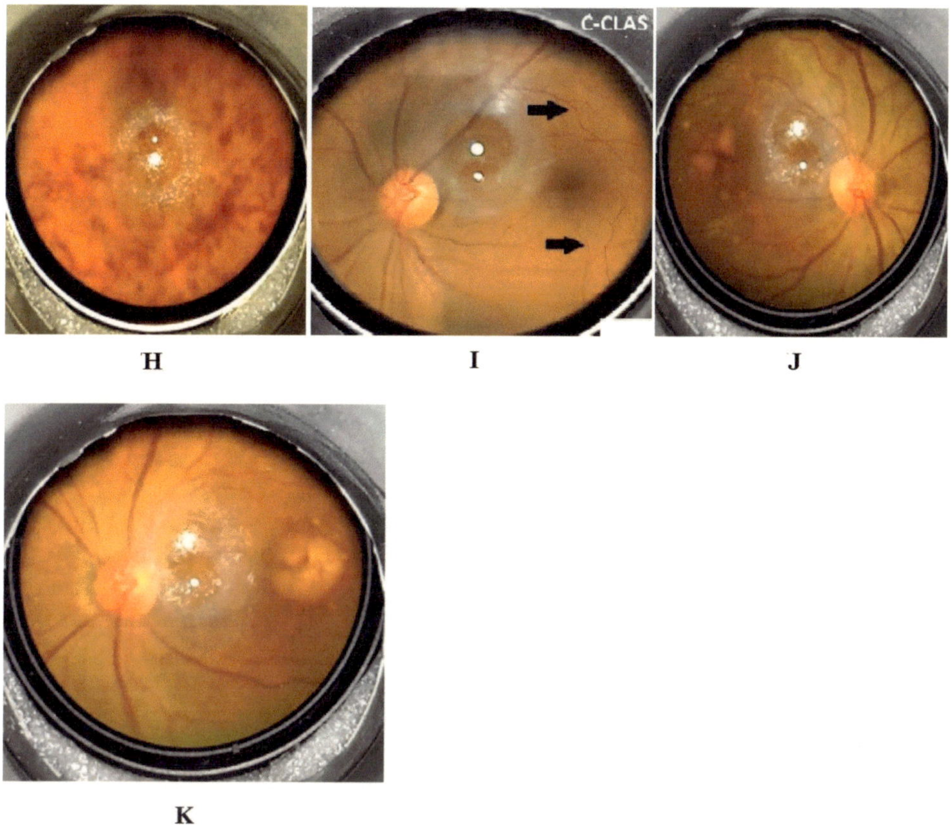

Figure 7.
(A–K) Pathologic fundus conditions; A—hypertensive retinopathy with hemorrhages (black arrow) and exudates (white arrow); B—macular involvement in same eye of the patient in A; C—florid drusen in a patient with dry age-related macular disease (ARMD); D—glaucomatous optic atrophy with vitreous floater; E—central retinal vein occlusion in the right eye of a woman with eclampsia; F—macular edema in left eye of a patient with diabetes mellitus; G—central retinal vein occlusion in right eye of a hypertensive patient; H—macular involvement in the same eye of the patient in G; I—Grade 1 hypertensive retinopathy with generalized arteriolar constriction (black arrows); J—large soft confluent drusen in right eye of a patient with dry ARMD; K—geographic atrophy in the left eye of a patient with dry ARMD (same patient in J).

gained traction among eye care providers— locally and internationally. This approach has become a standard examination technique reported by various ophthalmologists and has evolved over time [6–8, 13–16]. The first reported use of smartphones for fundus image capture was in 2010 by Lord et al. [15]. They demonstrated smartphone fundoscopy use for clinical and educational purposes, including capturing images of the eye, such as external photographs, fundus photographs, and slit-lamp photographs [15]. Since then, newer techniques and modifications have evolved, and resulted in the acquisition of high-quality images but with more expensive ophthalmic imaging devices such as the fundus camera.

Myung et al. [1], reported a three-dimensional printed lens holder attachment for an iPhone smartphone, as an improvement of the older technique by Lord et al. [15]. They reported that high-quality fundus images from normal and pathological findings were captured using their technology. Their adapter made the technique easier to master and reduced image acquisition time (**Figure 5**). Other 3D-printed adapters similar to that of Myung et al. [1], include: The ODocs (**Figure 6**) and Fundus

Variable	Frequency (N = 54)	Percentage (%)
Co-operation		
Co-operative	39	72
Unco-operative	15	28
Fundus findings		
Normal	15	28
Abnormal	24	44

Table 1.
Distribution of participants according to co-operation and fundus findings.

explorer (**Figure 7**). These devices coupled a condensing lens to the smartphone for fundus imaging; and also employed the use of a third-party apps to acquire better images including: ProCamera [Cocologics GmbH] for iOS only; and FiLMiC Pro [FiLMiCInc] for Android and iOS). Third-party apps regulate the flashlight during the procedure for adequate illumination of the fundus. This also helps to improve patients' comfort [17]. The FiLMiC Pro App was found to provide control of the light intensity and independent control of focus and exposure. The light levels of the iPhone 4 were tested by Kim et al. [16] and were found to be well within the safety standards for human eyes and 10 times less than the levels produced by the commercially available Keeler Vantage Plus LED indirect ophthalmoscope [17]. Other

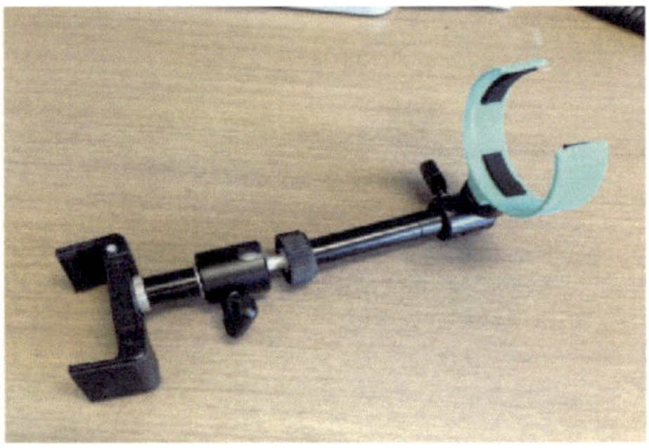

Figure 8.
3D-printed adapter by Myung et al. [1].

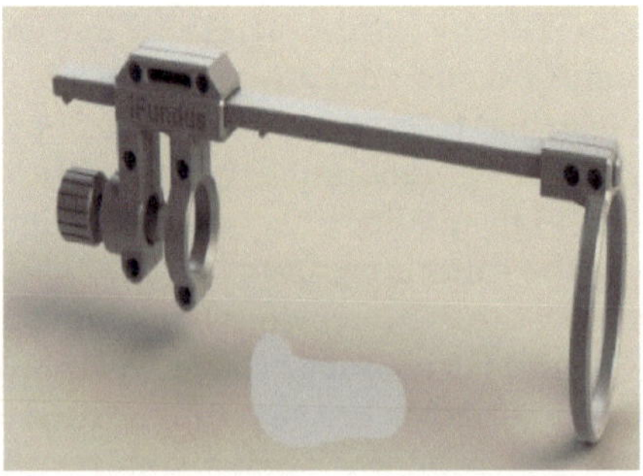

Figure 9.
The ODocs adapter.

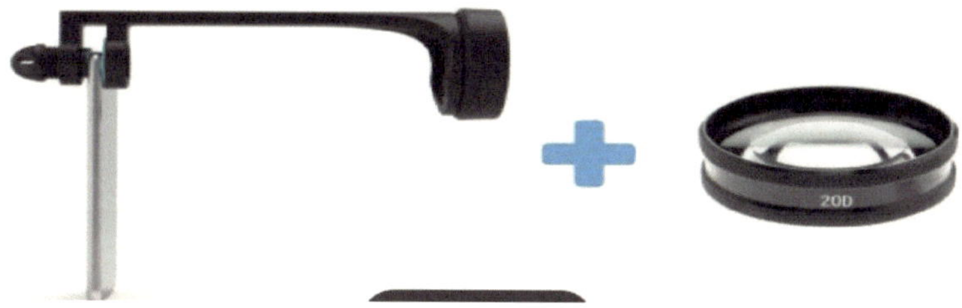

Figure 10.
The fundus explorer adapter.

third-party apps, such as Movie-To-Image or Video-2-Photo enable image extraction from the recorded videos (**Figures 8–10**) [16, 17].

Conceptually, different techniques have been reported for smartphone fundoscopy. Haddock et al. [17] noted the following functionalities and capabilities for smartphone fundoscopy. First, as a fundus camera without hardware attachments (smartphone indirect ophthalmoscopy). This approach was the earliest technique used and relies on the smartphone's native video recording app, flashlight app, and a condensing lens (+20D or +28D) to obtain fundus photographs. Fundus images are captured in the video mode, and still-images subsequently acquired from the videos [17]. Secondly, as an image transfer device, i.e., the image from a conventional fundus camera is transferred to the smartphone and sent to another site. This technique remains useful for imaging of the anterior segment of the eye. However, for fundus imaging, newer techniques have made imageacquisition simpler and of higher quality [18]. Thirdly, as a digital camera attached to an existing fundus-examination device, such as an ophthalmoscope or a slit lamp.

Following this, in January 2013, the United States Food and Drug Administration approved the iExaminer, which is a smartphone adapter system that attaches and aligns an iPhoneto Welch Allyn's PanOptic Ophthalmoscope (**Figure 11**). It uses the iPhone's camera to capture images of the retina and optic nerve and can capture fundus images without dilation of the pupil with 25° field of view [19]. Although good images of the optic nerve can be acquired with this device, yet, fundus imaging was limited by the narrow field of view. Various slit-lamp adapters have also been invented for ocular imaging with smartphones. Most of these adapters simplify attachment of the phone to available slit lamps and align the smartphone camera with the ocular

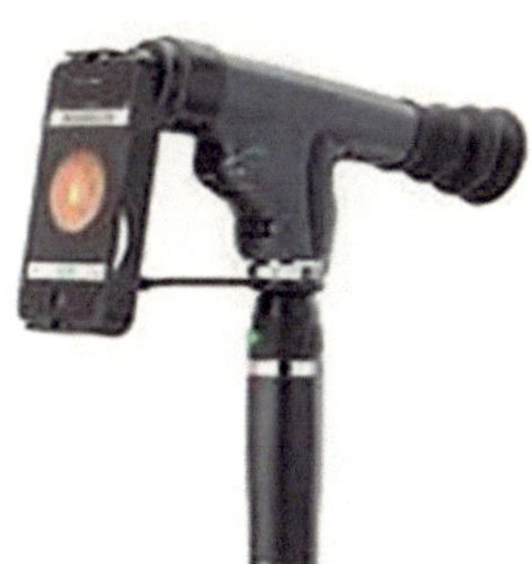

Figure 11.
Panoptic ophthalmoscope.

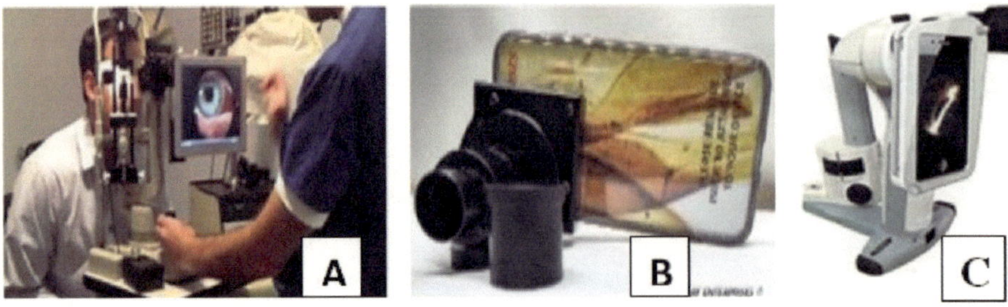

Figure 12.
(A) Eyephotodoc; (B) Zarf's adapter; (C) portable keeler adapter.

of the slit lamp. Most of these adapters are designed for anterior-segment imaging including EyePhotoDoc (Fullerton, CA), Zarf's (Spokane, WA) iPhone and slit-lamp adapters, and the Keeler's (Broomall, PA) Portable Slit Lamp iPhone 4 image adapter (**Figure 12A–C**) [20, 21].

Fourthly, as a fundus camera with hardware attachments that are smartphone specific (often referred to as hardware apps). Giardini et al. [22] documented an adapter for the Samsung Galaxy S III smartphone, which is a low-cost alternative to a direct ophthalmoscope and can capture high-quality fundus images, including the optic nerve [22, 23]. Russo et al. [23] also reported on the use of the D-Eye adapter (Padova, Italy), which magnetically attaches to the smartphone and can captures fundus images of an approximately 20° of field of view (**Figure 13**).

Recent publications have shown that more complex fundus imaging can be accomplished with smartphones. Suto et al. reported on a technique for performing fluorescein fundus angiography using a smartphone [9]. Smartphone fundus angiography could be beneficial for bedridden patients and infants in poor resource settings. Suto et al. were able to capture adequate images for diagnosing certain diseases, although they cautioned that subtle findings might be missed due to the quality of the images with the current technology [9]. In addition, Maamari et al. (described a prototype wide-field lens attachment for the smartphone called Ocular CellScope, which can slide into the phone and capture wide-field images using the phone's built-in camera [12]. Their technique could capture approximately 55° of the fundus in a single image. Additional software could be used to merge multiple images to create a montage.

Technically, the C-CLAS adapter is similar to the adapters invented in previous studies, such as the ODocs, Fundus explorer, and the 3D adapter by Myung et al. [1]. However, compared to the C-CLAS, these adapters are 3D-printed, relatively more

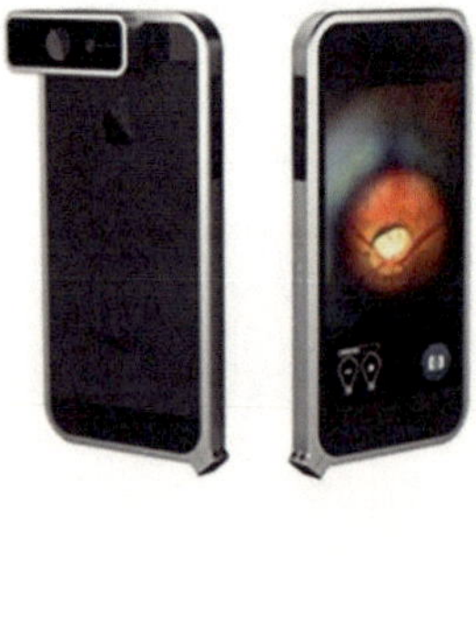

Figure 13.
D-eye smartphone adapter.

expensive and require both hands for stabilization. Functionally, they share the same optical principles with the C-CLAS. Compared to the Welch Allyn Panoptic ophthalmoscope which has a 25° field of view, the C-CLAS presents a 45° field of view with the +20D lens. Both systems are also portable. While the Panoptic ophthalmoscope is more complex, the C-CLAS offers greater working distance and simplicity. Though much more portable than the C-CLAS, D-Eye smartphone adapter has an approximately 20° field of view in a dilated eye, and 5–8° field of view in an un-dilated eye. This is lower, compared to the C-CLAS' 45° field of view.

The Keeler, Eyephotodoc, and Zarf's adapter are slit lamp-based platforms. They require a seated patient, and a stationary slit lamp biomicroscope for fundoscopy, which compromises portability of the entire system. In addition, the adapters are relatively expensive. The Ocular Cellscope comes with a 55° field of view; 10° higher than the C-CLAS, with a mobile application to capture retinal images and record patient information. The C-CLAS offers greater working distance than these adapters, and can be used with the patient seated, standing or supine. The C-CLAS is novel as it rendered the technique of coupling a lens to a smartphone hands-free, with the addition of the tripod; in stark contrast and refinement of the initial method by Lord et al. [15]. In addition, the initial method of placing a +20 D lens over the eye, and manually aligning it with the smartphone's light and camera as reported by Lord et al. [15] and other researchers had a steep learning curve [13, 24]. The 3D-printed lens adapters that directly and reversibly coupled an iPhone to a +20D lens aimed to address this challenge. It was a step forward, but had problems of weight balancing at increased working distances, which made the authors resort to a fixed working distance. Some of the adapters (ODocs, Fundus explorer) require the system to be stabilized with one hand, leaving the other hand to operate the smartphone. However, the design of the C-CLAS addresses this challenge, making it very easy to use with one hand.

Other systemic challenges noted with the technique of smartphone fundoscopy include the high intensity of the smartphone's light which was reported to be discomforting for some patients. Haddock et al. [24] reported an iPhone application that allows control of the native flash as an adjustable light-source. This reduced the light intensity to safe levels for indirect ophthalmoscopy [24, 25]. Myung et al. [1] used neutral density filters or polarizing filters to overcome discomforting high flashlight intensity. However, the C-CLAS used a readily available double-layer of yellow paper-tape, and was able to achieve comparable results in terms of comfort and image quality. Yellow filters are thought to improve patient comfort and are very affordable for resource-poor contexts [26].

The use of third-party apps has improved ease of image acquisition and processing. Haddock et al. [24] described the use of either the App Movie-To-Image or Video-2-Photo that enabled the still-images of interesting areas to be taken from the video clips [24, 25]. These applications were not used with the C-CLAS system as images were acquired directly as screenshots of the paused videos, making it simple and efficient to acquire images. Also, screen casting of the fundoscopy procedure on a large screen by the C-CLAS system made fundoscopy a fun-filled and interesting procedure, enabling patient relatives and eye team members to watch comfortably at spaced-out distance; in compliance to COVID-19 social distancing protocols.

The C-CLAS system addresses challenges related to cost and sophistication documented by other studies. The polyvinylchloride material used in designing the adapter is cheap, lightweight, readily available and does not require 3D printing. This makes it easy for mass production. Despite the incorporation of a tripod-stand, its portability was not compromised, as the tripod-stand can be extended or retracted.

This means that it can be carried to rural settings where fundus cameras are lacking, and images captured can be transmitted with the smartphone for telemedicine purposes. In addition, it requires no special training to use, making it easily usable by other members of the eye team. The simplicity in design of the C-CLAS, and the ability for self-image acquisition with the aid of a mirror means that patients can actually use it for self-screening and monitoring of select fundus pathologies with minimal training; thus making it a veritable tool of prevention in eye care.

While quality of smartphone-captured media cannot compare to higher-end fundus cameras [24, 27]. They are of sufficient quality to be interpreted, and recent studies have validated their potential for screening and telemedicine. Studies showed that smartphone fundoscopy images could be successfully used to screen for glaucoma and diabetic retinopathy. The results were comparable to standard images or examinations, and they could largely expand its utility in the community setting and in isolated rural areas with poor resources [22, 23].

2.4 Challenges

Despite interesting capabilities of the C-CLAS innovation, yet this study noted some limitations. The authors noted the presence of a white translucent ring artifact at the center of the images captured with the +20D Volks lens. However, when another Volks lens was used, the same artifact appeared on the images, though reduced. These artifacts came from the condensing lenses, but did not hamper the ability to interpret the images, as the original video showed different angles and views. We recommend future studies to explore other lens brands that can be used to address this challenge. In addition, high-fidelity artificial intelligence, can be incorporated to translate captured pathological conditions into the local language, for better understanding. The +20D Volk lenses used in this study had about 40°′ field of view, implying that peripheral view of the retina is limited. Future studies should explore the use of wide-field lenses for more peripheral views. The flashlight of the Infinix X650B smartphone is not dimmable, and luxmeter measurements of the flashlight intensity was not taken with a standard luxmeter. However, to ensure patient's safety, and eliminate risk of thermal and photochemical hazard, in-keeping with the limit set by the International Organization for Standardization (ISO 15004-2.2) [28], a double-layer of adhesive yellow paper-tape was placed over the flashlight of the smartphone. This significantly reduced the flashlight intensity, and improved patient's comfort without altering image quality. We recommended that future models of smartphones have adjustable control of the flashlight. A total of 54 patients were used in this study, and based on the projections from the findings, the utility of this hardware will remain unchanged, even when the patient number is called up significantly in the hundreds or thousands. Therefore, future studies can explore this factor. Lastly, the C-CLAS is not yet commercially available, however, efforts are in top gear towards making it available and affordable.

2.5 Conclusion

The C-CLAS system introduced another dimension to smartphone fundoscopy with the coupling of a tripod-stand to a smartphone adapter, and wireless screencasting of the fundoscopy procedure, while retaining simplicity. This innovation can leverage on the expanding mobile phone networks to advance digital health in ophthalmology among resource-poor settings. African governments should identify turn-around investment strategies for adopting and implementing simple mHealth

DOI: http://dx.doi.org/10.5772/intechopen.114207

innovations to improve population health, strengthen service delivery and advance ophthalmic health outcomes. Moving forward, the authors are hopeful that as the smartphone camera technology continues to evolve, better images with better resolution will be obtained.

Acknowledgements

We acknowledge the support from the staff and management of the Federal University Teaching Hospital, Owerri, Nigeria for their support during the Postgraduate training period. This research was completed during the Postgraduate training year as part of the requirements for completing the Medical Postgraduate Training in Nigeria. We also acknowledge the contributions and support from Cynthia Alozie during the Training year and in getting this manuscript ready. We are solely responsible for the views expressed in this manuscript, as it does not reflect the views and policies of authors' affiliated institutions.

Funding

Not applicable.

Competing interests

The authors declare that they have no competing interests.

Disclosure

The authors have completed the Unified Competing Interest form at www.icmje.org/coi_disclosure.pdf and have nothing to declare.

Author details

Alozie Emeonye[1], Florence Nkwogu[2], Joseph Okeibunor[3] and Sunny Ibeneme[4*]

1 Ophthalmology Department, Federal Teaching Hospital, Owerri, Nigeria

2 Ophthalmology Unit, Department of Surgery, College of Medicine, Imo State University, Nigeria

3 World Health Organization—African Regional Office, Brazzaville, Congo

4 UNICEF East Asia Pacific Regional Office, Bangkok, Thailand

*Address all correspondence to: sibeneme@unicef.org

References

[1] Myung D, Jais A, He L, Blumenkranz M, Chang RT. 3D printed smartphone indirect lens adapter for rapid, high quality retinal imaging. Journal MTM. 2014;**3**(1):9-15. DOI: 10.7309/jmtm.3.1.3

[2] Monjur M, Hoque IT, Hashem T, Rakib MA, Kim JE, Ahamed SI. Smartphone based fundus camera for the diagnosis of retinal diseases. Smart Health. 2021;**19**:100177

[3] World Health Organization. Health Systems in Africa; Community Perceptions and Perspectives - The Report of a Multi-Country Study. Brazzaville, Congo; 2012

[4] Ibeneme S, Karamagi H, Muneene D, Goswami K, Chisaka N, Okeibunor J. Strengthening health systems using innovative digital health Technologies in Africa. Frontiers in Digital Health. 2022;**4**:854339. DOI: 10.3389/fdgth.2022.854339

[5] World Health Organization. Regional Office for Africa. The Africa Health Transformation Programme 2015-2020: A Vision for Universal Health Coverage. World Health Organization. Brazzaville, Congo: Regional Office for Africa; 2015. Available from: https://apps.who.int/iris/handle/10665/206535

[6] World Health Statistics 2015. Geneva: World Health Organization; 2015

[7] Ibeneme S, Revere L, Hwang L, Rajan S, Okeibunor J, Muneene D, et al. Impact of information and communication technology diffusion on HIV and tuberculosis health outcomes among African health systems. Informatics. 2020;**7**(2):11. DOI: 10.3390/informatics7020011

[8] Ademola-Popoola DS, Olatunji VA. Retinal imaging with smartphone. Nigerian Journal of Clinical Practice. 2017;**20**:341-345

[9] Suto S, Hiraoka T, Okamoto Y, Okamoto F, Oshika T. Photography of anterior eye segment and fundus with smartphone. Nippon Ganka Gakkai Zasshi. 2014;**118**(1):7-14

[10] Stryjewski T, Mukai S. The retina selfie: A techniques video demonstrating smartphone ophthalmoscopy. Digital Journal of Ophthalmology. 2022;**22**(4). [Accessed: March 5, 2024]. Available from: https://djo.harvard.edu/index.php/djo/article/view/342

[11] Nazari Khanamiri H, Nakatsuka A, El-Annan J. Smartphone fundus photography. Journal of Visualized Experiments. 2017;**125**:55958

[12] Maamari RN, Keenan JD, Fletcher DA, Margolis TP. A mobile phone-based retinal camera for portable wide field imaging. The British Journal of Ophthalmology. 2014;**98**(4):438-441

[13] Oluleye TS. Mobile phones for fundus photography in Ibadan, sub-Sahara Africa. Advances in Ophthalmology & Visual System. 2018;**1**(4):0020. DOI: 1.15406/aovs.2014.01.00020

[14] Oluleye TS, Rotimi-Samuel A, Akinshola FB, Adefule-Ositelu OA, Onakoya OA, Aribaba OT, et al. Mobile phone fundoscopy screening for retinal manifestation of systemic disease in poor resource settings of sub-Sahara Africa. EC. Ophthalmology. 2015;**2**(4):131-136

[15] Lord RK, Shah VA, San Filippo AN, Krishna R. Novel uses of smartphones in ophthalmology. Ophthalmology. 2010;**117**(6):1274.e3

[16] Kim DY, Delori F, Mukai S. Smartphone photography safety.

Ophthalmology. 2012;**119**(10): 2200-2201

[17] Haddock LJ, Qian C. Smartphone Technology for Fundus Photography. Greater portability could mean greater versatility. Retinal Physician. 2015;**12**:51, 54-56, 58

[18] Kumar S, Wang EH, Pokabla MJ, Noecker RJ. Teleophthalmology assessment of diabetic retinopathy fundus images: Smartphone versus standard office computer workstation. Telemedicine Journal and E-Health. 2012;**18**:158-162

[19] WelchAllyn. iExaminer Eye Imaging for your iPhone. Available from: http://www.welchallyn.com/en/microsites/iexaminer.html [Accessed: Month 25, 2022]

[20] EyeWiki. Smartphone Fundoscopy - How to Use Smartphone to Take Fundus Photographs. Available from: http://eyewiki.org/Smartphone Fundoscopy - How to Use Smartphone to Take Fundus Photographs - EyeWiki [Accessed: October 31, 2022]

[21] Lee WW. Slit lamp adapters turn smartphones into clinical cameras. Ophthalmology Web. Available from: http://www.ophthalmologyweb.com/Featured-Articles/136817-Slit-Lamp-Adapters-turn-Smartphones-into-Clinical-Cameras/ [Accessed: January 31, 2022]

[22] Giardini ME, Livingstone IA, Jordan S, et al. A smartphone-based ophthalmoscope. Conference of the IEEE Engineering in Medicine and Biology Society. 2014;**2014**:2177-2180

[23] Russo A, Morescalchi F, Costagliola C, Delcassi L, Semeraro F. Comparison of smartphone ophthalmoscopy with slit-lamp biomicroscopy for grading diabetic retinopathy. American Journal of Ophthalmology. 2015;**159**:360-364

[24] Haddock LJ, Kim DY, Mukai S. Simple, inexpensive technique for high-quality smartphone fundus photography in human and animal eyes. Journal of Ophthalmology. 2013;**2013**:518479

[25] Chhablani J, Kaja S, Shah VA. Smartphones in ophthalmology. Indian Journal of Ophthalmology. 2012;**60**(2):127

[26] Kanski JJ, Bowling B. Clinical Ophthalmology – A Systematic Approach. 8th ed. Oxford: Butterworth Heinmann; 2016. p. 685

[27] Darma S, Zantvoord F, Verbraak FD. The quality and usability of smartphone and hand-held fundus photography, compared to standard fundus photography. Acta Ophthalmologica. 2015;**93**(4):e310-e311

[28] International Standard. ISO, 15004-2.2, Ophthalmic Instruments, Light Hazard Protection. In: International Standards Organization (ISO). Geneva, Switzerland; 2007

Chapter 11

Connecting Smiles: Bridging Gaps in Oral Health Access with Teledentistry

Radhika Thakkar, Shivani Karre, Abhishek Jahagirdar, Sunaina Swatantramath, Vikranth Ravipati, Digvijaysinh Parmar and Jitesh V. Pimpale

Abstract

This chapter "Bridging Gaps in Oral Health Access with Teledentistry" delves into the ways that teledentistry may be used to address oral health disparities amongst vulnerable populations, including elderly residents of nursing homes and patients with special needs. Teledentistry represents a revolutionary change with its integration of digital imaging, remote consultations, and advanced technology particularly for patients with complex medical history. The chapter also highlights examples of implementation of teledentistry at the global level. Furthermore, the chapter outlines the inevitable challenges, such as technology constraints, regulatory impediments, acceptability concerns, and geographic obstacles. Strategies for overcoming these challenges are put forth, emphasising teamwork, with a focus on enhanced regulatory structures and continuing training for dental practitioners to implement new technology. In order to satisfy the specific needs of these vulnerable populations, customised teledentistry focused on patient-centric approach is crucial. Looking ahead, the chapter describes future direction for growth, importance of collaborative approach, possible developments in technology and emphasises how important it is to carry out further research and work together. This chapter functions as a comprehensive guide, in reducing disparities in oral health amongst the underprivileged with the inclusion of teledentistry.

Keywords: teledentistry, special needs, oral health, telehealth, virtual consultation

1. Introduction

Teledentistry is a ray of hope that improves patient accessibility and comfort whilst also bridging regional divides. Teledentistry facilitates real-time contact between dental professionals and patients resulting in timely interventions and personalised care. With advancements in technology, telehealth services have strengthened patient accessibility and comfort whilst also bridging regional divides [1, 2]. It includes a broad range of services that may be provided virtually, such as remote consultation, evaluation of oral health lesions which does not require radiograph, primary diagnosis based on existing health records, treatment planning, and follow-up visits. All of these can be done without the requirement for in-person presence. This chapter aims to highlight the significant influence of teledentistry in addressing inequities in oral health by legislative progress, patient-centric care, collaborative approach, and raised consciousness in order to bridge the gap in oral health access. By exploring the history, applications, and challenges involved in the integration of digital tools and platforms, this chapter seeks to demonstrate the tremendous impact it has on mitigating disparities in oral health [3–5].

2. Teledentistry: a solution for the underserved population

Teledentistry fills critical gaps in oral healthcare access for marginalised groups, especially the elderly in nursing homes and people with special needs (**Figure 1**). Traditional dental appointments are sometimes hampered for these disadvantaged populations by obstacles like restricted mobility, remote location, and inadequate financial resources. By removing these obstacles and providing remote consultations, diagnostics, and customised care plans, teledentistry emerges as a lifeline, which contributes to the patients' overall well-being [6–8].

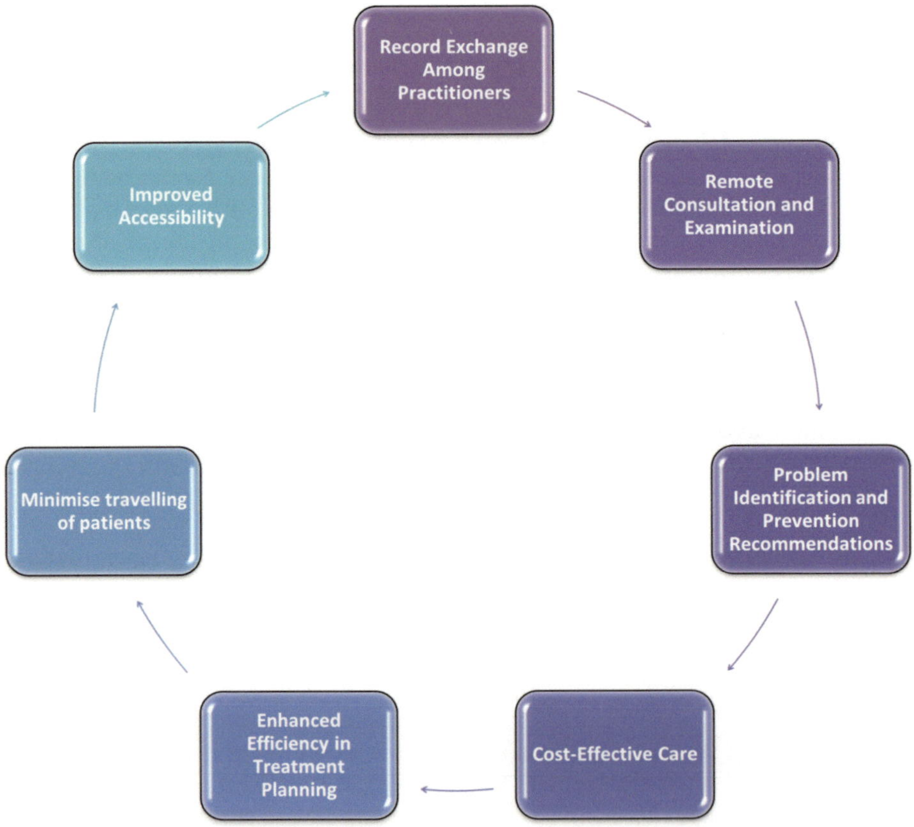

Figure 1.
Teledentistry: A solution for the underserved population.

2.1 Unique challenges facing impoverished populations in dental health

Oral health is a complex issue for underserved groups, made worse by things like financial hardships or restricted access to care owing to remote locations (**Figure 2**). Oral health problems are made worse for the elderly living in nursing homes and for those with special needs who frequently struggle with limited mobility, communication difficulties, and complicated medical conditions. These difficulties are further exacerbated by a lack of knowledge and instruction, which raises the prevalence of untreated oral issues. To close the gap and guarantee equitable oral healthcare delivery, these disadvantaged groups must overcome significant barriers to preventative and restorative dental services. One such alternative is teledentistry [9].

Teledentistry serves as an accessible platform which changes the way dental care is delivered for everyone, irrespective of geography or physical constraints aiming to achieve equitable oral health [10, 11].

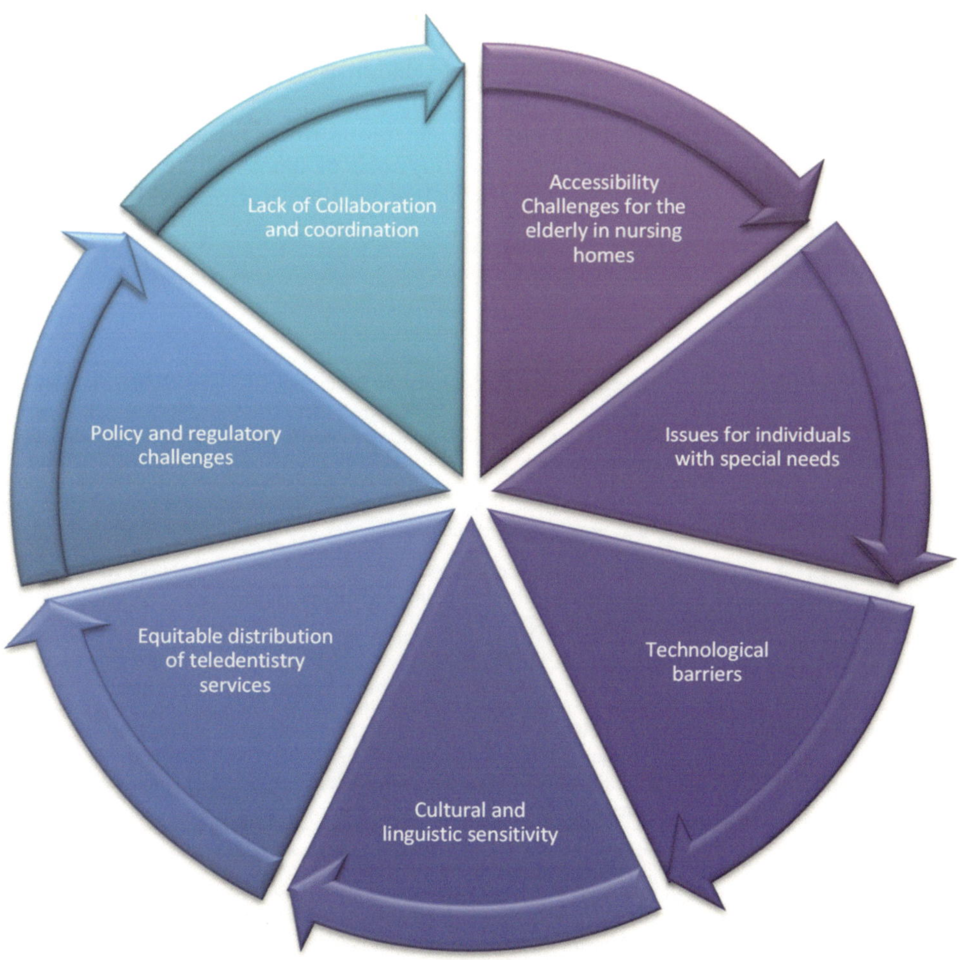

Figure 2.
Unique challenges facing impoverished populations in dental health.

3. Advancements in teledentistry technology

Remote consultations are made possible via teledentistry, which facilitates easy contact between dental specialists and patients (**Table 1**). Dental professionals do virtual examinations, address issues, and provide preliminary diagnosis via video conferencing and secure platforms. This strategy makes it easier for underprivileged populations—particularly those with restricted mobility or geographic restrictions—to quickly obtain professional counsel [12]. It lowers obstacles to care and improves early interventions for oral health concerns by enabling patients to get advice without needing to make in-person visits [13, 14].

High-resolution dental pictures are captured and sent for evaluation and diagnosis in teledentistry using digital imaging. With the use of these technologies, dental diseases may be evaluated remotely, which helps with treatment planning and progress tracking. With the use of telemonitoring equipment, continuous treatment may be provided remotely in real time by assessing indications of oral health. This innovation is especially helpful for vulnerable populations since it ensures fast treatment plan modifications and constant monitoring without requiring numerous in-person visits [15–17].

Modern technologies like 3D printing, intraoral scanners, and artificial intelligence are introduced by the development of teledentistry. These developments improve tailored care, accuracy of diagnosis, and precision of therapy [18]. Whilst 3D printing makes it easier to create customised dental items remotely, AI systems assist in the analysis of photographs for the diagnosis of disease. The precision of treatment planning and remote consultations has been revolutionised by intraoral scanners, which allow for exact digital impressions [19]. A new age in teledentistry

Advancements in Teledentistry Technology	Description
Development of ICT	Information and Communication Technology (ICT) is evolving continuously. Connects patients, dentists, and specialists globally, facilitating exchanges for health information and consultation directly from patients' homes, reducing healthcare costs.
Types of Interaction	Two main types: "Store-and-forward" (pre-recorded/asynchronous) and "real-time" (synchronous).
Store-and-Forward	Clinical information, including images, stored in a virtual place for diagnostic reference, treatment planning, and patient counselling.
Real-Time Methods	Consultation through video calling or conferencing for quick review of clinical information, medical history, radiographic images, and laboratory findings. Allows real-time interaction and understanding between parties.
3D printing, intraoral scanners, and artificial intelligence (AI)	These advancements enhance tailored care, accuracy of diagnosis, and precision of therapy. Revolutionises remote oral healthcare with the combination of 3D printing, AI image analysis, and intraoral scanners, promising more capabilities and better results.
Low-Bandwidth Internet	Suitable for store-and-forward systems, making remote exchanges and interactions feasible.
Mobile Communication Devices	Mobile devices, especially cell phones and tablets, gaining attention in public health education and promotion.

Table 1.
Advancements in Teledentistry technology.

is being ushered in by the combination of these cutting-edge technologies, one that promises more capabilities and better results in the provision of remote oral healthcare [20, 21].

4. Practical implications of teledentistry

When taken as a whole, these case studies highlight how teledentistry improves oral health results (**Figure 3**). They show a significant decline in untreated dental problems, a reduction in the incidence of oral illnesses, and an improvement in participants' general oral hygiene. Additionally, they show improved patient satisfaction, emphasising the practicality and simplicity of the use of remote dental services. The use of teledentistry not only helps with urgent dental requirements, but also promotes preventative treatment, which improves oral health and general well-being [22, 23]. Initiatives including teledentistry for people with special needs and in nursing homes have shown to be very effective in improving oral healthcare results and accessibility [24].

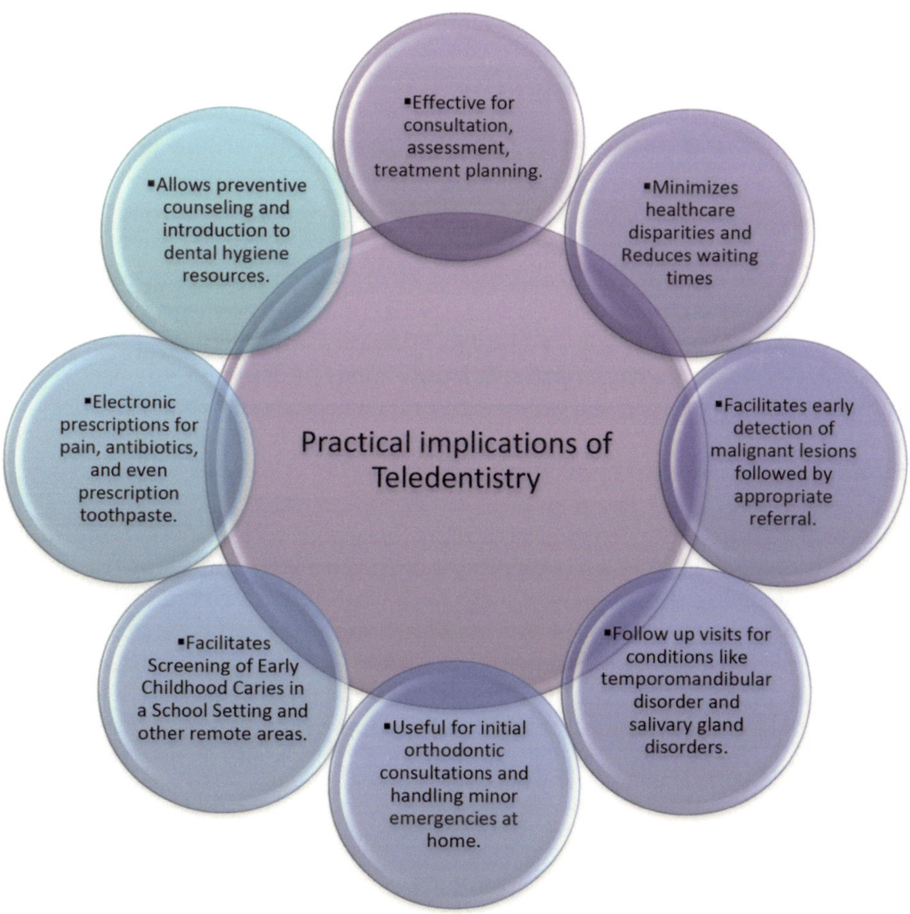

Figure 3.
Practical implications of teledentistry.

4.1 Customising teledentistry for elderly patients

The cognitive, physical, and technical constraints of older patients must be taken into account whilst designing teledentistry services to meet their needs. User-friendly platforms, aided technologies, and simplified interfaces address possible issues with dexterity or inexperience with digital instruments. During remote consultations, older patients can feel empowered and at ease by emphasising clear communication, patience, and support throughout the virtual treatment process. This encourages patients to take an active role in their oral healthcare [23–25].

4.2 Adapting services for people with special needs

Teledentistry needs to address the specific needs of those who are disabled. This entails using staff members who have been educated to handle a variety of demands, as well as adaptable technology and augmentative communication tools. During virtual consultations, tailored techniques take into account deficits related to sensory processing, cognition, or physical functioning, promoting pleasant and productive encounters. Incorporating diverse communication styles and offering substitute means of exchanging information guarantees inclusiveness and promotes a favourable encounter for patients with exceptional requirements [26].

4.3 Ensuring accessibility and inclusivity

A key component of patient-centred teledentistry is accessibility. Incorporating functionality like text-to-speech, captioning, and language translation services guarantees inclusion for a variety of language- and hearing-impaired groups. Moreover, accessibility is improved by guaranteeing compatibility with assistive technology. Inclusivity is further promoted by addressing socioeconomic differences by providing low-bandwidth alternatives or collaborating with community centres for technological access. By incorporating universal design principles into the development of teledentistry platforms, usability for patients from a range of demographic backgrounds is ensured, promoting fair access to superior oral healthcare services [27–29].

4.4 Examples of teledentistry programmes in foreign countries

Case studies highlight the transforming influence of teledentistry programmes conducted globally (**Table 2**). These programmes give senior citizens full dental treatment by utilising computerised diagnostics and remote consultations. These programmes address obstacles such as restricted mobility and transportation issues by forming relationships between dental practitioners and care institutions. By providing dental services to people directly, these programmes help to improve oral health outcomes for this vulnerable population by facilitating prompt treatments, preventative care, and early interventions specifically during the COVID pandemic [27, 28].

5. Barriers to teledentistry implementation

A number of obstacles impede the extensive acceptance and application of teledentistry, including technological, acceptance, and regulatory issues.

Country	Policies and Regulations	Projects
Bosnia and Herzegovina	Telemedicine introduced in the Law on Healthcare of the Republic of Srpska. No national policies/strategies for telemedicine, teledentistry, or E- health.	Electronic health record and E- prescription used. One platform for online consultations with healthcare professionals.
Finland	National Patient Data Repository (Kanta) for archiving electronic patient data. Municipal health centres use six different Health Information Systems (HIS).	HIS utilised by oral healthcare sector. Teledentistry programs established during the COVID-19 pandemic.
France	French law defines telemedicine as a remote medical activity using ICT. - Dentists allowed to practice teledentistry under the law.	e-DENT project in Montpellier. - Teledentistry programs: asynchronous dental consultation, telepathology, synchronous dental consultations, mobile applications for monitoring orthodontic procedures.
Italy	National Recovery and Resilience Plan (NRRP) with a telemedicine program. - No laws regulating teledentistry currently.	Teledentistry facilitated remote management of dental emergencies during the COVID-19 pandemic.
United Kingdom	Teledentistry occasionally used before 2020, mostly for orthodontic consultations.	Nationwide Attend Anywhere service introduced for video consultations. Teledentistry used for virtual training of dental students. - Positive feedback from patients, dentists, and dental students.

Table 2.
Examples of Teledentistry Programmes in foreign countries.

5.1 Regulatory challenges and compliance

Regulatory obstacles for teledentistry include those related to licensure, privacy, and telehealth rules, which differ by location. The scalability of services is impacted by the frequent complexity of interstate practice caused by compliance with disparate state requirements [30].

5.2 Technological limitations

It is difficult to provide high-quality technological infrastructure in underserved or distant locations when there is a lack of sufficient digital resources or reliable internet access. Its application is further constrained by the lack of interoperability with current dental software and the availability of advanced diagnostic equipment, requiring significant investments in technological improvements [21].

5.3 Patient and provider acceptance

Both patients and dental professionals are resistant to the use of teledentistry. Patients who prefer in-person visits to online treatment may display scepticism owing to worries over the quality of virtual care. At the same time, dentists may be reluctant to accept teledentistry because they believe that it will be difficult to do thorough examinations or provide practical treatments from a distance [31].

5.4 Insurance and reimbursement issues

The lack of uniformity in compensation schemes and coverage gaps for virtual consultations makes teledentistry practices financially unviable. Encouraging the widespread adoption and sustainability of teledentistry projects requires addressing these payment gaps and pushing for fair compensation for remote dental treatments [31, 32].

6. Teledentistry in the United States

In order to effectively overcome teledentistry challenges, a variety of tactics and best practices including community participation, legislative advocacy, education, and teamwork are needed (**Table 3**). This table highlights implications of teledentistry in the USA [21, 30–33].

7. Future trends and opportunities

Future directions for research, service extension, and cooperative projects are presented by anticipated developments and possibilities in teledentistry, which will influence the provision of remote oral healthcare.

7.1 Collaborative approaches to teledentistry implementation

It is essential to promote joint ventures between dental practitioners, medical facilities, and technological specialists. Working with legislators to develop uniform

CDT codes	Platforms	Teledentistry initiatives
These codes are used in conjunction with another code, typically an exam • D9995 synchronous; real-time encounter. • D9996 asynchronous; information stored and forwarded to dentist for subsequent review.	• Sesame • Live Dentist • DentalChat • Denteractive • Virtudent, Inc. • Aspen Dental • Toothpic • The TeleDentists • Dentulu • Smile Virtual • Alpha Dental Excellence	• **Colorado** Building Equity Through Telehealth Reach (BETTR). University of Colorado School of Dental Medicine
		• **California** The Virtual Dental Home System of Care (VDH). Pacific Center for Special Care at the University of the Pacific, Arthur A. Dugoni School of Dentistry (Pacific)
		• **New York** Eastman Institute for Oral Health at the University of Rochester
		• **Arizona** Text2Floss and PH2OH Apps. Arizona School of Dental and Oral Health.
		• **Alaska** Dental Health Aid Therapist (DHAT) System.

Table 3.
Teledentistry in United States.

standards for privacy laws, telehealth reimbursement, and licencing promotes uniformity and clarity between jurisdictions. In addition, resolving legal obstacles, advancing telemedicine-friendly legislation, and compensation for services are also important areas of advocacy work. Collaboration allows for the sharing of infrastructure, knowledge, and resources, which promotes creative thinking. Opportunities for synergy are revealed through collaboration amongst stakeholders, including lawmakers, healthcare institutions, dentistry experts, and tech developers [34].

7.2 Community engagement and outreach

Engagement with the community and outreach programmes are essential to promoting acceptability and use of teledentistry. Outreach programmes may be more effectively tailored to cater to the requirements, languages, and cultural sensitivities of a varied community. Forming alliances with neighbourhood groups bolsters outreach initiatives and encourages participation and ownership in the teledentistry-based promotion of oral health [34, 35].

7.3 Training and education for dental professionals

In-depth training courses and ongoing education are essential for giving dental practitioners the skills they need to implement teledentistry. Improvements in machine learning algorithms, remote imaging methods, and artificial intelligence hold the potential to improve precision [35].

8. Conclusion

With all the technical advancements in teledentistry, dentists may ultimately connect to online dental health clinics, ushering in a completely new age in dentistry. Traditional dental appointments are sometimes hampered for these disadvantaged populations by obstacles like restricted mobility, remote location, and inadequate financial resources. However, there are a number of challenges associated with legal frameworks including licensure, remuneration, malpractice liability, patient privacy, jurisdiction, electronic commerce, and fiscal and taxation guidelines, which necessitate further improvements in order to ensure seamless implementation. Validating the many facets of teledentistry applications will require larger-scale research with more participants. In order to create a future where everyone, regardless of their circumstances, has access to oral health, teledentistry must be progressively integrated into the healthcare system. On a broader level, Teledentistry is more than just a technology; it is a tool that empowers communities.

Author details

Radhika Thakkar[1*], Shivani Karre[2], Abhishek Jahagirdar[3], Sunaina Swatantramath[4], Vikranth Ravipati[5], Digvijaysinh Parmar[6] and Jitesh V. Pimpale[7]

1 Graduate Medical Education (GME) Residency Program, Eastman Institute for Oral Health, University of Rochester, NY, USA

2 Division of General Dentistry, Loma Linda University School of Dentistry, CA, USA

3 Brownfield Dental, Lubbock, Texas, USA

4 Oral Medicine and Maxillofacial Radiology, Sinhgad Dental College, Pune, India

5 Orofacial Pain Residency Program, Eastman Institute for Oral Health, University of Rochester, NY, USA

6 Dental Public Health (DPH) Residency Program, University of California, San Francisco, CA, USA

7 Community Health Systems, Beloit, Wisconsin, USA

*Address all correspondence to: radhika_thakkar@urmc.rochester.edu

References

[1] Khan SA, Omar H. Teledentistry in practice: Literature review. Telemedicine e-Health [Internet]. 2013;**19**:565-567. DOI: 10.1089/tmj.2012.0200

[2] Mariño R, Ghanim A. Teledentistry: A systematic review of the literature. Journal of Telemedicine and Telecare. 2013;**19**:179-183

[3] Daniel SJ, Wu L, Kumar S. Teledentistry: A systematic review of clinical outcomes, utilization and costs. The Journal of Dental Hygiene [Internet]. 2013;**87**(6):345-352. Available from: https://api.semanticscholar.org/CorpusID:41246006

[4] Talla PK, Bussières A, Giraudeau N, Komarova S, Basiren Q, Bergeron F, et al. Teledentistry for improving access to, and quality of oral health care: A protocol for an overview of systematic reviews and meta-analyses. PLoS One. 2024;**19**:1-11

[5] Daniel SJ, Kumar S. Teledentistry: A key component in access to care. Journal of Evidence-Based Dental Practice [Internet]. 2014;**14**:201-208. Available from: https://www.sciencedirect.com/science/article/pii/S1532338214000517

[6] Park JH, Rogowski L, Kim JH, Al Shami S, Howell SEI. Teledentistry platforms for orthodontics. The Journal of Clinical Pediatric Dentistry. 2021;**45**:48-53

[7] Howell SEI, Fukuoka B. Teledentistry for patient-centered screening and assessment. Dental Clinic [Internet]. 2022;**66**:195-208. DOI: 10.1016/j.cden.2022.01.002

[8] Fornaini C, Rocca J-P. Relevance of teledentistry: Brief report and future perspectives. Frontiers in Dental Medicine [Internet]. 2022;**19**:25. Available from: https://fid.tums.ac.ir/index.php/fid/article/view/4370

[9] Minervini G, Russo D, Herford AS, Gorassini F, Meto A, D'Amico C, et al. Teledentistry in the management of patients with dental and temporomandibular disorders. BioMed Research International. 2022;**2022**:7091153

[10] Park JH, Kim JH, Rogowski L, Al Shami S, Howell SEI. Implementation of teledentistry for orthodontic practices. Journal of the World Federation of Orthodontists. 2021;**10**:9-13

[11] Sharma H, Suprabha BS, Rao A. Teledentistry and its applications in paediatric dentistry: A literature review. Pediatric Dental Journal. 2021;**31**:203-215

[12] Kirkwood B. Development of military teledentistry. Medical Journal (Fort Sam Houston, Tex). 2021;**2**:33-39

[13] Islam MRR, Islam R, Ferdous S, Watanabe C, Yamauti M, Alam MK, et al. Teledentistry as an effective tool for the communication improvement between dentists and patients: An overview. Healthcare (Basel, Switzerland). 2022;**10**:1586

[14] Batra P, Tagra H, Katyal S. Artificial intelligence in teledentistry. Discoveries (Craiova, Rom). 2022;**10**:153

[15] Estai M, Kanagasingam Y, Tennant M, Bunt S. A systematic review of the research evidence for the benefits of teledentistry. Journal of Telemedicine and Telecare [Internet]. 2017;**24**:147-156. DOI: 10.1177/1357633X16689433

[16] Ghai S. Teledentistry during COVID-19 pandemic. Diabetes and Metabolic Syndrome: Clinical Research and Reviews. 2020;**14**:933-935

[17] Menhadji P, Oberai K. Teledentistry safeguards. British Dental Journal England. 2020;**229**:635-636

[18] Kumar G, Rehman F, Al-Muzian L, Farsi D, Hiremath S. Global scenario of teledentistry during COVID-19 pandemic: An insight. International Journal of Clinical Pediatric Dentistry. 2021;**14**:426-429

[19] Ben-Omran MO, Livinski AA, Kopycka-Kedzierawski DT, Boroumand S, Williams D, Weatherspoon DJ, et al. The use of teledentistry in facilitating oral health for older adults: A scoping review. Journal of the American Dental Association (1939). 2021;**152**:998-1011.e17

[20] Deshpande S, Patil D, Dhokar A, Bhanushali P, Katge F. Teledentistry: A boon amidst COVID-19 lockdown-A narrative review. International Journal of Telemedicine and Applications. 2021;**2021**:8859746

[21] Hung M, Lipsky MS, Phuatrakoon TN, Nguyen M, Licari FW, Unni EJ. Teledentistry implementation during the COVID-19 pandemic: Scoping review. Interactive Journal of Medical Research. 2022;**11**:e39955

[22] Singhal S, Mohapatra S, Quiñonez C. Reviewing teledentistry usage in Canada during COVID-19 to determine possible future opportunities. International Journal of Environmental Research and Public Health. 2021;**19**:31

[23] Gryglewska B, Perera I, Klimek E, Fedyk-łukasik M, Piotrowicz K, Mocanu I, et al. Teledentistry and oral health in older adults — Aspects for implementation of the "patient centric solution for smart and sustainable healthcare (ACESO)" project. Folia Medica Cracoviensia. 2022;**62**:5-16

[24] Wolf TG, Schulze RKW, Ramos-Gomez F, Campus G. Effectiveness of telemedicine and teledentistry after the COVID-19 pandemic. International Journal of Environmental Research and Public Health. 2022;**19**:13857

[25] Gurgel-Juarez N, Torres-Pereira C, Haddad AE, Sheehy L, Finestone H, Mallet K, et al. Accuracy and effectiveness of teledentistry: A systematic review of systematic reviews. Evidence-Based Dentistry. 2022;**24**(8):639-648

[26] Kui A, Popescu C, Labuneț A, Almășan O, Petruțiu A, Păcurar M, et al. Is teledentistry a method for optimizing dental practice, even in the post-pandemic period? An integrative review. International Journal of Environmental Research and Public Health. 2022;**19**:7609

[27] El Tantawi M, Lam WYH, Giraudeau N, Virtanen JI, Matanhire C, Chifamba T, et al. Teledentistry from research to practice: A tale of nineteen countries. Frontiers in Oral Health. 2023;**4**:1188557

[28] Nichols K. Teledentistry overview: United States of America. Journal of the International Society for Telemedicine and eHealth. 2019;**7**:e9-e1

[29] Daniel SJ, Kumar S. Teledentistry: A key component in access to care. Journal of Evidence Based Dental Practice. 2014;**14**:201-208

[30] Estai M, Kanagasingam Y, Tennant M, Bunt S. A systematic review of the research evidence for the benefits of teledentistry. Journal of Telemedicine and Telecare. 2018;**24**(3):147-156

[31] Tiwari T, Diep V, Tranby E, Thakkar-Samtani M, Frantsve-Hawley J. Dentist perceptions about the value of teledentistry. BMC Oral Health. 2022;**22**(1):176

[32] Bahanan L, Alsharif M. Factors affecting the acceptance of teledentistry determined using the technology acceptance model: A cross-sectional study. Digital Health. 2023;**9**:20552076231158034

[33] Fortich-Mesa N, Hoyos-Hoyos V. Applications of teledentistry in dental practice: A systematic review. Revista Facultad de Odontología Universidad de Antioquia. 2020;**32**(1):77-88

[34] da Costa CB, Peralta FDS, Ferreira de Mello ALS. How has teledentistry been applied in public dental health services? An integrative review. Telemedicine and E-Health. 2020;**26**(7):945-954

[35] Amin M, Lai JY, Lindauer PA, McPherson K, Qari H. Should dental schools adopt teledentistry in their curricula? Two viewpoints. Journal of Dental Education. 2021;**85**(7):1238-1244

Section 4

Future Directions

Chapter 12

Remote Monitoring in Telehealth: Advancements, Feasibility and Implications

Muhuntha Sri-Ganeshan and Peter Cameron

Abstract

Over the past several decades, telehealth has evolved within various medical fields, gaining momentum with sequential technological advancements. The development of remote monitoring specifically expands the function of telehealth by facilitating the ongoing review of patients remotely. Through leveraging of technologies such as wearable sensors, mobile apps, and implantable devices, remote patient monitoring (RPM) enables the collection of biometric data for clinical decision-making. The utilisation of decision-making algorithms in addition to this can flag patient deterioration prompting for a clinician review. This narrative review summarises disease-specific applications, patient and clinician perspectives, and potential future acute care applications, highlighting RPM as a promising tool that, when combined with telehealth, could revolutionise healthcare delivery in the near future.

Keywords: remote monitoring, tele-monitoring, virtual wards, wearable devices, m-health

1. Introduction

Telehealth has been used for several decades within various fields of medical practice. However, progressive technological advancements, particularly in the development of secure videoconferencing, the Internet of Things and cloud computing now provide us with the option of managing appropriately selected patients outside the traditional hospital or clinic setting. This, in combination with demand pressures exerted by the COVID-19 pandemic, has facilitated a greater acceptance of remote delivery of care by both clinicians and patients and has paved the way for more sophisticated telehealth care models.

Leveraging these technologies presents not only the opportunity to enhance patient experience by facilitating hospital level care at a patient's residence but also potentially leads to improved patient outcomes, because of better access to a wide range of expertise. Telehealth also potentially reduces the negative consequences of hospital admissions (e.g. nosocomial infections, delirium in the patient with cognitive impairments). Further, by mitigating the barriers of distance on a health service level, the integration of these tools allows for operational efficiency and greater scalability opportunities.

Previous experience suggests that the use of these technologies is a safe means of delivering care. This narrative review aims to provide some insight into the potential applications of remote patient monitoring in conjunction with telehealth, based on current published literature.

2. Remote patient monitoring interventions

Remote patient monitoring (RPM) refers to the collection of biometric data without an in-person clinical team present, to inform clinical decision-making. Utilising technology, health-related data from an individual patient can be transferred from their location to a healthcare provider situated elsewhere. This process employs various devices, such as wearable sensors, mobile apps, or medical instruments to track vital signs and other health metrics. RPM facilitates early detection of deterioration, thus enabling the initiation of timely care.

2.1 Self-monitoring

Self-monitoring refers to technologies that enable patients to manually record clinical parameters. A patient may receive a monitoring device and is then prompted to record data. Objective variables such as heart rate and weight have been utilised as clinical parameters [1]. Additionally, teleconsultation may be used in conjunction with self-monitoring, by requesting patients to report data as part of the consultation.

2.2 Non-invasive monitoring

Non-invasive continuous monitoring encompasses technologies or devices that monitor one or more clinical parameters and transmit this data to treating teams. These teams may either review the data regularly or be alerted when a variable sits outside a specified range.

Wearable technologies capable of such monitoring include smartwatches, handheld devices and skin patches. A diverse range of parameters can be measured using remote non-invasive monitoring, with the most common being vital signs such as oxygen saturations, heart rate, blood pressure.

2.3 Invasive monitoring

Invasive monitoring involves devices which have been implanted within the patient. A notable example is implantable haemodynamic monitors. Elevations in left ventricular filling pressures and pulmonary artery pressures are closely correlated with clinical congestion, functional limitation and prognosis in patients with heart failure [2]. Invasive continuous monitoring devices can be integrated into other devices already used for managing heart failure, such as cardiac resynchronisation therapy devices and pacemakers. Additionally, these monitors can also be employed for heart rhythm monitoring.

3. Decision making algorithms

Remote monitoring frequently employs algorithms to support data analysis. These algorithms can be divided into two categories. Firstly, pre-processing algorithms extract meaningful information from physiological signals (such as removing erratic spikes in heart rate data caused my movement artefacts or identifying patterns indicating irregular heartbeats). Secondly, inference algorithms convert clinical variables into alarms and determine risk probabilities [3].

Inference algorithms are further categorised into three types:

- *Heuristic threshold-based algorithms*: these use predefined thresholds or rules to detect anomalies or trigger alerts based on specific criteria (e.g. a range of acceptable heart rates). While simple and easy to implement, they lack adaptability to individual patients and may miss complex patterns or gradual changes.

- *Non-sequential models*: employing machine learning, these algorithms analyse data without considering the sequential order of events. They predict outcomes or infer patterns without taking time dependencies into account. Capable of handling complex relationships between various patient parameters, they offer predictions on outcomes but may not capture changing trends associated with clinical deterioration.

- *Sequential models*: utilising machine learning in a more sophisticated manner, these models specifically analyse time-dependent patterns and relationships. While they can be more complex to implement, they offer a more nuanced analysis of sequential data.

Inference algorithms can be employed to trigger alerts about patient decompensation by analysing the physiological data obtained from remote patient monitoring devices.

4. Disease specific applications

4.1 Cardiac applications

The cardiac diseases most extensively evaluated to date in the context of remote monitoring are arrhythmias and heart failure [4]. The capability to measure respiratory rate, heart rate, electrocardiogaphy (ECG) and oxygen saturations through remote monitoring broadens the application to a variety of cardiac conditions.

4.1.1 Arrhythmias

Remote monitoring for arrhythmias has existed for some time, initially with Holter monitors and then implantable loop recorders. Recently, developments include mobile phone-based photoplethysmography (PPG) and hand-held ECG recorders, which are used to monitor heart rate and heart rate variability.

PPG sensors detect variations in light intensity through transmission or reflection from tissue, with these variations correlating to changes in blood perfusion. Hand-held ECG recorders require an additional external sensor unit and enable recording of a standard lead I ECG.

The most studied devices for arrythmia monitoring are handheld ECG recorders and mobile phone-based PPG which yield sensitivities and specificities of over 90% in detecting atrial fibrillation [5, 6]. Some devices have yielded particularly impressive results. For instance, a study by Lau et al. involving the AliveCor ECG recorder reported a sensitivity of 87% and a specificity of 97% in detecting atrial fibrillation, compared with a cardiologist's interpretation. Modifying the algorithm to emphasise the absence of P waves improved sensitivity to 97%, maintaining the same level of specificity [7].

The Apple Heart Study, involving 419,297 self-enrolled participants, utilised the Apple Watch and Heart Study iOS app. Notifications were based on irregular pulse detection via PPG. Subjects were notified to contact the study physician via telehealth to determine the necessity of further arrhythmia work up. Those with urgent symptoms were directed to attend in person emergency care, however those that were felt to not require urgent treatment were sent an ECG patch to wear for 7 days which was subsequently reviewed by trained technicians. 0.52% of participants received a notification and of the 450 participants who returned ECG patches, 34% of participants were found to have atrial fibrillation. Notably, in those who had been notified of an irregular pulse, the positive predictive value was 0.84 for observing atrial fibrillation on the ECG simultaneously when a subsequent irregular pulse was picked up by PPG [8]. Only half of those who had been notified of an irregular rhythm failed to contact the study clinician. This study highlighted the need for accessible follow-up care to enhance the utility of remote monitoring in screening.

Many cardiac implantable electronic devices (CIED) like permanent pacemakers, implantable cardioverter-defibrillators (ICDs) and implantable cardiac monitors are now able to provide remote monitoring, enabling the detection of life-threatening arrhythmias such as ventricular tachyarrhythmias, along with enabling a timely reaction to shocks delivered by ICDs (be they appropriate or inappropriate). Pacemaker and ICD rhythms can be monitored through sensing electrical activity by leads attached to cardiac tissue. With insertable cardiac monitors (ICM), far field subcutaneous electrocardiograms are obtained by sensing from a subcutaneous electrode.

Dual chamber devices can facilitate the early recognition of atrial fibrillation (AF) or atrial flutter in those at risk, such as patients with heart failure. Atrial arrhythmias pose a risk in heart failure patients with CIEDs due to risks of systemic thromboembolism, inappropriate shocks, or decompensation [9]. Episodes picked up as potentially being AF or Atrial Flutter are termed Atrial High-Rate episodes (AHREs). Among 2718 individuals with heart failure and CIEDs, AHREs were picked up in 34.8% of patients, with 91% of these being confirmed as AF [10]. Similarly, in a observational study involving 304 heart failure patients with CRT, 57.9% of patients had AHREs detected within 2.5 years post implantation, with 89.2% of these being confirmed as AF on follow up [11]. However, there is the potential to pick up short "sub-clinical" episodes of AF and the risk of thromboembolic events with such episodes has yet to be comprehensively evaluated. Consequently, a consensus on the appropriate timing for anticoagulation in such cases has yet to be established [12].

The traditional management of patients with CIEDs involves scheduled in-person device interrogation combined with the event-triggered alerts from the device. Advanced adaptations in CIEDs now allow remote interrogation through wand-based radiofrequency data transfer via home transceivers through phone lines or cellular connections to a remote server. Most recently low-energy Bluetooth allows coupling the CIED with the patient's smartphone, allowing the smartphone to act as the transceiver [13]. This not only facilitates data transmission but also provides information on device functionality, such as battery status or electrode function [13].

4.1.2 Heart failure

Early iterations of remote monitoring in heart failure primarily focused on non-invasive methods, especially monitoring vital parameters such as weight, blood pressure and heart rate [14]. However, CIEDs now have the capability to monitor parameters like intracardiac filling pressures or their surrogates, detecting haemodynamic congestion before clinical decompensation occurs.

Weight gain is a well-established clinical parameter for monitoring exacerbations of heart failure, with guidelines [15, 16] recommending daily body weight monitoring for these patients. Educating patients on the importance of daily weight recordings and encouraging regular compliance has long been considered crucial.

External blood pressure monitoring alone has not shown accuracy in predicting heart failure exacerbation [17–20]. However, some studies [21, 22], have demonstrated that combining blood pressure data with weight measurements can yield more accurate predictive models.

Heart rate and respiratory rate monitoring are standard practices for heart failure patients. A higher heart rate has been associated with increased hospitalizations due to heart failure [23] and Goetze et al. [24] reported significant increases in daily minimum, maximum, and median respiratory rates in the 30 days preceding a heart failure decompensation event.

Studies using multiple non-invasive parameters to predict decompensation have shown varied performances. Differences in the parameters used and associated algorithms contribute to some heterogeneity. The effectiveness of these monitoring systems is significantly influenced by patient compliance with self-monitoring [25]. Mobile technologies could aid compliance through programmed reminders and electronic charting of measurements via Bluetooth-capable devices.

Expert consensus recommends remote follow up with CIEDs for all patients with devices implanted for heart failure [26]. A recent meta-analysis compared the outcomes of remote haemodynamic assessment versus standard care in patients with heart failure [27]. It found that in the remote monitoring group containing 7733 patients compared to the control group of 7567 there was a 32% lower risk of CHF-related hospitalisation (RR 0.68, 95% CI 0.87–1.07, $p < 0.001$), however there was no significant difference between the group in terms of all cause mortality (RR 0.97, 95% CI 0.87–1.07, $p = 0.53$). These results did not specify the outcomes for those receiving both non-invasive and haemodynamic monitoring simultaneously. Further assessment of trend detection algorithms utilising a combination of invasive and non-invasive parameters might offer greater predictive accuracy for decompensation episodes.

4.1.3 Myocardial infarction

The ALERTS trial [28] employed an implanted device connected to a right ventricle apical pacemaker lead. The system was designed to store and capture electrocardiogram data and detect rapid progressive ST-segment shifts relative to a subjected baseline. Upon detecting changes, the device would alert the patient to seek medical attention through a vibratory alarm, along with a visual and auditory alarm transmitted wirelessly to a pager. When comparing outcomes for patients who had active alerts turned on compared to controls who had alerts disabled, there was no significant difference in the occurrence of pre-set primary endpoints (cardiac or unexplained death, new Q-wave myocardial infarction or detection to presentations > 2 hours). This result may be partly attributed to the low number of cardiac events in the study.

However, 96.7% of the participants experienced no system related complications, suggesting that early detection of myocardial infarction could be another potential safe application for implantable devices.

4.2 Respiratory applications

4.2.1 Chronic Obstructive Pulmonary Disease (COPD)

Early recognition of exacerbations in Chronic Obstructive Pulmonary Disease (COPD) can potentially reduce hospitalisations through prompt initiation of treatment. A change in respiratory effort has been shown to be a strong indicator of exacerbations [29] and can be detected through impedance pneumography. This method involves injecting current into the chest tissue using two drive electrodes and measuring the potential difference between them. The difference in potential varies with the impendence of the tissue, which changes with respiration. Alternatively, respiratory rate can be assessed using stretch sensors that detect chest wall movements, or flow thermography, which identifies temperature differences between inhaled and exhaled air.

Pulse oximetry, which provides continuous measurement of peripheral oxygen saturation (SpO_2), is a well-established practice in medicine. The market offers numerous inexpensive and user-friendly devices.

Diagnostic spirometry measures the volumes of air inspired and expired by the lungs. The forced expiratory volume in one second (FEV1 can be a useful indicator in assessing COPD exacerbations. Portable handheld spirometers, now available for remote monitoring, are considered less useful during acute exacerbations [30].

Peak expiratory flow metres are simpler and cheaper than spirometers and determine the maximum speed of forced expiration, rather than the volume of expired air. Low readings from these metres could indicate an acute COPD exacerbation.

A recent systematic review highlighted that most telemonitoring intervention studies for COPD utilised online platforms connected to devices that collect and transmit various parameters such as clinical symptoms and vital signs [31]. Compared to usual care, telemonitoring did not reduce hospital admissions for COPD but did decrease emergency department presentations.

A scoping review focused on telemedicine applications in managing patients post-hospitalisation for COPD exacerbations. The reviewed studies employed varied strategies, combining phone or video consultations with a nurse and ongoing symptom and vital sign monitoring. Out of 27 studies examining hospital readmissions, 18 indicated a reduction, but only 13 of these were statistically significant [32].

4.2.2 Asthma

In asthma management, wearable home monitors can longitudinally measure symptoms, physiological parameters, and assess risk factors. Focusing on environmental triggers such as allergens (e.g., pollen, dust), air pollution, and weather (known exacerbators of asthma) wearable devices equipped with sensors have been developed [33, 34]. These devices detect levels of specific triggers and integrate additional data to alert patients about the risk of an exacerbation. However, there is currently a lack of intervention studies involving such devices.

The use of peak flow meters in asthma management is a topic of ongoing discussion. Peak flow monitoring can potentially enhance self-management, improve trigger identification, and decrease emergency department presentations and hospital admissions [35]. While some guidelines [36] consider peak flow measurements appropriate for confirming asthma exacerbations, reliance on this method alone is generally cautioned against [37]. Remote spirometry systems that record and transmit peak expiratory flow (PEF) readings have been developed and may play a role in remote monitoring [38].

Patient engagement is crucial for effective asthma control. Mobile health applications (apps) are considered useful tools for helping patients monitor symptoms and medication use, as well as for providing education. There are numerous apps designed for self-monitoring, but more sophisticated versions can communicate with inhaler sensors via Bluetooth. These apps collect data on medication usage, which can then be transmitted to healthcare providers [39]. Additionally, they can remind patients to take preventive inhalers [40]. The use of such technology has been shown to improve medication adherence, increase symptom-free days, and has received positive patient feedback [41].

Asthma exacerbations are complex and multidimensional phenomena. Predicting an individual patient's risk depends on factors like history of exacerbations, lung function, smoking status, and environmental exposures. Machine learning, using data from patient cohorts with previous exacerbations, can develop algorithms to predict exacerbation risks in the near future. A recent meta-analysis [42] looked at 11 studies including 23 prediction models designed to determine if individual patients were at risk of asthma exacerbations. The pooled area under the curve of receiver operating characteristics (AUROC) of 11 studies was 0.80 (95% CI 0.77–0.83). The most common important predictors were systemic steroid use, short acting beta2-agonist use, emergency department visits, age and exacerbation history. Boosting, Logistic regression (LR) and Random Forest (RF) were the top three popular machine learning methods for asthma exacerbation prediction. Boosting was the best performing algorithm with the overall pooled AUROC of boosting being 0.84 (95% CI 0.81–0.87). These results suggest that machine learning models for asthma exacerbation prediction can achieve good discrimination. Applying this to data from remote monitoring could help identify patients requiring closer follow-up and more regular reviews.

4.3 Early post-operative period

In the post-operative phase, patients experience a potent stress response and, during convalescence, often have decreased mobility and are subject to the side effects of medications, such as opioids. Consequently, post-operative patients are at an increased risk of complications including falls, myocardial infarction, and pneumonia. Traditionally, post-operative monitoring has included regular reviews of pain, mood, wound healing, oral intake, fluid balance, and bowel movements. With an increasing focus on facilitating shorter hospital stays, telemedicine combined with remote monitoring offers an opportunity to extend this approach to a broader patient population.

A scoping review by Amin et al. [43] explored published research on the use of wearable devices for remote patient monitoring across a range of surgical disciplines, including general, cardiac, orthopaedic and obstetric procedures. In most of the studies reviewed (23 out of 24), devices employing either accelerometry or pedometer functions were utilised to track physical activity thereby serving as markers of postoperative function. The potential development of remote ambulatory monitoring in this context could enable earlier hospital discharge and improve continuity of care at home, thereby enhancing support during the rehabilitation period.

4.4 Other disease applications for remote patient monitoring

In the existing literature, a significant focus of remote patient monitoring (RPM) lies in cardio-pulmonary diseases. However, RPM has also shown promise in managing other conditions. Beyond monitoring for deterioration, RPM can assist in enhancing control of chronic conditions like diabetes and hypertension. This is achieved by facilitating data collection (e.g., blood sugar or blood pressure readings), which can then be reported back to clinicians or patients themselves [44]. More regular intervention theoretically enables better disease control and improved long-term outcomes [45].

In geriatric care, RPM can play a crucial role in fall detection. Falls among the elderly are a major cause of morbidity and mortality, and early detection may mitigate harm by flagging patients for welfare checks, potentially initially through teleconferencing. These systems often use accelerometers to detect movement patterns associated with falls, such as sudden increases in acceleration followed by rapid deceleration upon impact [46]. Machine learning could further enhance the accuracy of fall detection by analysing accelerometer data.

In obstetric care, especially during the later stages of pregnancy, a high degree of self-monitoring is necessary to identify maternal and fetal complications, such as pre-eclampsia or fetal distress. RPM may improve both safety and convenience in this context. Proposed external devices for monitoring pregnant patients include blood pressure monitors, electronic scales for weight tracking, and electrodes for monitoring uterine contractions and fetal electrocardiography [47].

This review has outlined just a few applications of RPM. The technology holds the potential to assist in managing a variety of conditions beyond the traditional healthcare setting. By tracking vital signs, physical activity, symptom monitoring, and medication adherence, RPM can facilitate care in a patient's usual residence. This not only enhances convenience from the patient's perspective but also provides superior care across a broad spectrum of diseases and patient populations. The utility of RPM is further amplified when combined with teleconferencing. As technology advances, additional applications of RPM with more sophisticated models of care are likely to emerge in the near future.

5. Patient and clinician perspectives

Qualitative studies, involving structured interviews with clinicians and patients engaged in telemonitoring for chronic conditions [48, 49] and those in "virtual wards" [50], have provided valuable insights into the patient journey. These insights are crucial for developing more patient-centered interventions. The studies have identified themes highlighting both the benefits and potential drawbacks of remote care via telemonitoring from a patient perspective.

In managing chronic conditions, patients have reported an increased sense of security with telemonitoring. They feel more visible to the healthcare system and safer, knowing that their condition is being monitored and help is available if needed. Despite the initial burden of self-monitoring and reporting, many patients find that these activities become routine and part of their daily schedule over time. In some patient groups there is a potential for apprehension regarding the use of technology if they are unfamiliar, however some are able to overcome this with experience. Patients have reported that whilst they felt that telemonitoring provided better access to care, they have some concerns that over reliance on technology might reduce direct clinician contact and that the desire to interact with a professional remains.

Both clinicians and patients report that the process of self-monitoring helps patients understand their conditions better, empowering them to manage their own health more effectively. In particular it enabled them to identify and mitigate deteriorations in their conditions. Nonetheless, some patients have experienced anxiety due to alerts, in particular when there were notifications of deterioration.

Regarding the "virtual ward" model, patients have expressed greater satisfaction due to proximity to friends and family. This model is especially beneficial for those with access to informal social support. Conversely, the virtual ward model was perceived to be more challenging to patients lacking such support. Caution must be taken when admitting patients to virtual wards, particularly if they might find using the required technology difficult.

6. Potential future acute care applications

While the majority of existing literature on remote patient monitoring (RPM) focuses on chronic condition management, the COVID-19 pandemic has highlighted its potential in acute care. The strain on healthcare resources, including a lack of inpatient bed capacity and heightened risk of disease transmission, led to an expansion in the use of "virtual wards," where patients remain in their usual residence and are monitored through online platforms, telephone calls and wearable sensors. COVID-19 has been the acute condition to which virtual wards have been applied most commonly [51]. These wards enable monitoring for patient deterioration, triggering unscheduled tele-conferencing reviews and decisions about inpatient admission or alternative care escalation (e.g., community outreach teams, medication dispensing). Although this model of care has yet to be extensively applied to other conditions, it does provide a potential means to address some of the issues facing healthcare systems worldwide.

Applying this model to other conditions could address some global healthcare system challenges. Emergency Department overcrowding is a widespread problem and the associated effects on morbidity and mortality as well as staff burnout are well documented. Boarding is largely driven by "access block" or the inability to access an appropriate hospital bed for an admitted patient. Telehealth in combination with RPM would allow more patients to be managed at home, without the need to take up an inpatient bed, thus potentially reducing the strain on the healthcare system as a whole.

RPM could also enhance care in lower acuity settings, such as rural hospitals or residential aged care facilities. By remotely monitoring patients, the burden of observations on local staff is reduced, thereby easing their workload and enabling the care of higher acuity patients within these environments. Telehealth also allows such centres to access expertise that might otherwise only be available in urban centres, this prevents the need for costly transfers for some patients.

In urban centers, RPM can be beneficial not only in lower acuity areas but also in high-demand situations where patient safety is at risk. Emergency Department waiting rooms might be made safer through being able to continuously monitor patient's vital signs with wearable devices.

7. Future research priorities

New remote patient monitoring devices continue to be developed however the utility of such technology in a real-world setting is dependent on multiple factors, including the reliability of network coverage, user acceptability and cost-effectiveness. Wearable devices, particularly in the form of smart watches may be appropriate devices for the purposes of remote patient monitoring. The latest commercially available smart watches are able to measure oxygen saturations, heart rate, ECGs, blood pressure and alert for falls using built in accelerometers and gyroscopes. If reliable, these provide the means to assess patients and detect deterioration in the same what that conventionally obtained patient vital signs might do in the hospital setting.

Whilst there have been some studies looking into the accuracy of such devices [52], there has been little done to look into their reliability when being used in a clinical setting and little research into the ability of these devices to improve patient outcomes [53].

Future research should be focused on translational research looking into the application of these technologies into models of care which supplement monitoring with ongoing remote consultations. Implementation of such technology should be accompanied by robust, well rounded evaluations which include both qualitative and quantitative components assessing patient and clinician experience as well as determining patient outcomes. Validation of the reliability of data obtained from wearable devices in the clinical setting would be the first step prior to utilisation within a pilot. Graded expansion of telehealth systems making use of remote patient monitoring can then progress if evaluations are shown to be of benefit, again accompanied by robust evaluation with each stage of expansion. In this way, mature telehealth systems can be developed which can gradually increase the range of conditions covered in both the acute and outpatient setting, whilst also providing the infrastructure to which more sophisticated remote monitoring technologies might be introduced, making use of more complex decision-making algorithms and additional sensors.

8. Conclusions

There has been a significant increase in literature surrounding the use of remote patient monitoring (RPM). These studies have focused on chronic disease management and a limited range of medical conditions. RPM has demonstrated a facility to enhance tighter control of chronic diseases by allowing more regular review of relevant parameters. It also has been shown to be effective in early detection of deterioration allowing for timely intervention. To date a majority of studies related to RPM are proof of concept or pilot studies with relatively few studies operating within mature telehealth models of care.

In conjunction with telehealth, developments in remote monitoring devices hold the potential to cause a paradigm shift in health care. Many conditions that would have traditionally required inpatient care can be managed safely within a patient's own residence. However, aside from management of COVID-19, the literature has not concentrated on the application of RPM to acute conditions. Given the current strain on many health systems, further research into the utility of virtual wards is warranted. Future analyses should not only consider patient outcomes but also encompass patient satisfaction and cost analysis to justify the implementation of such care models.

RPM represents an exciting and evolving tool in healthcare delivery. While further studies looking into patient outcomes as well as the broader application of RPM are required, existing literature shows significant promise and the technology has the potential to revolutionise the delivery of healthcare going forward.

Conflict of interest

The authors declare no conflict of interest.

Author details

Muhuntha Sri-Ganeshan* and Peter Cameron
School of Public Health and Preventive Medicine, Monash University, Melbourne, Australia

*Address all correspondence to: myles.sri-ganeshan@monash.edu

References

[1] Senarath S, Fernie G, Roshan FA. Influential factors in remote monitoring of heart failure patients: A review of the literature and direction for future research. Sensors. 2021;**21**:3575

[2] Sousa C, Leite S, Lagido R, et al. Telemonitoring in heart failure: A state-of-the-art review. Revista Portuguesa de Cardiologia (English Edition). 2014;**33**:229-239

[3] Castelyn G, Laranjo L, Schreier G, et al. Predictive performance and impact of algorithms in remote monitoring of chronic conditions: A systematic review and meta-analysis. International Journal of Medical Informatics. 2021;**156**:104620

[4] Singhal A, Cowie MR. Digital health: Implications for heart failure management. Cardiac Failure Review. 2021:7:e08

[5] Li KHC, White FA, Tipoe T, et al. The current state of Mobile phone apps for monitoring heart rate, heart rate variability, and atrial fibrillation: Narrative review. JMIR mHealth and uHealth. 2019;**7**:e11606

[6] MacKinnon GE, Brittain EL. Mobile health technologies in cardiopulmonary disease. Chest. 2020;**157**:654-664

[7] Lau JK, Lowres N, Neubeck L, et al. iPhone ECG application for community screening to detect silent atrial fibrillation: A novel technology to prevent stroke. International Journal of Cardiology. 2013;**165**:193-194

[8] Perez MV, Mahaffey KW, Hedlin, et al. Apple heart study investigators. Large-scale assessment of a smartwatch to identify atrial fibrillation. The New England Journal of Medicine. 2019;**381**:1909-1917

[9] Ono M, Varma N. Remote monitoring for chronic disease management: Atrial fibrillation and heart failure. Cardiac Electrophysiology Clinics. 2018;**10**:43-58

[10] Jędrzejczyk-Patej E, Lenarczyk R, Mazurek M, et al. Can we rely on machines? Device-detected atrial high rates correspond well with atrial arrhythmias in cardiac resynchronization recipients. Europace. 2016;**18**:436-444

[11] Gorenek B, Bax J, Boriani G, et al. Device-detected subclinical atrial tachyarrhythmias: Definition, implications and management. Europace. 2017;**19**:1556-1578

[12] Perino AC, Fan J, Askari M. et al, Practice variation in anticoagulation prescription and outcomes after device-detected atrial fibrillation. Circulation. 2019;**139**:2502-2512

[13] Varma N, Braunschweig F, Burri H. Remote monitoring of cardiac implantable electronic devices and disease management. Europace. Online. 2023;**25**

[14] Inglis SC, Clark RA, Dierckx R, et al. Structured telephone support or non-invasive telemonitoring for patients with heart failure. Cochrane Database of Systematic Reviews. 2017;**103**:255-257

[15] Ezekowitz JA, O'Meara E, McDonald MA, et al. Comprehensive update of the Canadian cardiovascular society guidelines for the management of heart failure. The Canadian Journal of Cardiology. 2017;**33**:1342-1433

[16] McMurray JJ, Adamopoulos S, Anker SD, et al. ESC guidelines for the diagnosis and treatment of acute and

chronic heart failure 2012: The Task Force for the Diagnosis and Treatment of Acute and Chronic Heart Failure 2012 of the European Society of Cardiology. Developed in collaboration with the Heart Failure Association (HFA) of the ESC. European Heart Journal. 2012;**33**:1787-1847

[17] Koulaouzidis G, Iakovidis DK, Clark AL. Telemonitoring predicts in advance heart failure admissions. International Journal of Cardiology. 2016;**216**:78-84

[18] Worley SL. Experts provide a glimpse of the new post-SPRINT era of hypertension. Pharmacology & Therapeutics. 2017;**42**:118-123

[19] Fonarow GC, Heywood JT, Heidenreich PA, ADHERE Scientific Advisory Committee and Investigators. Temporal trends in clinical characteristics, treatments, and outcomes for heart failure hospitalizations, 2002 to 2004: Findings from Acute Decompensated Heart Failure National Registry (ADHERE). American Heart Journal. 2007;**153**:1021-1028

[20] Lieback A, Proff J, Wessel K, et al. Remote monitoring of heart failure patients using implantable cardiac pacing devices and external sensors: Results of the Insight-HF study. Clinical Research in Cardiology. 2012;**101**:101-107

[21] Joshi R, Gyllensten IC. Changes in daily measures of blood pressure and heart rate improve weight-based detection of heart failure deterioration in patients on telemonitoring. IEEE Journal of Biomedical and Health Informatics. 2018;**23**:1041-1048

[22] Koulaouzidis G, Iakovidis DK, Clark AL. Telemonitoring predicts in advance heart failure admissions. International Journal of Cardiology. 2016;**216**:78-84

[23] Fox K, Ford I, Steg PG, et al. Heart rate as a prognostic risk factor in patients with coronary artery disease and left-ventricular systolic dysfunction (BEAUTIFUL): A subgroup analysis of a randomised controlled trial. Lancet. 2008;**372**:817-821

[24] Goetze S, Zhang Y, An Q, et al. Ambulatory respiratory rate trends identify patients at higher risk of worsening heart failure in implantable cardioverter defibrillator and biventricular device recipients: A novel ambulatory parameter to optimize heart failure management. Journal of Interventional Cardiac Electrophysiology. 2015;**43**:21-29

[25] Dickinson MG, Allen LA, Albert NA, et al. Remote monitoring of patients with heart failure: A white paper from the Heart Failure Society of America Scientific Statements Committee. Journal of Cardiac Failure. 2018;**24**:682-694

[26] Slotwiner D, Varma N, Akar JG, et al. HRS expert consensus statement on remote interrogation and monitoring for cardiovascular implantable electronic devices. Hear Rhythm. 2015;**12**:e69-e100

[27] Buttar C, Lakhdar S, Nso N, et al. Meta-analysis comparing outcomes of remote hemodynamic assessment versus standard care in patients with heart failure. The American Journal of Cardiology. 2023;**192**:79-87

[28] Gibson C, Holmes D, Mikdadi G, et al. Implantable cardiac alert system for early recognition of ST-segment elevation myocardial infarction. Journal of the American College of Cardiology. 2019;**73**:1919-1927

[29] Yañez AM, Guerrero D, Pérez De Alejo R, et al. Monitoring breathing rate at home allows early identification

of COPD exacerbations. Chest. 2012;**142**:1524-1529

[30] Vestbo J, Hurd SS, Agustí AG, et al. Global strategy for the diagnosis, management, and prevention of chronic obstructive pulmonary disease GOLD executive summary. American Journal of Respiratory and Critical Care Medicine. 2013;**187**:347-365

[31] Jang S, Kim Y, Cho WK. A systematic review and meta-analysis of telemonitoring interventions on severe COPD exacerbations. International Journal of Environmental Research and Public Health. 2021;**18**:6757

[32] Rezende LC, Ribeiro EG, Parreiras LC, et al. Telehealth and telemedicine in the management of adult patients after hospitalization for COPD exacerbation: A scoping review. Jornal Brasileiro de Pneumologia. 2023;**49**:e20220067

[33] Hosseini A, Buonocore C, Hashemzadeh S, et al. HIPAA compliant wireless sensing smartwatch application for the self-management of pediatric asthma. In: International Conference on Wearable and Implantable Body Sensor Networks. San Francisco, USA: IEEE; 2016. pp. 49-54

[34] Fletcher R, Oreskovic N, Robinson A. Design and clinical feasibility of personal wearable monitor for measurement of activity and environmental exposure. In: Annual International Conference of the IEEE Engineering in Medicine and Biology Society. Chicago, USA: IEEE; 2014. pp. 874-877

[35] van der Kamp MR, Hengeveld VS, Brusse-Keizer MGJ, et al. eHealth technologies for monitoring pediatric asthma at home: Scoping review. Journal of Medical Internet Research. 2023;**25**:e45896

[36] Barnard A. Management of an acute asthma attack. Australian Family Physician. 2005;**34**:531-534

[37] The Royal Children's Hospital Melbourne Clinical Guideline: Acute Asthma[Internet]. [cited 13 Mar, 2024]. Available from: https://www.rch.org.au/clinicalguide/guideline_index/asthma_acute/

[38] Liao CA, Young TH, Cheng CT, et al. The feasibility and efficiency of remote spirometry system on the pulmonary function for multiple ribs fracture patients. Journal of Personalized Medicine. 2021;**11**:1067

[39] Merchant RK, Inamdar R, Quade RC. Effectiveness of population health management using the propeller health asthma platform: A randomized clinical trial. The Journal of Allergy and Clinical Immunology in Practice. 2016;**4**:455-463

[40] Kenyon CC, Sundar KG, Gruschow SM. Tailored medication adherence incentives for high-risk children with asthma: A pilot study. Journal of Asthma. 2020;**57**(12):1372-1378

[41] Nguyen E, Miao B, Pugliese N. Systematic review of mHealth applications that interface with inhaler sensors in asthma. The Journal of Allergy and Clinical Immunology: In Practice. 2021;**9**:844-852

[42] Xiong S, Chen W, Jia X, et al. Machine learning for prediction of asthma exacerbations among asthmatic patients: A systematic review and meta-analysis. BMC Pulmonary Medicine. 2023;**23**:278

[43] Amin T, Mobbs RJ, Mostafa N, et al. Wearable devices for patient monitoring in the early postoperative period: A literature review. Mhealth. 2021;**7**:50

[44] Lundell S, Modig M, Holmner Å, et al. Perceptions of home telemonitoring use among patients with chronic obstructive pulmonary disease: Qualitative study. JMIR mHealth and uHealth. 2020;**8**:e16343

[45] Ekstedt M, Nordheim ES, Hellström A, et al. Patient safety and sense of security when telemonitoring chronic conditions at home: The views of patients and healthcare professionals - A qualitative study. BMC Health Services Research. 2023;**23**:581

[46] Ko SQ, Chua CMS, Koh SH. Experiences of patients and their caregivers in a virtual Ward in Singapore: A descriptive qualitative study. International Journal of Medical Informatics. 2023;**177**:105111

[47] Farias FA, Dagostini CM, Bicca YD, et al. Remote patient monitoring: A systematic review. Telemedicine and e-Health. 2020;**26**:576-583

[48] Lee SG, Blood AJ, Cannon CP. remote cardiovascular hypertension program enhanced blood pressure control during the COVID-19 pandemic. Journal of the American Heart Association. 2023;**12**:e027296

[49] Ajerla D, Mahfuz S, Zulkernine F. A real-time patient monitoring framework for fall detection. Wireless Communications and Mobile Computing. 2019;**2019**:1-3

[50] Alves DS, Times VC, da Silva ÉM, et al. Advances in obstetric telemonitoring: A systematic review. International Journal of Medical Informatics. 2020;**134**:104004

[51] Vindrola-Padros C, Singh KE, Sidhu MS, et al. Remote home monitoring (virtual wards) during the COVID-19 pandemic: A systematic review. MedRxiv. 2020;**2020**:10

[52] Khushhal A, Nichols S, Evans W, et al. Validity and reliability of the apple watch for measuring heart rate during exercise. Sports Medicine International Open. 2017;**1**:E206-E211

[53] Masoumian Hosseini M, Masoumian Hosseini ST, Qayumi K, et al. Smartwatches in healthcare medicine: Assistance and monitoring; a scoping review. BMC Medical Informatics and Decision Making. 2023;**23**:248

Chapter 13

Telemedicine in Africa: Applications, Opportunities, and Challenges

Simon Onsongo and Elizabeth Kagotho

Abstract

Telemedicine is the delivery of healthcare services remotely through information and communication technology (ICT) devices. Telemedicine offers a promising solution to address unmet healthcare needs across the African continent. This review explores the current state, opportunities, and challenges of telemedicine in this context. While growth has been significant in recent decades, access remains limited in many rural and underserved regions due to numerous barriers. Despite these limitations, telemedicine has demonstrated its great potential to improve healthcare delivery, particularly in primary care, chronic disease management, specialist consultations, and remote education and training. As new technologies emerge, the scope of services will expand. When used effectively, telemedicine not only improves patient outcomes and healthcare efficiency but also enables collaboration among healthcare professionals, fostering knowledge sharing, and capacity building across geographical barriers. To increase effective utilization across African states, access barriers such as limited internet connectivity, inadequate infrastructure, regulatory hurdles, cultural beliefs, and individual (patient/provider) concerns must be addressed. This requires a multifaceted approach involving various stakeholders supporting healthcare service delivery in the continent.

Keywords: telemedicine, telehealth, e-health, healthcare access, Africa

1. Introduction

Throughout the history of mankind, people have used various tools such as drums, smoke, and horns to communicate over considerable distances [1]. In the 1700s and 1800s, various groundbreaking electrical inventions such as telephones and telegraphs allowed for almost instantaneous communication over long distances and gave birth to the information and communication age [1]. Information and communication technologies are increasingly being used across all facets of our lives today. These technologies have great potential to address some of our pressing healthcare needs, particularly in Africa and other developing countries.

The word 'telemedicine' is derived from the Greek word 'tele,' meaning 'at a distance,' and the word 'medicine,' which has its roots in the Latin word 'medicina,' meaning 'to heal.' This translates to 'healing at a distance' [2]. Telemedicine is both the art and science of diagnosing, treating, and managing patients and providing healthcare services over a distance using information and communication technology.

2. History of telemedicine

Telemedicine's history stretches back over a century ago. As early as 1879, an article in The Lancet envisioned the use of telephones to decrease unnecessary hospital visits, foreshadowing telemedicine's potential to improve healthcare accessibility [3]. The invention of the electrocardiogram (ECG) in 1906 enabled the transmission of medical data across distances in the Netherlands, and by the 1920s, radio consultation centers had sprouted across Europe [4]. In the 1940s, Pennsylvanian cities successfully transferred radiographic images by telephone, showcasing the increasing possibilities of remote diagnosis and consultation [4].

The United States has played a key role in telemedicine's evolution and expansion through supporting innovation in telemedicine. In 1960, the National Aeronautics and Space Administration (NASA) pioneered using telemedicine technologies to monitor astronauts during space missions [5, 6]. Use of such technologies allows physicians to monitor and manage astronauts through Mission Control, and the scope has expanded due to advancement in satellite communications and connectivity. Soon after NASA piloted the use of telemedicine, its application spread quickly to other areas beyond space science. In the Space Technology Applied to Rural Papago Advanced Health Care (STARPAHC) project, two-way radio, television, and telemetry to provide care to remote regions over 100 miles away in Southern Arizona [7], greatly increasing access to care for rural communities in the served areas.

Concurrently, between the 1950s and early 1960s, closed-circuit television facilitated psychiatric consultations between the Nebraska Psychiatric Institute and Norfolk State Hospital [8]. Technological advancements continued to propel progress in telemedicine, particularly in teleradiology, which has gained widespread global adoption. Radiologists were early adopters and embraced standards like the Digital Imaging and Communications in Medicine (DICOM) for efficient transmission and storage of medical images worldwide, allowing for connectivity, interoperability, and scale-up [9, 10].

The past three decades have seen a surge in telemedicine adoption, fueled by the rise of the internet and mobile technologies. The COVID-19 pandemic further accelerated its growth, highlighting its critical role in maintaining healthcare access while safeguarding safety [11–13]. By necessitating social distancing measures, the pandemic drove healthcare providers to utilize telemedicine to ensure continuity of care while minimizing the risk of coronavirus transmission. Governments relaxed regulations, insurers expanded coverage, and healthcare systems invested in telehealth infrastructure to meet the increasing demand for remote healthcare services [14–16]. Telemedicine is undergoing continual evolution, marked by the expanding application of technologies like artificial intelligence, wearable devices, cloud computing, blockchain, 5G networks, remote monitoring devices, and numerous others. These technological advancements hold the potential to enhance access to quality healthcare, improve patient outcomes, and hopefully reduce healthcare costs.

3. Definitions

In 2007, The World Health Organization (WHO) defines telemedicine as '*the delivery of health care services, where distance is a critical factor, by all health care professionals using information and communication technologies for the exchange of valid information for diagnosis, treatment and prevention of disease and injuries, research and evaluation, and for the continuing education of health care providers, all in the interests of advancing the health of individuals and their communities*' [17]. The WHO also specifies that for a service to qualify as telemedicine, it must have four key features, namely offering clinical support, overcoming geographical barriers, or being delivered remotely, utilizing information and communication devices, and increasing accessibility, utilization, efficiency, and effectiveness of healthcare services and a reasonable or affordable cost [18].

While many authors use 'telehealth' and 'telemedicine' interchangeably, others distinguish them by defining telemedicine as a specific subset of telehealth focused on direct clinical care delivery through telecommunications technology. This contrasts with the broader definition of telehealth, which encompasses all uses of telecommunication technology in healthcare such as prevention, diagnostics, treatments, and healthcare administration including information sharing and education between patients and providers [19].

Telemedicine employs a variety of information and communication technologies, such as phone calls, virtual video-based communication platforms, smartphone applications, wearable technologies, remote diagnostic devices, and telehealth carts that bring mobile clinics to underserved areas. Additionally, dedicated platforms integrate various tools like video calls, messaging, appointment scheduling, and electronic health records (EHR) management. Newer technologies such as chatbots, Internet of Things (IoT), Virtual Reality systems, ultrafast connectivity, computer vision, machine learning algorithms, and natural Large Language Models (LLMs) such as ChatGPT will support a wider scale and scope of applications in telemedicine and beyond [18, 20]. Increased integration of artificial intelligence (AI models) into healthcare systems will support patients and clinicians, allowing for more personalized patient care, increased access, and better population health, while hopefully with affordable costs.

4. Types of telemedicine

There are three main types of telemedicine, categorized by the timing of information exchange:

1. Store-and-forward: patient data is stored before transmitting it to a healthcare provider for later review. There is no simultaneous interaction between sender and receiver.

2. Remote monitoring: this method employs various technological devices to remotely track a patient's health and clinical signs. This is frequently utilized in management of chronic conditions like cardiovascular disease and diabetes.

3. Synchronous/real-time interactive services: this telemedicine approach features live, face-to-face communication between patients and healthcare providers. It encompasses activities like taking medical history, consultations, discussing treatment plans, and offering counseling.

5. Disease burden in Africa

Compared to other world regions, Africa's healthcare system faces numerous challenges and lags behind other continents on almost all health indicators [21]. The African continent also lags in human development partly due to high disease burden. With an increasing population (11–13%) and high disease burden of disease contributing to 25% of global disease burden, Africa's spending is less than 1% of the global budget for health, shows the need for further investment to improve access [21]. The high burden of infectious diseases like HIV/AIDS, malaria, and tuberculosis, coupled with significant maternal, neonatal, and childhood illness and mortality and the rapid rise of chronic non-communicable diseases, severely strain African healthcare systems. Urgent action is needed to bridge care gaps across the continent and reverse these negative health trends, aligning with the United Nation's (UN) Sustainable Development Goals (SDGs) launched in 2015.

The 2022 WHO survey revealed a region-wide average of only 1.55 health workers per 1000 people, far below the recommended 4.45 [22]. This translates to just 2.3 healthcare workers per 1000 in Africa compared to 24.8 in the Americas, leaving only 1.3% of global health workers to shoulder 25% of the global disease burden [21]. Many countries do not meet the WHO's recommended density of 2.5 per 1000, with half having fewer than 10 physicians per 100,000 people (compared to 250 or more in developed nations). These gaps significantly hinder essential healthcare delivery and achieving universal health coverage across the continent.

With the increasing adoption and use of technological devices around the world, the use of telemedicine has the potential to revolutionize healthcare delivery in Africa and other low- and middle-income countries (LMICs) and bridge the healthcare gap. Telemedicine can offer a wide range of services, including preventive/health promotive, curative, diagnostic, monitoring, and health educational services. In this chapter, we will explore the application/opportunities and barriers to telemedicine in Africa.

6. History of telemedicine in Africa

Although telemedicine is considered to be in its infancy in Africa, it is not new in the continent. Africa's adoption of telemedicine has been marked by innovation, but uneven infrastructure and resource limitations have made progress slow and geographically patchy. Despite these challenges, several countries have pioneered successful telemedicine programs, offering hope for the future of healthcare delivery on the continent.

The early 1980s saw Ethiopia and, later, Sudan in the 2010s, take the first tentative steps, using telecommunications to bridge the gap between remote communities and healthcare specialists in areas like obstetrics, pediatrics, and family medicine [23, 24]. These pilot projects offered hope for the continent but also brought forth the harsh realities that exist in the diverse continent of Africa. Below are some of the successful telemedicine projects across the continent:

6.1 Gezira family medicine project

One of the earliest telemedicine projects was in Sudan. This explored the use of telemedicine and e-learning in a primary care context. Over 3800 online consultations and 165,000 new patient records were created by doctors enrolled in the program. Participants found both telemedicine and electronic medical records (EMRs). Nearly all participants emphasized the value of telemedicine and electronic records, and trainees highly appreciated the great value of online learning despite logistical challenges. This study demonstrates the potential of information and communication technology (ICT) for both training and healthcare delivery in primary care settings [24].

6.2 RAFT

In 2001, the Réseau en Afrique Francophone pour la Télémédecine (RAFT) network was established by the University Hospitals and the University of Geneva in French-speaking Africa. Initially targeting 15 countries and focusing on medical education, the project faced challenges with high operational costs. However, it successfully connected hundreds of healthcare professionals, offered teleconsultations, implemented clinical information systems, and even deployed mHealth projects. Since 2010, RAFT has expanded its reach to Bolivia and Nepal [25].

6.3 iPath

Launched in 2001, the University of Basel's iPath telemedicine platform was a point-to-point telepathology system. This web-based platform facilitated online case discussions, real-time telepathology, and case repository access. Within 4 years, the network boasted over 700 users and diagnosed over 6300 cases, transforming into a global pathology network [26].

6.4 African teledermatology project

This collaboration between various institutions, including the University of Pennsylvania and African universities, used store-and-forward telemedicine to provide consultations for dermatological conditions in 13 Sub-Saharan African nations including Uganda, Botswana, Malawi, Swaziland, Burkina Faso, and Lesotho. From 2007 to 2009, it processed over 345 consultations, addressing various skin concerns like adverse drug reactions and HIV/AIDS-related diseases [27, 28].

6.5 The Swinfen charitable trust network

This innovative telemedicine system employed a low-cost, store-and-forward approach to connect healthcare workers in developing countries with a global network of volunteer consulting specialists. Launched in 1999, the program had grown to encompass over 163 hospitals across 60+ countries. Communication initially relied on email but later transitioned to a secure, web-based messaging platform accessible through any internet connection, eliminating the need for specialized software. Central to the program was a secure, centralized system where healthcare workers share anonymized clinical case details when requesting specialist advice. These volunteer specialists would offer their expertise free of charge. Despite its success, the network faces some challenges, including outdated equipment, unreliable internet access in some regions, navigating medicolegal considerations, and ensuring consistent specialist quality. Additionally, the network's rapid expansion has presented sustainability concerns [29–32].

6.6 Pan-African E-network

This ambitious project, a collaboration between India and Africa, aimed to build capacity through quality education and tele-expertise. It provided consultations by Indian medical institutions to African Union member states. While it successfully delivered degrees, telemedicine consultations, and continuous medical education sessions, the project was discontinued in 2017, with the infrastructure handed over to the African Union Commission [33].

These are just a few examples of the many telemedicine projects that have shaped the landscape in Sub-Saharan Africa. While challenges remain, such as digital divides, data security, and skilled personnel, the potential for telemedicine to revolutionize healthcare access and quality in the region is undeniable. With continued collaboration, innovation, and clear strategies for integration and sustainability, this technology can truly bridge the gap and bring vital healthcare services closer to those who need them most.

7. Application of telemedicine technologies in Africa

Telemedicine offers a variety of technologies, like video conferencing, mobile health apps, remote monitoring devices, electronic health records (EHRs) and wearable technologies. These technologies allow healthcare professionals to remotely consult with patients, manage and monitor their health, and manage records effectively. In Africa, mobile health applications have seen particular growth due to the continent's widespread smartphone use and expanding cellular and connectivity networks. As reported by GSMA Intelligence, 46% of the population in Sub-Saharan Africa were mobile phone subscribers in 2024, with smartphone adoption reaching 64%. GSMA predicts that Africa will gain 120 million new mobile subscribers by 2025, bringing the total to 615 million [34]. These applications empower patients to consult healthcare providers, schedule appointments, and access medical information directly from their mobile devices, offering convenient and accessible healthcare solutions.

Below are some of the applications of telemedicine in the continent:

7.1 Remote/virtual consultations

Remote or virtual consultations emerged in the 1980s and 1990s as a powerful tool connecting patients in remote locations with healthcare providers [1]. These consultations served as valuable tools in expanding and improving healthcare access, especially for patients with limited mobility or residing in resource-limited, geographically isolated areas. Remote consultations enabled consultations, diagnoses, and follow-up appointments, leading to improved access and outcomes [35]. The coronavirus pandemic further accelerated the adoption of remote consultations, normalizing their use and demonstrating their feasibility, safety, and effectiveness through initiatives like the Cabo Verde Telemedicine program [36], Réseau Afrique Francophone de Télémédecine (RAFT) [37] and REaCH studies in Tanzania and Nigeria [38]. Remote consultations can be used to support primary care providers by linking hospital-based physicians, enhancing integrated healthcare service delivery over a distance.

While ethical considerations regarding high-risk conditions, vulnerable populations, and technology access require careful attention, many regulatory bodies, such as the General Medical Council (GMC) in the United Kingdom, Health Education, and Improvement Wales, and the Health Professions Council of South Africa, recommend healthcare providers adopt the following high-level principles when conducting remote consultations. These principles ensure patient safety and quality care in a virtual or remote setting [39–41]:

1. Healthcare providers (HCP) must always prioritize patient safety. Concerns should be raised if the platform or system lacks adequate safeguards, including secure patient identification and verification protocols.

2. HCP should be capable of identifying vulnerable patients and taking appropriate steps to ensure their safety and well-being during the consultation.

3. Both the HCP and patients and others present should introduce themselves and their roles/titles at the start of the consultation. The HCP should explain the remote consultation process and address any concerns the patient may have.

4. Obtain informed consent from the patient, adhering to relevant mental capacity laws and applicable ethical codes.

5. The HCP should conduct a comprehensive clinical assessment, utilizing available or previous medical records and, if necessary, performing virtual examinations or requesting additional tests as required.

6. HCP should clearly explain all available options, including the right to decline treatment, in a language understandable to the patient.

7. The HCP should summarize the agreed treatment or action plans, highlighting any timelines and opportunities for further questions.

8. The HCP should update patient records accurately and immediately after the consultation.

9. The HCP should arrange for appropriate aftercare and, with the patient's consent, share relevant information with other healthcare providers involved in their care.

Table 1 shows some of the potential benefits and limitations of using telemedicine for remote or virtual consultations. Adopted from Khanji et al. [42].

7.2 Chronic disease management

Africa's healthcare systems, already grappling with infectious diseases like malaria, HIV/AIDS, and tuberculosis, face a growing threat from chronic illnesses like diabetes, heart failure, COPD, and autoimmune diseases [43]. In Tanzania, for instance, the prevalence of diabetes is on the increase, straining an already understaffed healthcare system with an 87.5% and 67% doctor shortage in the private and public sectors, respectively [44]. In SSA, about 24 million people were living with diabetes in Africa in 2021, predicted to increase by 129% to 55 million by 2045, according to the World Health Organization [45]. The same reports also note that more than half (54%) of people living with diabetes in the African Region remain undiagnosed.

	Potential benefits of remote consultations	Potential limitations of remote consultations
Patient	Real-time interaction over a distance	Inability to express symptoms or problems effectively, Limited access to technology, and internet connectivity
	Enhanced access to specialist expertise	Language barriers and cultural differences
	Convenience (e.g., for those with children elderly, immobilized, or those with disabilities etc.)	Privacy and data protection breaches
	Save travel costs	Reduced satisfaction from less clinical interaction (physical contact, body language, examination, clinic investigations, etc.)
	Saves time since no need for travel	Inability to conduct physical examination, Challenges with accurate diagnosis and treatment without physical examination
	Greater access to services	Peri-visit tests less readily available (blood, X-ray, ECG, etc.)
	Reduced risk of exposure to infectious diseases	Lack of trust in remote consultations
Healthcare system	Greater flexibility in service delivery models	Limited ability to provide urgent prescriptions
	Reduced requirement for hospital waiting areas	Need for staff training for effective delivery
	Increased efficiencies in cost	Potential for clinical risk from reduced ability to identify deteriorating patient's need for appropriate training and support for healthcare workers
	Reduced risk of nosocomial infection	Need for robust, potentially costly, clinical governance and local data protection systems
Other (environment/ societal)	Reduced pollution from vehicle travel	Higher energy consumption from internet data use/ storage with potential impact on environment and climate change
	Potential for innovation and software development	High cost of technology, interoperability challenges between different applications

Table 1.
Potential benefits and limitations of remote consultations.

Traditional healthcare delivery models struggle to keep pace with this rising burden, potentially leading to poor health outcomes. Innovative solutions are urgently needed. Telemedicine offers a promising approach to managing chronic diseases and alleviates pressure on healthcare systems. By enabling remote monitoring, medication reminders, and virtual support groups, among other telemedicine applications, it empowers patients to actively participate in their health management.

In Rwanda, a telemedicine program for diabetes patients using smartphones in primary health care settings showed a significant reduction in blood sugar levels compared to traditional care [46, 47]. During the COVID-19 pandemic, many providers across Africa adopted mental health tech startups like Wazi (Kenya), PsyndUp (Nigeria), MindIT (Ghana), and the MEGA project (South Africa and Zambia) to offer free virtual consultations, thereby facilitating easier and quicker access to mental health services [13, 48]. In Cameroon, TELEMED-CAM study assessed the role of telemedicine in controlling hypertension in rural villages. Cardiologists at a central hospital remotely connected with rural healthcare workers (nurses). After 24 weeks of follow-up, patients receiving telemedicine support, especially those at high risk, saw significantly better blood pressure control. This suggests telemedicine could be a valuable tool to improve chronic disease management in resource-limited regions [49].

Such programs not only free up healthcare workers for critical tasks but also improve patient engagement and access to specialist care and form part of an integrated healthcare delivery ecosystem. Investing in telemedicine technologies can significantly enhance existing healthcare systems and optimize the utilization of their limited workforce. This can also reduce travel costs by reducing the need to travel to seek specialist care and help break geographical barriers to access. Patients can also benefit from second opinions that were previously hard to obtain and make informed decisions about their health.

7.3 Medical education

Across Africa, a critical need exists to bolster human resources for health (HRH) to keep pace with growing demands. Advances in technology affect healthcare delivery and healthcare education in equal measure. With rapid advances in technology, we need to constantly evolve, adapt, and incorporate new and emerging technologies into the future healthcare worker. Medical institutions can leverage the power of technology to train, connect, and upskill healthcare professionals more effectively to meet pressing needs. Though new technologies are still emerging and evolving, changes such as asynchronous, 'on demand educational content,' learner-directed content, humanistic educational methods, use of artificial intelligence and large language model, and globally diverse learning communities with greater diversity are anticipated [50]. Newer technologies can offer more opportunities for distance learning in a more collaborative and personalized learning environment.

The coronavirus disease pandemic (COVID-19) pandemic served as a catalyst for technology adoption, demonstrating its crucial role in ensuring uninterrupted learning, fostering innovation, and wide-scale technology diffusion [51]. The rapid spread of coronavirus around the world and the need for social distancing coupled with the need to continue learning and carrying out required tasks enabled rapid adoption of technologies at an extraordinarily rapid pace. Experiences from the COVID-19 pandemic showed that telemedicine and tele-education offer scalability and overcome geographical barriers, minimizing the need for physical travel, though initial capital costs can be prohibitive. Further complicating the issue are reduced funding, budget cuts in medical education, and 'brain drain.' Embracing cutting-edge technologies like 3D printing, virtual reality, and real-time video simulations is crucial for driving innovation and tackling these challenges [52].

However, several hurdles need to be addressed:

1. Africa's ICT infrastructure lags behind, limiting access to technology.

2. Limited Internet speeds: poor download speeds hinder online learning

3. Unreliable electricity: erratic electricity supply disrupts technology-based learning.

4. High Internet COSTS: EXPENSIVE internet access creates another barrier.

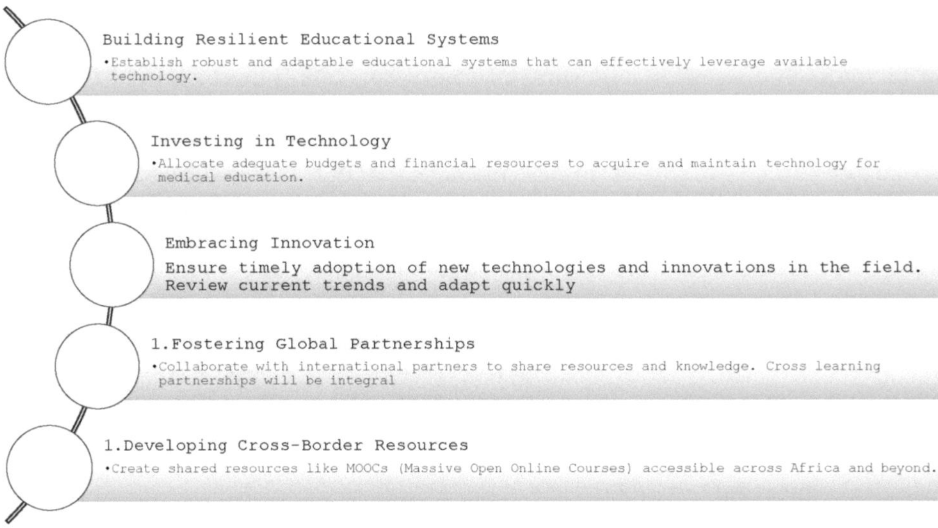

Table 2.
Multi-pronged approach needed to unlock telemedicine's potential in medical education across Africa.

To maximize the future of medical technology and education in Africa, a multi-pronged approach is necessary, as shown in **Table 2**.

8. Telemedicine: bridging the gap in healthcare access

Advancements in technology offer significant opportunities to revolutionize healthcare delivery in Africa. In many developing countries, both within and beyond the continent, these technologies can bridge the gap between existing services and unmet healthcare needs [4]. With rising disease burdens and growing populations amidst constrained healthcare budgets, technology offers a cost-effective solution to address these challenges. Increasing internet connectivity and mobile phone penetration across Africa empower individuals to actively participate in health promotion activities [34]. Access to tertiary medical care in underserved regions, made possible by telemedicine, allows scarce medical specialists to reach a wider patient population, improving quality of life and disease management. Telemedicine fosters continuous learning and skill development for both patients and healthcare providers [9, 50]. Additionally, it reduces the need for long-distance travel to access specialist care, saving valuable time and resources for patients and healthcare systems. By enabling simultaneous consultations across multiple regions, telemedicine further optimizes efficiency and resource utilization [10]. With the increasing use of mobile telephone devices, it is possible to provide care even in conflict zones or disaster hit areas where access to care may be difficult or unavailable in a timely manner [3]. If implemented well and supported, telemedicine programs may have far greater impact and success in Africa and other developing countries than in developed countries.

8.1 Benefits of telemedicine

See **Table 3**. Advances in technologies offer great opportunities for the advancement of healthcare services in Africa. In many developing countries in Africa and

Patients

□Access to care including specialist care or service.
•Improved early detection and intervention.
•Enhanced mental health support.
•Reduced stigma associated with certain conditions.
•Increased adherence to treatment plans
•Empowerment through health education
•Saves costs and time.
•Can be used in conflict or disaster hit areas.

Healthcare providers

□Improved efficiency and productivity
•Enhanced collaboration and consultation
•Reduced burden on healthcare systems
•Support for continuing medical education.
•Expansion of reach and impact

Health systems

•Reduced environmental impact- reducedcarbon foot print
•Empowerment of rural communities
□Economic opportunities: New jobs and new businesses
□Bridge the gaps in healthcare service delivery
□Improve public health outcomes

Table 3.
Investment in telemedicine brings numerous benefits to all stakeholders in the healthcare sector, including patients, providers, systems, and governments. Various stakeholders can collectively work toward achieving the shared vision of improving healthcare access, enhancing patient outcomes, and building more resilient and sustainable healthcare systems for the future.

beyond, technologies offer opportunities to bridge the gaps and fulfill the unmet healthcare needs of their citizens. With increasing disease burden and growing population amidst meager or reducing healthcare budgets, efficient application and use of technology may bridge some of the unmet health needs around the world.

Increased investment in internet connectivity through 4G, 5G, and cable connections coupled with increased smartphone penetration in many countries in Africa will provide opportunities to utilize these emerging technologies to reach millions of people across Africa [34]. With reduced end to end latency, faster bandwidths and reduced congestion will enhance seamless connectivity will enhance user experience and increased adoption [53–55]. Access to tertiary medical care in underserved regions in Africa providing opportunities for very few medical specialists to serve deserving patients overcome physical and geographical barriers [14]. Access of specialist services through telemedicine also reduces the need for patients to travel over long distances for the search of specialist care, hence saving valuable time and money.

9. Telemedicine barriers

Successful implementation and utilization of telemedicine in Africa depends on understanding and addressing its various barriers. Here are some of the most common barriers faced in Africa:

9.1 Infrastructure technology

Limited access to electricity and unreliable grids in many regions frequently disrupt vital telemedicine communications due to power outages. Additionally, across much of Africa, internet connectivity is either absent or slow, hindering the quality of services offered. The high cost of equipment and software creates a significant barrier to entry, as highlighted in a recent Kenyan survey [56]. A functional telemedicine unit requires various functional equipment, including video conferencing rooms, video cameras, and electronic stethoscopes, which may not be readily available or accessible, particularly in rural Africa, where these services are urgently required [57]. Fortunately, increasing Internet and grid connectivity across many parts of Africa promises to break these access barriers. However, it is important to note that these changes remain unevenly distributed across the continent, with remote and rural localities experiencing the most need and often the least progress.

9.2 Organizational barriers

Organizations play a crucial role in shaping culture and societal norms, including in areas related to healthcare. However, the widespread adoption of telemedicine in Africa faces challenges due to limited expertise and experience within both staff, who ultimately shape organizational culture across the continent. This limited knowledge and inadequate training can lead to reduced professional competency in using or applying available telemedicine applications and technologies [58]. Such shortcomings can have a negative impact on adoption, restricting the potential benefits of the technology and even fostering negative attitudes. Additionally, a lack of understanding about telemedicine services and their potential impact can exacerbate resistance to this new technology, leading to reduced motivation and delayed adoption. Models such as the Systems Engineering Initiative for Patient Safety (SEIPS) can provide organizations with useful frameworks that help in better adoption of new technologies [59]. The SEIPS model ensures healthcare systems or technologies through multiple lenses, namely person, technologies, environment, tasks, and organization. Such a model can outline various system components and how they interact and ultimately contribute to the successful implementation of telemedicine (**Table 4**).

9.3 Legal and regulatory hurdles

Widespread adoption of telemedicine requires a comprehensive legal and regulatory framework [60]. Governments across Africa are providing the required legal and policy frameworks to support the uptake and growth of telemedicine. Such frameworks facilitate the seamless integration and dissemination of technologies across both private and public sectors. Establishing clear policies and regulations is crucial to ensure meticulous handling of patient data, required security measures, licensures, approved funding models, quality standards, and confidentiality requirements [1, 2, 61]. Implementing robust data protection regulations Health Insurance Portability and Accountability Act of 1996 in the United States of America (HIPAA or the Kennedy–Kassebaum Act) ensures compliance, strengthens patient trust, and fosters an environment of secure and responsible data handling, protection of individual's health records and continued medical care [62]. It is also important to emphasize that the legal and regulatory landscape should be adapted to local context for ease of adoption and to serve local needs. Successful policies from the West may not be effective in Africa [53].

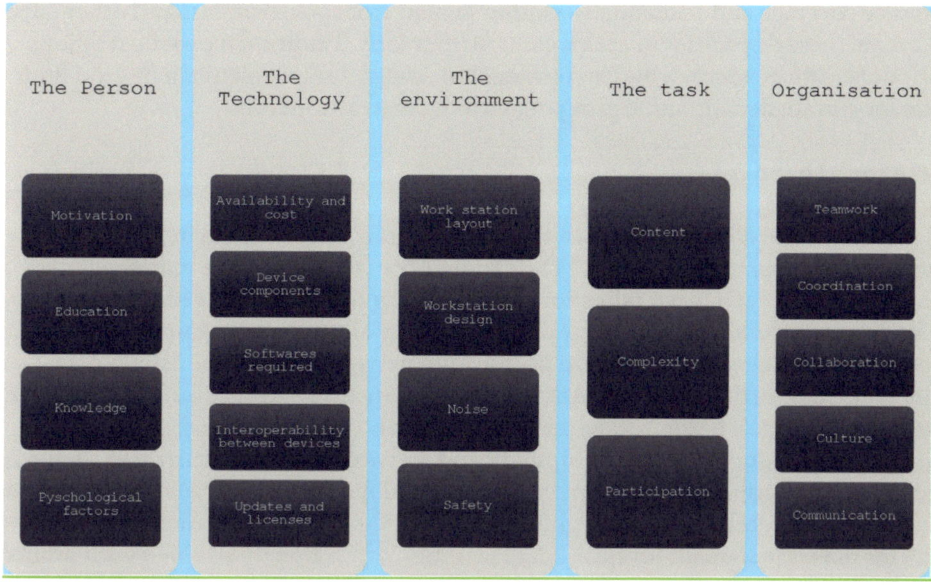

Table 4.
Illustrating the SEIPS model highlighting the key to successful telemedicine implementation and the role of understanding the interconnectedness of patients, technologies, networks, practices, and healthcare institutions, modified from T. Zhang et al. [59].

9.4 Individual barriers to telemedicine

These barriers encompass various factors affecting both patients and providers. Healthcare providers may perceive telemedicine as a threat to their professional autonomy due to fears of misdiagnosis, litigation, and loss of control over patient care.

This resistance to change can stem from concerns about conflict of interest, increased workload, limited information and technology infrastructure, technophobia, difficulty understanding the technology, and anxiety about using new technologies [63, 64]. Limited or lack of integration of telemedicine services into daily workflow and low motivation for compliance can affect adoption by healthcare providers. Lack of physical examination or face-to-face contact with patients diminishes the personal touch, leading to some physician skepticism toward the effectiveness of telemedicine [63]. This can make healthcare providers fear litigation for fear of misdiagnosis. Clear guidelines for prompt referral to a hospital need to be provided to ensure the risk of adverse events is minimized.

Both healthcare providers and patients may have concerns regarding the secure handling of sensitive medical information and the protection of data privacy and confidentiality during telemedicine consultations. Clear communication of data protection mechanisms in place in telemedicine platforms should be emphasized. Factoring the recent adoption of new and emerging technologies in telemedicine in the continent, digital illiteracy presents as an important barrier for both patients and providers. Digital illiteracy can hinder their ability to effectively engage with telemedicine platforms and technologies [56, 57]. Poverty and low socioeconomic status significantly limit access to technology gadgets such as mobile phones and internet connectivity, creating substantial barriers for patients seeking to utilize telemedicine services. Moreover, lack of insurance coverage and inadequate reimbursement from governments and other payers exacerbate these disparities in access even further [56]. Traditional beliefs, religious restrictions, and gender norms can influence attitudes toward telemedicine and limit access for certain demographic groups such as women and elderly.

9.5 Financial barriers

Limited budget allocation for health infrastructure and telemedicine support remains an important barrier [63]. While some African nations have increased healthcare spending, it often falls short of addressing the required needs of widescale telemedicine implementation. The lack of budgetary allocation for training healthcare professionals, developing robust communication networks, and establishing data centers impedes further progress. Additionally, reliance on external funding and grants creates uncertainties, hinders long-term planning, and raises sustainability concerns [65]. High costs associated with equipment and software are a particularly challenging issue in African nations. The continent's fragmented market, with numerous countries and diverse needs, often leads to higher prices for specialized telemedicine technologies. This makes it difficult for healthcare facilities, often already strained with limited resources, to invest in necessary hardware and software. Furthermore, the need for reliable technical support and maintenance further adds to the financial burden. High electricity costs and erratic power supplies often create disruptions and hinder access to telemedicine services. Unequal access to electricity across urban and rural areas exacerbates existing disparities, leaving remote and rural communities further marginalized [63]. While internet penetration is increasing, affordability and reliability continue to be major concerns. Rural areas often lack access to broadband connections, and mobile data costs can be exorbitant for many individuals across many countries. This creates a barrier, particularly for those who could benefit most from the convenience and accessibility of telemedicine. High taxation tariffs on telemedicine equipment, software, and other supplies significantly increase procurement and operational costs for healthcare providers, ultimately discouraging adoption and hindering access to services in Africa.

Increasing telemedicine penetration across Africa requires significant and sustained financial investment. Governments must take the lead by increasing budgetary allocations. Budgetary allocations will support the development of critical telemedicine physical infrastructure, the acquisition of essential equipment and technology, and ongoing training and capacity building for healthcare professionals. Efforts to expand insurance coverage and revise/review reimbursement rates should be supported. Expanding health insurance schemes, particularly for low-income populations, would make telemedicine a more viable option for accessing healthcare. Furthermore, establishing fair reimbursement rates for virtual consultations will incentivize both patients and providers to utilize telemedicine. Exploring alternative financial models should be considered. Public-private partnerships can leverage the expertise and resources of both the public and private sectors to accelerate the adoption and use of telemedicine. This collaborative approach can unlock the potential of telemedicine and expedite its widespread adoption across the continent.

10. Conclusion

Telemedicine, the use of information and communication technologies to provide healthcare services remotely, is emerging as a promising solution to address unmet healthcare needs in Africa. With the increasing availability and adoption of various mobile and fixed technologies, coupled with growing electrification and internet connectivity across the continent, the potential for telemedicine remains immense. It promises to bridge the unmet healthcare needs in an acceptable, cost-effective, and sustainable manner. While tremendous progress has been made in recent years, accelerated by the 2019 COVID-19 pandemic, several challenges limit access for those in urgent need. These challenges include the persistent digital divide, particularly between rural and urban areas, the lack of comprehensive legal and policy frameworks, provider and patient barriers, cultural beliefs that may hinder adoption, and concerns regarding data protection and safety. Unlocking telemedicine requires a concerted multifaceted approach involving stakeholders across various sectors in Africa to address barriers while nurturing the role of telemedicine across the continent.

Author details

Simon Onsongo[1*] and Elizabeth Kagotho[2]

1 Aga Khan Hospital, Kisumu, Kenya

2 Aga Khan University Hospital, Nairobi, Kenya

*Address all correspondence to: simonya@live.com

References

[1] Telemedicine I of M (US) C on ECA of, Field MJ. Evolution and Current Applications of Telemedicine. 1996. Available from: https://www.ncbi.nlm.nih.gov/books/NBK45445/ [Accessed: February 11, 2024]

[2] Okoroafor IJ, Chukwuneke FN, Ifebunandu N, et al. Telemedicine and biomedical care in Africa: Prospects and challenges. Nigerian Journal of Clinical Practice. 2017;**20**:1-5

[3] Eikelboom RH. The telegraph and the beginnings of telemedicine in Australia. Studies in Health Technology and Informatics. 2012;**182**:67-72

[4] Services B on HC, Medicine I of. The Evolution of Telehealth: Where Have We Been and Where Are We Going? 2012. Available from: https://www.ncbi.nlm.nih.gov/books/NBK207141/ [Accessed: February 17, 2024]

[5] Nicogossian AE, Pober DF, Roy SA. Evolution of telemedicine in the space program and earth applications. Telemedicine Journal and E-Health. 2001;7:1-15

[6] Doarn CR, Nicogossian AE, Merrell RC. Applications of telemedicine in the United States space program. Telemedicine Journal. 1998;**4**:19-30

[7] Freiburger G, Holcomb M, Piper D. The STARPAHC collection: Part of an archive of the history of telemedicine. Journal of Telemedicine and Telecare. 2007;**13**:221-223

[8] Brown FW. Rural telepsychiatry. Psychiatric Services. 1998;**49**:963-964

[9] Thrall JH. Teleradiology. Part I. History and clinical applications. Radiology. 2007;**243**:613-617

[10] Norris TG. Telemedicine and teleradiology. Radiologic Technology. Nov-Dec 1999;**71**(2):139-164

[11] Rosen R, Wieringa S, Greenhalgh T, et al. Clinical risk in remote consultations in general practice: Findings from in-COVID-19 pandemic qualitative research. BJGP Open. 2022. DOI: 10.3399/BJGPO.2021.0204;**6**. Epub ahead of print 1 September 2022

[12] Raju AS, le Roux HE, Pretorius PJ, et al. Psychologists' experiences with telepsychology during the COVID-19 pandemic in South Africa. Health SA. 2024;**29**:2392

[13] Jaguga F, Kwobah E. Mental health response to the COVID-19 pandemic in Kenya: A review. International Journal of Mental Health Systems. 2020;**14**. Epub ahead of print 18 August 2020. DOI: 10.1186/S13033-020-00400-8

[14] Cahan EM, Maturi J, Bailey P, et al. The impact of telehealth adoption during COVID-19 pandemic on patterns of Pediatric subspecialty care utilization. Academic Pediatrics. 2022;**22**:1375-1383

[15] Nguyen OT, Watson AK, Motwani K, et al. Patient-level factors associated with utilization of telemedicine services from a free clinic during COVID-19. Telemedicine and e-Health. 2022;**28**:526-534

[16] Ye S, Kronish I, Fleck E, et al. Telemedicine expansion during the COVID-19 pandemic and the potential for technology-driven disparities. Journal of General Internal Medicine. 2021;**36**:256-258

[17] World Health Organization. The Global Health Observatory. 2022.

Available from: https://www.who.int/data/gho/data/themes/hiv-aids/data-on-the-size-of-the-hiv-aids-epidemic [Accessed: August 12, 2022]

[18] van Dyk L. A review of telehealth service implementation frameworks. International Journal of Environmental Research and Public Health. 2014;**11**:1279-1298

[19] Gajarawala SN, Pelkowski JN. Telehealth benefits and barriers. The Journal for Nurse Practitioners. 2021;**17**:218

[20] Wójcik S, Rulkiewicz A, Pruszczyk P, et al. Beyond ChatGPT: What does GPT-4 add to healthcare? The dawn of a new era. Cardiology Journal. 2023;**30**:1018

[21] Azevedo MJ. The state of health system(s) in Africa: Challenges and opportunities. In: Historical Perspectives on the State of Health and Health Systems in Africa. Vol. II. United States: American Society of Radiologic Technologists; 2017. p. 1. Available from: http://www.radiologictechnology.org/

[22] Chronic staff shortfalls stifle Africa's health systems: WHO study | WHO | Regional Office for Africa. Available from: https://www.afro.who.int/news/chronic-staff-shortfalls-stifle-africas-health-systems-who-study [Accessed: February 11, 2024]

[23] Shiferaw F, Zolfo M. The role of information communication technology (ICT) towards universal health coverage: The first steps of a telemedicine project in Ethiopia. Global Health Action. 2012;**5**:15

[24] Mohamed KG, Hunskaar S, Abdelrahman SH, et al. Telemedicine and E-learning in a primary care setting in Sudan: The experience of the Gezira family medicine project. International Journal of Family Medicine. 2015;**2015**:1-7

[25] Bediang G, Perrin C, de Castañeda RR, et al. The RAFT telemedicine network: Lessons learnt and perspectives from a decade of educational and clinical Services in low- and middle-incomes Countries. Frontiers in Public Health. 2014;**2**. Epub ahead of print 7 October 2014. DOI: 10.3389/FPUBH.2014.00180

[26] Brauchli K, Oberholzer M. The iPath telemedicine platform. Journal of Telemedicine and Telecare. 2005;**11**(Suppl 2). Epub ahead of print December 2005. DOI: 10.1258/135763305775124795

[27] telederm.org Africa. Available from: http://africa.telederm.org/ [Accessed: February 13, 2024]

[28] Weinberg J, Kaddu S, Gabler G, et al. The African Teledermatology project: Providing access to dermatologic care and education in sub-Saharan Africa. The Pan African Medical Journal. 2009;**3**:16

[29] Patterson V, Swinfen P, Swinfen R, et al. Supporting hospital doctors in the Middle East by email telemedicine: Something the industrialized world can do to help. Journal of Medical Internet Research. 2007;**9**. Epub ahead of print 2007 10.2196/JMIR.9.4.E30

[30] Swinfen Telemedicine. 2024. Available from: https://www.swinfentelemed.org/ [Accessed: February 14, 2024]

[31] Swinfen R, Swinfen P. Low-cost telemedicine in the developing world. Journal of Telemedicine and Telecare. 2002;**8**:63-65

[32] Vassallo DJ, Swinfen P, Swinfen R, et al. Experience with a low-cost telemedicine system in three developing

countries. Journal of Telemedicine and Telecare. 2001;7:56-58

[33] Pan-African E-Network. 2024. Available from: https://www.nepad.org/agenda-2063/flagship-project/pan-african-e-network [Accessed: February 13, 2024]

[34] Sub-Saharan Africa: mobile penetration 2021-2025* | Statista. Available from: https://www.statista.com/statistics/1133365/mobile-penetration-sub-saharan-africa/ [Accessed: February 17, 2024]

[35] Vodička S, Zelko E. Remote consultations in general practice – A systematic review. Slovenian Journal of Public Health. 2022;**61**:224

[36] Azevedo V, Latifi R, Parsikia A, et al. Cabo Verde telemedicine program: An update report and analysis of 2,442 teleconsultations. Telemedicine Journal and e-health: The Official Journal of the American Telemedicine Association (Larchmont, NY, United States: Mary Ann Liebert, Inc.). 2021;**27**:172-177. Available from: http://online.liebertpub.com/loi/tmj. ISSN: 1078-3024

[37] Bagayoko CO, Müller H, Geissbuhler A. Assessment of Internet-based tele-medicine in Africa (the RAFT project). Computerized Medical Imaging and Graphics. 2006;**30**:407-416

[38] Sturt J, Griffiths F, Ajisola M, et al. Safety and upscaling of remote consulting for long-term conditions in primary health care in Nigeria and Tanzania (REaCH trials): Stepped-wedge trials of training, mobile data allowance, and implementation. The Lancet Global Health. 2023;**11**:e1753-e1764

[39] HEIW. Remote Consultation Principles. 2024. Available from: https://heiw.nhs.wales/workforce/workforce-development/remote-consultation-principles/ [Accessed: February 11, 2024]

[40] GMC. Remote Consultations. 2024. Available from: https://www.gmc-uk.org/professional-standards/ethical-hub/remote-consultations [Accessed: February 11, 2024]

[41] Rabe M. Telehealth in South Africa: A guide for healthcare practitioners in primary care. South African Family Practice. 2022;**64**. Epub ahead of print 2022. DOI: 10.4102/SAFP.V64I1.5533

[42] Khanji MY, Gallagher AM, Rehill N, et al. Remote consultations: Review of guiding themes for equitable and effective delivery. Current Problems in Cardiology. 2023;**48**:101736

[43] Achieng MS, Ogundaini OO, Achieng M. Digital health and self-management of chronic diseases in sub-Saharan Africa: A scoping review. South African Journal of Information Management. 2022;**24**:8

[44] Sirili N, Kiwara A, Nyongole O, et al. Addressing the human resource for health crisis in Tanzania: The lost in transition syndrome. Tanzania Journal of Health Research. 2014;**16**. Epub ahead of print 2014. DOI: 10.4314/THRB.V16I2.6

[45] Africa | Regions | International Diabetes Federation. 2024. Available from: https://idf.org/our-network/regions-and-members/africa/ [Accessed: February 12, 2024]

[46] Lygidakis C, Uwizihiwe JP, Kallestrup P, et al. Community- and mHealth-based integrated management of diabetes in primary healthcare in Rwanda (D^2Rwanda): The protocol of a mixed-methods study including a cluster randomised controlled trial. BMJ

Open. 2019;**9**. Epub ahead of print 1 July. DOI: 10.1136/BMJOPEN-2018-028427

[47] Roodenbeke E de, Lucas S, Rouzaut A, et al. eHealth in Rwanda. 2011. Available from: https://www.ncbi.nlm.nih.gov/books/NBK310723/ [Accessed: February 12, 2024]

[48] Adepoju P. Africa turns to telemedicine to close mental health gap. Lancet Digital Health. 2020;**2**:e571-e572

[49] Kingue S, Angandji P, Menanga AP, et al. Efficiency of an intervention package for arterial hypertension comprising telemanagement in a Cameroonian rural setting: The TELEMED-CAM study. The Pan African Medical Journal. 2013;**15**. Epub ahead of print 29 August 2013. DOI: 10.11604/PAMJ.2013.15.153.2655

[50] Tokuç B, Varol G. Medical education in the era of advancing technology. Balkan Medical Journal. 2023;**40**:395

[51] Owolabi J, Bekele A. Medical educators' reflection on how technology sustained medical education in the most critical times and the lessons learnt: Insights from an African medical school. Digital Health. 2021;**7**. Epub ahead of print 16 November 2021. DOI: 10.1177/20552076211059358/ASSET/IMAGES/LARGE/10.1177_20552076211059358-FIG1.JPEG

[52] Olatunji G, Osaghae OW, Aderinto N. Exploring the transformative role of 3D printing in advancing medical education in Africa: A review. Annals of Medicine and Surgery. 2023;**85**:4913

[53] Chitungo I, Mhango M, Mbunge E, et al. Digital technologies and COVID-19: Reconsidering lockdown exit strategies for Africa. The Pan African Medical Journal. 2021;**39**. Epub ahead of print 2021. DOI: 10.11604/PAMJ.2021.39.93.29773

[54] Ogbodo EU, Abu-Mahfouz AM, Kurien AM. A survey on 5G and LPWAN-IoT for improved smart cities and remote area applications: From the aspect of architecture and security. Sensors (Basel). 2022;**22**. Epub ahead of print 1 August 2022. DOI: 10.3390/S22166313

[55] Chávez-Santiago R, Szydełko M, Kliks A, et al. 5G: The convergence of wireless communications. Wireless Personal Communications. 2015;**83**:1617-1642

[56] Onsongo S, Kamotho C, Rinke de Wit TF, Lowrie K. Experiences on the utility and barriers of telemedicine in healthcare delivery in Kenya. International Journal of Telemedicine and Applications. 2023;**2023**:1487245, 1-10. DOI: 10.1155/2023/1487245v

[57] Telemedicine I of M (US) C on ECA of, Field MJ. The Technical and Human Context of Telemedicine. 1996. Available from: https://www.ncbi.nlm.nih.gov/books/NBK45449/ [Accessed: February 19, 2024]

[58] Dodoo JE, Al-Samarraie H, Alzahrani AI. Telemedicine use in sub-Saharan Africa: Barriers and policy recommendations for Covid-19 and beyond. International Journal of Medical Informatics. 2021;**151**:104467

[59] Carayon P, Schoofs Hundt A, Karsh BT, et al. Work system design for patient safety: The SEIPS model. Quality & Safety in Health Care. 2006;**15**:i50

[60] Dodoo JE, Al-Samarraie H, Alsswey A. The development of telemedicine programs in sub-Saharan Africa: Progress and associated challenges. Health and Technology (Berl). 2022;**12**:33

[61] Haleem A, Javaid M, Singh RP, et al. Telemedicine for healthcare: Capabilities, features, barriers, and applications. Sensors International. 2021;**2**:100117

[62] Edemekong PF, Annamaraju P, Haydel MJ. Health insurance portability and accountability act. Encyclopedia of Information Assurance. 2022:1299-1309. Available from: https://www.ncbi.nlm.nih.gov/books/NBK500019/

[63] Dhyani VS, Krishnan JB, Mathias EG, et al. Barriers and facilitators for the adoption of telemedicine services in low-income and middle-income countries: A rapid overview of reviews. BMJ Innovations. 2023;**9**:215-225

[64] Borges do Nascimento IJ, Abdulazeem H, Vasanthan LT, et al. Barriers and facilitators to utilizing digital health technologies by healthcare professionals. npj Digital Medicine. 2023;**6**:1-28

[65] Karamagi HC, Njuguna D, Kidane SN, et al. Financing health system elements in Africa: A scoping review. PLoS One. 2023;**18**. Epub ahead of print 1 September 2023. DOI: 10.1371/JOURNAL.PONE.0291371

Chapter 14

Innovations to Enhance Engagement and Efficacy in a mHealth Psychological Intervention Targeting Grief: Lessons Learned and Future Directions

Liliane Efinger, Maya Kheyar, Valentino Pomini, Laurent Berthoud, Robin Wicki and Anik Debrot

Abstract

mHealth psychological interventions have gained popularity among both researchers and the general public as a means to address a variety of psychological problems or disorders. However, despite the increasing use of these interventions, there is a lack of clear guidelines on how to implement them successfully. This chapter focuses on LIVIA 2.0, a mHealth psychological intervention developed to address prolonged grief symptoms experienced after bereavement or romantic dissolution. Drawing on empirical sources, the program included several innovations aimed at improving engagement and outcomes compared to its former version, LIVIA-FR. These innovations included providing guidance on demand, sending automated reminders, tailoring the intervention to the specific needs of each user, assessing and promoting personal resources, and targeting autobiographical memory and identity adjustment. This chapter describes each innovation and presents the descriptive results regarding the usefulness of each strategy that were obtained within a randomized controlled trial. The chapter concludes by examining the outcomes of these innovations and provides practical recommendations for researchers looking to develop mHealth psychological interventions.

Keywords: mHealth, psychological interventions, tailoring, innovations, engagement, grief

1. Introduction

Mental health issues are a significant challenge worldwide, with an estimate of one in every eight people, or 970 million people around the world, experiencing a mental disorder during their lifetime [1]. The digital revolution has opened new avenues for delivering psychological interventions to improve mental health issues *via* the internet. Internet-based psychological interventions (IBIs) are a type of mHealth interventions and are defined as "treatments that are mainly delivered via the internet with at least some therapeutic tasks delegated to the computer" [2]. Cognitive behavioral therapy (CBT) is the most employed and researched type of IBI (ICBT) [3, 4].

Even though IBIs may encounter certain challenges and barriers [5], they offer numerous advantages over conventional face-to-face interventions such as cost-effectiveness, accessibility, flexibility in time and place of delivery [6–9], and even anonymity [10]. Indeed, mHealth psychological interventions can be accessed from any location with an internet connection and can be delivered at a lower cost, making them more accessible to those with limited financial resources or underserved populations, particularly in rural areas [11]. Moreover, they allow both patients and clinicians to work at their own pace and reduce the stigma of having a mental disorder or going to a psychologist or therapist [6, 12].

IBIs can be classified into three categories based on their format and delivery mode: Self-guided, therapist-guided, and blended interventions [13]. Self-guided interventions are fully automated and designed to be self-administered without therapist support. Therapist-guided interventions involve a trained mental health professional who provides different levels of support and feedback through e-mail, brief phone calls, or short messages [14] on top of the online program. Finally, blended interventions combine face-to-face sessions with internet-based sessions into one integrated treatment [15, 16].

A large amount of randomized controlled trials (RCTs) [17, 18] and meta-analyses suggest that IBIs are effective for treating a wide range of mental health conditions [19–21]. However, most studies in this field show that therapist-guided interventions report a higher efficacy compared to self-guided ones and achieve equivalent effects to face-to-face therapy psychotherapies [22–25].

However, despite the evidence supporting the effectiveness of IBIs, their implementation can be challenging. A significant problem that arises in IBIs is high dropout rates, particularly in self-guided interventions [26, 27]. Indeed, engagement tends to be highly variable and inconsistent, leading to problems in retention, data quality, and clinical impact [28]. Evidence suggests that attrition rates for IBIs are quite high with an average dropout rate around 40% [26, 29]. Research on non-usage attrition has demonstrated an initial rapid decline in program use over the first few weeks, with most attrition occurring within the first month of the intervention [30]. Eysenbach [31] proposed the term "law of attrition" to describe the phenomenon of participants dropping out of IBIs at a higher rate. Self-administered IBIs suffer from higher attrition than guided IBIs [22]. The reasons are complex and multifaceted [22, 32].

Several factors to improve adherence to IBIs have been identified, such as reminders to visit or return to the website or to complete research data [31, 33–35]. Adherence operates on two levels: (1) within the IBI itself and (2) within the research project [31, 36]. Adherence to the IBI refers to the extent to which participants comply with and follow the guidelines and recommendations of the internet-based treatment or program [32]. This includes their willingness to engage with the intervention, their level of completion of the recommended activities, and their overall commitment to the program. Adherence to the research project refers to the extent to which participants adhere to established procedures during a study, including their commitment to completing questionnaires and providing feedback at different stages of the study.

Adherence is essential for ensuring that research findings are reliable and valid and can inform clinical practice and policy [28]. Moreover, adherence to the program is crucial for maximizing the effect of the intervention, the primary objective of which is to improve mental health [37, 38].

Given the importance of adherence for the success of IBIs, it is crucial to design interventions that are user-friendly and engaging and that address the challenges faced by individuals seeking mental health care. By doing so, we can improve adherence rates and therefore maximize the potential impact of such interventions. However, despite the increasing use of IBIs, guidelines for successful implementation are lacking [39].

1.1 Our project

Hereafter, we present our experience with LIVIA 2.0, a cognitive behavioral online program for prolonged grief symptoms after bereavement or romantic dissolution. LIVIA 2.0 was developed with the aim to include several innovations to LIVIA, the original program for grief-related symptoms after bereavement or separation, which demonstrated its efficacy in German and in therapist-guided format *via* an RCT for both bereaved and separated individuals [40]. LIVIA consisted of ten text-based sessions and covered topics such as emotional reactions in the context of interpersonal loss, obstacles to successful adaptation, and possibilities for overcoming them. For more information on the program's content, please refer to Brodbeck et al. [40].

Given that no empirically-assessed IBI for grief existed in French [41], we translated the original LIVIA program from German into French and adapted it into a self-guided program (LIVIA-FR) [42]. Results from a pilot study showed that out of 148 interested individuals, 41 participants completed the pretest and 29 completed the post-test questionnaire. With 12 people dropping out of the study between pretest and posttest, the attrition rate was 29.2% for our self-guided program LIVIA-FR compared to the original German program, which offered guidance by a therapist, which had an attrition rate of 13.6%. In terms of psychopathological symptoms, the results showed a significant reduction in grief symptoms ($d = 0.66$) and in avoidance strategies ($d = 0.69$). Satisfaction with the program was good with more than two-thirds of participants giving a positive or neutral assessment. The results of our pilot study highlighted a promising tool but also showed weaknesses, which led us to develop an upgraded version called LIVIA 2.0.

LIVIA 2.0 was, therefore, developed based on theoretical and empirical findings on grief processes and IBIs to improve users' adherence and program efficacy compared to its original version, LIVIA-FR. Regarding the content, LIVIA 2.0 consists of 10 sessions. These include an introductory session, a closing session, and eight sessions in between belonging to four modules. Theoretically anchored in the dual process model of coping (DPM) [43, 44], one of the most influential models of coping with loss, each module features a session focused on loss and another on restoration. Indeed, according to the DPM, coping with loss involves two separate and interacting processes: A loss- and restoration-oriented process. The loss-oriented process involves facing the reality of the loss and the restoration-oriented process involves adjusting to an environment without the lost person. The DPM postulates that to efficiently cope with the loss people oscillate between the two processes. Therefore, LIVIA 2.0 imitates the oscillation process in the DPM by alternating between loss- and restoration-focused sessions.

The modules have the following main themes: cognitions, emotions, behaviors, and identity. The sessions involving these modules are composed of psychoeducational information and exercises. In each session, participants can choose between three variations of an exercise (some exercises vary in content, others in duration). They are expected to complete one exercise per session but can complete all three available exercises if they wish to. LIVIA 2.0 also contains texts, audio and video files, and interactive quizzes. Participants were able to contact a health professional upon request through a contact button on the program's homepage. For more details about the content of each session, please refer to the study protocol [45]. A total of 62 individuals participated in the trial, with 29 participants assigned to LIVIA 2.0 and 33 participants assigned to LIVIA 1. The results showed that 37.9% of the participants in LIVIA 2.0 failed to complete the posttest and dropped out of the program, while 42.4% of the participants in LIVIA 1 dropped out [46].

This chapter will provide an overview of the five innovations implemented in LIVIA 2.0 and examine their success and relevance for the future of mHealth psychological interventions. It will also present descriptive results regarding their implementation to shed light on the potential benefits they may bring to the field.

2. Innovations implemented in LIVIA 2.0

2.1 Guidance on demand

Recent research has shown that adding guidance to an IBI improves effectiveness and retention rates [38]. However, additional research has nuanced this finding. Indeed, in their meta-analytic review, Moshe et al. [25] showed that guidance has less benefits when implemented in more interactive IBI. Moreover, as shown hereafter, several studies indicate that optional guidance might be a reasonable alternative to weekly guidance. In a large, naturalistic trial testing the effectiveness of five self-help cognitive behavior e-therapy programs for different anxiety disorders. Klein et al. showed that, out of 2660 people who subscribed for an anxiety-oriented online intervention, only 75 (2.8%) chose to have a weekly e-mail guidance, whereas the rest chose a fully automated program. Additionally, a few studies have implemented guidance on demand and compared it to weekly per default guidance. In a RCT assessing the effectiveness of an IBI for social phobia, Berger et al. [17] compared a self-guided intervention group to a weekly therapist-guided intervention group and to a therapist-guided on-demand group. The intervention was equally efficient for all groups. In a RCT of an iCBT program for anxiety and depression symptoms, Hadjistavropoulos et al. [47] showed that participants send half as many messages with optional guidance compared to weekly guidance. Moreover, even if optional guidance was associated with more dropouts, the effectiveness was similar to that of the weekly guidance group. Finally, in an uncontrolled trial with a similar program, Hadjistavropoulos et al. [48] showed that, even if only 22% of participants chose optional (vs. weekly) support, both groups achieved similar symptom reduction. This encouraged us to propose a guidance on demand (and not a default weekly guidance) to the participants in our study.

In both our control (LIVIA-FR) and experimental interventions (LIVIA 2.0), participants had continuous access to a contact form when they were logged into their accounts. We informed them during the introduction session that they could contact our team of psychologists whenever they felt the need. In LIVIA 2.0, they were additionally reminded on several occasions within the program that they could contact us. We committed to providing an answer within three working days. To analyze the requests for the present paper, we counted as one conversation a request by a participant, the answer from our team, and the potential answer of the participant. Two members of our team independently coded the requests according to a predefined coding scheme with the following categories: (1) "technical problem," (2) "understanding problem," (3) "need for support," and (4) "announcing the withdrawal from the program.". For e-mails from category 3, we applied the motive-oriented therapeutic relationship (MOTR), an approach that relies on the underlying motives of the patient to guide the therapeutic interventions [49] and has been argued to have the potential to boost the efficiency of the guidance within IBIs [50]. Hence, before responding to the participant, we conducted a Plan Analysis [51], a case formulation method that allows to identify the potential underlying motives of the participant at play based not only on the content of the e-mail but also on the responses to the pre-test questionnaires and to the program exercises (when available).

We received an e-mail from 15 of the 29 participants (52%) for a total of 29 conversations. When coding the content of the e-mails, we achieved an interrater reliability of $\kappa = 0.94$. Most requests (12 requests, 57%) concerned technical issues. No participant contacted us for an understanding problem and four (19%) announced their withdrawal from the program. Five requests (24%) concerned specifically a guidance request, stemming from a single participant.

For this participant, we first conducted a Plan Analysis within our team, which revealed two main themes: (1) "*Avoid putting your activities on pause,*" which satisfied the plan "*Avoid feeling loneliness and your husband's absence,*" and (2) "*Do your best,*" which fulfilled the plan "*Avoid showing your vulnerability.*" We tailored our response to their initial e-mail to consider these plans. The participant's response was enthusiastic, and they followed our recommendations while also sharing more intimate feelings. Afterward, they contacted us several times during the program, either to ask other questions related to the completion of the program or to share intimate thoughts that the program and our exchange had stimulated.

These results indicate that, when completing LIVIA 2.0, only very few participants asked for support. Only a small percentage of participants contacted us for guidance, and most of the requests were related to technical issues rather than emotional difficulties or program completion problems. While the percentage of participants requiring guidance corresponds to previous studies that reported 48–60% of the participants requiring guidance [17, 47], the content of the requests differs with the majority of participants contacting our team for technical support. One possible explanation for this low rate of proper guidance requests might be that we did not remind participants often enough that they could request guidance, contrary to Berger et al. [17]. Upon detailed consideration, the results of previous studies indicate that participants who are least in need of support are the ones benefiting from a guidance-on-demand format. Indeed, Berger et al. [17] showed that those requesting guidance were the ones most involved in the use of the program. Moreover, Hadjistavropoulos et al. [48] found that only people who had lower levels of symptoms chose a guidance on demand over a weekly guidance. It might be that our sample was in higher need of support be it because of the nature of the symptoms (grief symptoms are associated with more isolation) [52–54], because of the symptom load of the sample, or because of the timing of the research, which occurred after the COVID-19 crisis [41]. Indeed, COVID-19-related isolation was shown to predict poorer cognitive and mental health outcomes, as well as less healthy behaviors [55].

Nevertheless, our experience with applying MOTR to our IBI, even though limited, was satisfactory and showed potential to increase alliance and engagement within the program. In summary, relying on the present evidence, we recommend using a default weekly guidance and applying MOTR in IBIs targeting grief symptoms.

2.2 Automated reminders

Several studies have highlighted the positive aspects of using reminders in the context of IBIs. Ritterbrand et al. [56] found that e-mail reminders increased by 45% program logins, while Hutchesson et al. [57] found that enhanced program features, including reminders and tailored feedback, facilitated greater adherence to their web-based program. Additionally, when given the choice, people prefer to receive reminders to use programs and applications [34, 35, 58]. Other researchers have found no significant difference between phone and postcard reminders in terms of login frequency, making e-mail reminders a particularly appealing option as they require fewer resources and are cheap and easy to disseminate [33, 59]. Christensen et al. [60] conducted a RCT to evaluate the effectiveness of different types of reminders for an internet-based mental health intervention. Their study included five groups in total: Three treatment groups and two control groups. The treatment groups received either e-mail reminders, telephone reminders, or combined e-mail and telephone reminders, while one control group received a placebo website without any reminders and the other control group received the placebo website with telephone calls. Participants in the website condition with e-mail reminders group had the highest login frequency of 6.8 times per week, followed by the combined e-mail and telephone reminder group with 4.8 times per week, the telephone reminder groups with 4.4 times per week, the control group with the placebo website without reminders with 3.6 times per week, and the control group with calls reminders had the lowest login frequency with 3.3 times per week. In sum, the researchers of the study found that e-mail reminders were the most effective and efficient way to promote adherence to the IBI. Additionally, the website with e-mail reminders was the most preferred program among all conditions. These results highlighted the importance of considering participants' preferences and the use of cost-effective methods in the design of IBIs to enhance adherence [60].

Regarding the frequency of reminder delivery, Fry and Neff's [61] systematic review uncovered that reminder sent at a periodic interval minimized the use of assistance from a health professional resource. Schneider et al. [30, 62] also highlighted the importance of temporality by showing that reminders sent at the beginning of the intervention are the most relevant. Indeed, they noted that participants who received an e-mail 2 weeks after their first visit logged in to the program significantly more often compared to participants receiving the e-mail after 6 weeks.

For LIVIA 2.0, in an effort to enhance participant retention, automated e-mails were sent (a) when a new session becomes available and (b) if the participant has not logged into LIVIA 2.0 for seven consecutive days. Regarding adherence to the research project, a total of six reminders could be sent per participant during the study, including three reminders e-mails at each stage (pretest and posttest) before they were deemed to have dropped out. For the present paper, we counted the number of reminders e-mails that each participant received directly from LIVIA 2.0. The e-mails function was to notify either: (a) the opening of a new session, or (b) the observation of a nonconnection to the program. For the automated research e-mails, we also counted the number of e-mails sent per participant at each stage of the research project.

Regarding e-mails sent to increase program adherence, the LIVIA 2.0 program automatically sent 231 e-mails in total to 27 participants to notify them that the new session was available. More precisely, out of eight people who completed the entire study, an average of 17.75 (min = 17 and max = 19) e-mails were sent. For the remaining 19 participants, an average of 4.68 (min = 1 and max = 16) e-mails were sent for an average of 2.26 (min = 0 and max = 5) modules completed. In addition, 107 e-mails in total were sent to 27 participants to notify them that they had not logged in in seven consecutive days. More precisely, out of eight people who completed the entire study, an average of 6.88 (min = 2 and max = 14) e-mails were sent. For the remaining 19 participants, an average of 2.89 (min = 1 and max = 8) e-mails were sent.

Regarding adherence to the research project, at the pre-test stage, we sent five reminders to five different participants. Twenty-two participants needed no reminders to fulfill the pre-test questionnaire. In summary, 27 participants completed the pretest after receiving at the most one reminder. For the most committed participants in the project and program, eight participants, who completed the entire program (all modules), needed no reminders to complete the pre-test questionnaires. At the post-test stage, we sent 36 automated reminders to 27 participants. A total of 11 participants needed no reminders to complete the post-test questionnaires, five participants needed one reminder, two participants needed two reminders, and nine participants received three reminder e-mails and did not complete the post-test questionnaires. In summary, 18 participants completed the posttest after receiving at the most two reminders. Out of eight participants who completed both the post-test questionnaires and all the modules of LIVIA 2.0, 5 of them did not need any reminders, two participants needed one reminder and one participant needed two reminders. Importantly, one participant decided to stop participating in the project, mentioning that they felt pressured because of the multiple e-mails they were receiving.

The analyses have led us to make several conclusions regarding the use of automated reminders to increase adherence to IBIs. Firstly, the results indicate that a substantial number of reminders were sent to participants, with varying effects on adherence. While some participants completed the program successfully without any reminders, others required multiple reminders. It is, therefore, important to strike a balance in the frequency of reminders to avoid overwhelming participants and potential negative effects. Our study acknowledges that it is difficult to determine the exact impact of reminders on completion rates within the LIVIA 2.0 program. Limited information is provided on the individual responses and experiences of participants, except for one participant who mentioned feeling pressured due to multiple e-mails. Further, research is needed to gain a better understanding of the specific impact of reminders on adherence and participant experiences. Despite the potential negative effects experienced by a minority of participants, the cost-effectiveness ratio of implementing automated reminder e-mails remains attractive. The majority of participants appeared to benefit from reminders. Researchers are encouraged to consider the overall positive impact of reminders while being mindful of potential negative effects and participant experiences. Finally, it is strongly recommended to monitor the frequency of e-mails received by participants from different sources. Tracking the number of reminders and the sources they originate from can help researchers ensure that participants are not overwhelmed with excessive reminders. Monitoring the frequency will also help identify patterns and optimize the reminder strategy for better participant engagement.

2.3 Tailored recommendations and exercise selection

Tailoring is the process of designing customized communications by collecting and evaluating personal data to determine the most appropriate information or strategies to meet an individual's specific needs, preferences, and characteristics [63]. It has been found that tailoring individualized messages for each participant can be more effective than presenting generic information in terms of program engagement, self-efficacy, and health behavior improvement [64]. Tailored information is more likely to be processed more intensively, remembered, and perceived as personally meaningful than generic information [65]. It could be argued that some degree of tailoring may be needed for people suffering from the loss of a loved one as each significant relationship and path with the grieving process is unique.

To enhance program adherence and to address the observation that participants tend to open most of the modules at the beginning of the program to see what it offers before selecting which module they want to start with,[1] we developed personalized recommendations about the order in which to complete the modules in LIVIA 2.0. Automatic and personalized recommendations (e.g., start with the "emotion" module, followed by the "behavior" module, etc.) were made based on a questionnaire in which each participant had reported their program goals and priorities in the introduction module (see **Table 1**). The program recommended the modules in order of their importance for each participant. Regardless of their answers to the questionnaire, participants were able to choose the completion order freely. This implies that all participants did not experience the same navigation journey to complete LIVIA 2.0. The aim of this innovation was to evaluate the tailored recommendations based on participant goals and priorities, hypothesizing it would enhance program adherence.

Moreover, another level of tailoring was applied within the navigation of each module, where three choices of exercises were offered so that participants could select the exercise they felt suited their needs the most. For instance, in the loss-focused session in the emotion module, participants had the choice between three audio exercises: (1) a 5-minute self-compassion break, (2) a 12-minute acceptance exercise, and (3) a 20-minute emotion awareness exercise. The answers generated by the program were different according to the exercise chosen and the participants' answers.

Results showed that of the 29 LIVIA 2.0 participants, eight (27.6%) completely finished the program and 21 (72.4%) did not, six (20.7%) followed the module recommendation order, eight (27.6%) did not, and the data for 15 (51.7%) were not available as the participants did not pursue the program far enough to extract this information. Regarding dropouts, these happened for 11 participants during the introduction session, for four during the emotion module (all occurred during the session dealing with loss), for three during the behavior module (1 occurred during the session dealing with loss, two during the restoration session), for two during the cognition module (one occurred at the very beginning of the module, one occurred during the session dealing with restoration), and for one during the identity session dealing with loss.

The module recommendation order was very diversified among the 17 participants for whom the recommendation order was provided, with 10 different orders established. The most common orders were "cognition-emotion-identity-behavior" and "cognition-identity-emotion-behavior," both of which were the recommendation

---

[1] We made this observation in our pilot study with the LIVIA-FR program [42].

It is important for me...	Not at all 1	2	3	4	5	6	7	8	9	Very 10	Related module
... to be able to do the things (activities) that give me satisfaction											Behavior
... to better understand who I am today (my identity)											Identity
... to be able to confront situations that remind me of the person lost											Behavior
... to feel and accept my negative emotions (e.g., anger, sadness, guilt)											Emotions
... not to let my negative thoughts overwhelm me											Thoughts
... project myself into a future that makes sense to me											Identity
... allow myself to experience positive emotions (e.g., pleasure, joy, peacefulness)											Emotions
... develop more positive ways of thinking											Thoughts

Table 1.
Questions asked to establish order of modules recommendations for sessions 2–9.

order for three participants. The cognition module was suggested most frequently as the first choice for nine participants, followed by the emotion (5), behavior (2), and identity (1) modules. The behavior module was most frequently recommended as the last module to be completed for 10 participants, followed by the cognition (3), emotion (2), and identity (2) modules.

Regarding the selection of the exercises within a session, 67% of the participants completed one exercise, 16% completed two, and 16% completed all three. Generally, the first exercise proposed was the most often selected in every session.

The recommendation order was very diversified among participants, even with a sample size as small as ours. Therefore, no specific participant profiles or individual differences may be extracted. Nevertheless, this indicates that participants have a great diversity in their priorities when completing an IBI. However, some tendencies can be outlined. For more than half of the sample, the cognition and behavior modules were recommended as the modules to start and finish with, respectively. Approximately, half of the participants (42.8%) followed the recommended order. Future research could help better understand how participants experience this specific kind of tailoring. For example, why did some participants not follow the recommended order? Is the endorsement of the recommendation associated with the outcome?

Finally, regarding the selection of the choice of exercises within a session, the experience of the present study indicates that most participants selected only one exercise and chose the first one available. Thus, if program developers have limited means to develop the content, we would recommend proposing a single exercise per session.

2.4 Assessment and promotion of personal resources

Clinical psychology and psychotherapy have long offered methods based on the principle of resource activation in patient assessment, treatment planning, and psychological interventions [66, 67]. Problem-solving techniques and solution-focused approaches are two classic examples of effective psychotherapeutic interventions that build on this paradigm in individual and family psychotherapy [68–70]. Picked up in particular by the positive psychology approach, identifying and especially mobilizing people's resources are seen as important vectors for change and well-being [71]. These principles are also echoed in internet therapies and chatbots [72].

There are few psychometric instruments, especially in French, that provide a broad profile of a person's individual resources (psychological and social), which do not focus on specific positive skills or dispositions (coping, optimism, creativity, gratitude, forgiveness, etc.) or which does not rely on very long inventories to assess a full range of resources, such as Seligman's values in action assessing character strengths [73, 74].

The tool, known as AERES (from French "Auto-Evaluation des RESsources": resources self-evaluation) [75] addresses these gaps, offering a tailored approach to assess and activate patients' resources, contributing to symptom alleviation and enhanced quality of life. It is a resource self-assessment instrument based on card sorts and a semi-structured interview, initially developed and validated with a population of patients with chronic psychiatric disorders [75]. AERES covers 31 domains under three dimensions of resources: The individual's personal qualities, their leisure activities and passions, and their external resources (social and environmental). The sorting is done for each type of resource in two steps: First, the person selects all the resources they believe they have, and then they take each resource and evaluate its effectiveness for their personal recovery. For each selected resource, the person indicates the extent to which it contributes to their well-being, and whether it is useful, especially when they are not feeling well. This evaluation allows to distinguish the present/absent resources and, among the present resources, the ones that can be mobilized and the ones that are effectively mobilized for the recovery or restoration of well-being.

We integrated a computerized version of AERES in LIVIA 2.0, whereby participants completed it during the introductory session. The self-assessment of resources process was simplified to reduce its duration and thus limit the length of the first program session. Nevertheless, it pursues the usual goals of this type of task: Firstly, to complement an otherwise problem- and symptom-focused clinical assessment with a more positive view of oneself; secondly, to encourage the use of personal resources to cope constructively with negative events or challenges; and thirdly to stimulate the use of resources in case of difficulties encountered during an intervention (e.g., a tedious, painful, or stressful exercise in the program). For this reason, participants were able to access their personal resource profile at any time by clicking on a dedicated button.

A computerized version of AERES was developed within the LIVIA 2.0 program and was proposed in the introductory session. Compared to the original tool, only the sorting of cards illustrating the resources was retained. As the computer tool obviously does not allow to carry out a semi-structured clinical interview, this part of the AERES was removed. The instruction on the usefulness of each resource was adapted to focus attention on grief management (and not recovery in the more general sense of the term). The sorting of the cards was expected to take 3–5 minutes. It resulted in a personal profile that was presented in three independent sections (leisure and passions, social and environmental resources, and personal qualities). In each section, the participant could see all the cards that they considered as personal resources and then their classification according to their usefulness in the management of grief. No comments or graphics accompanied this pictorial and synthetic presentation.

Of the 29 participants, 17 people completed the AERES in the introductory session (the 12 who did not also did not go further in the program). Eleven people reported having a total of more than 20 resources, four people between 18 and 20, and three between 14 and 16. Except for one person who indicated having only three personal qualities, there were at least four resources listed in each of the three areas. On average, the participants checked off 6.7 leisure/passions resources (SD = 1.7, min. 4, max. 9), 6.2 socio-environmental resources (SD = 1.2; min. 4, max. 8), and 8.9 personal qualities (SD = 2.8; min. = 3, max. = 12).

As shown in **Table 2**, the most cited personal qualities are humor (16×), courage, curiosity, perseverance (15×), reflection, gratitude, and hope (14×). The least cited resources are optimism (7×) and self-confidence (9×). Regarding socio-environmental resources, family and nature (16×) along with acquaintances and friends (15×) are the most selected ones; health professionals are the least cited (3×) with romantic relationships (7× anyway) and pets (6×). Playing sports (16×), traveling (15×), and watching TV/listening to the radio/surfing the internet (15×) are the most frequently mentioned leisure activities. Creative activities (plastic arts, 7×), playing games, and singing/playing music (8×) are the least frequently reported of this category. Compared to the data collected from 213 psychiatric patients [76], the profiles observed here show that our participants have more resources overall. In terms of personal qualities, our participants mentioned more often than the psychiatric patients having humor, courage, curiosity, perseverance, reflection, or spirituality;

	Resources	N (max = 17)	Percent	Psychiatric sample (%)*
Personal qualities	Humor	16	94.1	82.2
	Self-esteem	9	52.9	51.6
	Courage	15	88.2	76.5
	Curiosity/love of exploration	15	88.2	80.3
	Perseverance	15	88.2	73.2
	Wonder/savoring	11	64.7	66.7
	Body consciousness	11	64.7	62.0
	Reflectiveness	14	82.4	75.1
	Optimism	7	41.2	62.4
	Gratitude	14	82.4	92.0
	Spirituality	11	64.7	78.4
	Hope	14	82.4	56.3
Leisure activities and passions	Acquaintances	15	88.2	70.0
	Work	11	64.7	45.1
	Family	16	94.1	77.9
	Friends	15	88.2	76.5
	Romantic relationships	7	41.2	38.5
	Professional healthcare	3	17.6	85.9
	Living place	15	88.2	81.7
	Pet	6	35.3	39.0
	Nature	16	94.1	79.3
External resources	Cooking	9	52.9	63.8
	Sports	16	94.1	52.6
	Singing/playing an instrument	8	47.1	36.6
	Plastic arts	7	41.2	45.5
	Gardening/home repairing	10	58.8	37.1
	Reading/writing	13	76.5	70.0
	Going to a show	13	76.5	57.3
	Music/radio/TV/internet	15	88.2	93.0
	Traveling/visiting/ excursions	15	88.2	58.7
	Playing games	8	47.1	56.8

**Percentage of the selected resources by a psychiatric sample of N = 218 [76].*

Table 2.
Cumulative frequencies of resources considered present by the participants.

they reported as much self-confidence, wonder, and listening to one's body or hope but less optimism and gratitude. We also observed significant differences in the socio-environmental resources, where our sample ticked off more of these resources than the psychiatric patients, except for health professionals (who were naturally less present because the people receiving therapy could not take part in the study), romantic relationships, or pets. In terms of hobbies/passions, the differences are mainly in favor of our sample, except for cooking and games, which seem to be less practiced.

Once the AERES was completed, seven of the 17 people clicked at least once on their resource profile during the program: three returned once, one twice, and four three times. Unfortunately, it is not possible to know at what times and for what reasons these participants revisited their resource profile, knowing that this could have been part of one or another LIVIA 2.0 exercise or a tip given by the program in case of difficulty in completing an exercise.

Once the AERES was completed at the beginning of the program, it must be noted that the personal resource profile was consulted rather rarely by the participants. Even though the principle of providing a reminder of one's own resources at any given time could have been considered relevant, particularly in the case of difficulty in accomplishing certain tasks, its implementation remained unsatisfactory in view of the low number of times that participants explicitly and purposefully called upon their personal resources. Should we conclude that the self-assessment of personal resources is not relevant in this context and may not be included in an IBI?

In clinical practice, the original AERES is supplemented by a semi-structured interview that is particularly important because it stimulates recovery by focusing attention on new perspectives that are not necessarily focused on difficulties or problems. Points not retained in the computerized form are the selection of resources that the person wishes to develop or discover, which opens up a whole field of positive recovery-oriented interventions. The standardized nature of LIVIA 2.0 obviously did not allow this option to be explored. Apart from the few exercises that mobilize the results of the AERES, the availability of this inventory, therefore, remains largely unused and does not resolve the paradox associated with all resource-based interventions; if people are able to identify and mobilize their resources to solve their difficulties, they do not need the help of a therapist. It is doubtful that a relatively standardized program that simply brings out a list of resources is sufficient to bring about significant change. In this sense, it would probably have been more relevant to have the profile carried out at the same time as the exercises significantly require the use of personal resources, in order to optimize the profiles obtained from the outset. The exercise could also be split up to better focus attention on each of the resource areas. By being briefer, and more focused on a particular aspect of one's own resources, the person may have more opportunity to reflect on the presence and mobilization of their strengths to better deal with both the painful aspects of the loss and the new perspectives that it opens up in their life.

2.5 A module focused on identity and autobiographical memory

Autobiographical memory, which refers to memories from the past personal experiences, plays a crucial role in social interactions [77], helps us plan the future [78], and shapes our emotional experiences [79]. Our personal memories are also intertwined with our sense of self and help us understand who we are [80, 81]. Autobiographical memory disturbances can manifest in different ways according to the psychological disorder [82]. For people experiencing prolonged grief disorder, the image of the lost person remains central to the person's sense of self; they have what they called a merged identity. In these people, the image of the lost person continues to fuel personal goals, motivations, and future plans, as if detachment could not be achieved. This has implications for autobiographical memory retrieval and goal development [83]. Indeed, individuals with prolonged grief disorder are more likely to recall past memories related to the lost person and have difficulties recalling specific and positive past events or envisioning future events without the lost person [84, 85].

Therapies that employ cognitive-behavioral techniques are efficacious in ameliorating the symptoms of prolonged grief [86] such as exposure to memories of the death, behavioral activation, and restructuring of maladaptive appraisals. However, up to 50% of individuals do not respond to treatment and it is possible that these people are those characterized by a merged self-identity, for which the mere idea of doing better might imply a threatening de-merging from the lost person [83]. By addressing identity and autobiographical memory disturbances, patients with prolonged grief symptoms may benefit further from existing CBT programs. To our knowledge, no intervention for grief-related symptoms has specifically focused on these elements. To address this gap, we developed an innovative online module focused specifically on identity and autobiographical memory.

The identity module, such as the other three modules in LIVIA 2.0, consists of two sessions. In this module, the loss-oriented session aimed to help individuals process and integrate their experience of loss into their autobiographical memory. The participants could choose up to three exercises designed to help individuals revisit memories with and without the lost person, in order to explore the relationship between these memories and their sense of self. This session aims to support the development of a more congruent sense of self. In the restoration-oriented session, the focus lay on specific adaptive autobiographical memories and on specific adaptive future projections, for example, about pleasant activities or personal qualities. The session offered three exercises for individuals to choose from, aiming to help them identify and envision future goals that are meaningful and rewarding, and in harmony with their values and interests. By helping individuals develop positive and adaptive future goals, this session aims to support the maintenance of a positive and coherent sense of self over time. After finishing each exercise in LIVIA 2.0, participants were asked to complete an online evaluation containing an assessment of the utility of the exercise on a scale of zero (not at all) to five (extremely). Participants who answered 0 or 1 were required to explain why they found the exercise unhelpful, while those who answered between two and five were asked to elaborate on how the exercise proved useful. Based on this assessment, we collected quantitative and qualitative data from 14 participants about the usefulness of the different exercises proposed in the identity module. We used a thematic content analysis method [87], which involved coding and categorizing the data to identify key themes related to the usefulness of the different exercises proposed.

First results indicated high levels of utility, $M = 3.13$ on a scale ranging from zero (not at all) to five (extremely) for the six exercises included in the module. The thematic content analysis of participants' responses highlighted six main themes:

1. Self-reflection and identity: participants found value in exploring their own values, positive qualities, and independent activities.

   It made me realize that I have given up activities that I used to enjoy and that I need to focus more on group activities. (ID 9)

2. Future orientation: participants appreciated thinking about the future and setting goals, which helped them find direction and envision a life beyond the loss.

   It is useful to project into the future because I am stuck in my present sadness and regrets of having lost Harry. (ID 1)

3. Memory exploration: participants found it useful to recall different memories that they may not be used to remember, such as positive memories of the deceased or memories unrelated to the lost person.

   Reading this part of the module, I realize that I think all the time of my life with Harry, as described for the selective autobiographical memory. By doing this exercise, it is the first time that I look for memories elsewhere and it makes me think a lot. (ID1)

4. Positive mindset and personal growth: participants enjoyed focusing on the positive aspects of life and adopting a more optimistic perspective.

   I can see the positive side of my life. (ID4)

5. Progress monitoring: participants found beneficial that the exercises helped them monitor their progress in coping with grief and identify areas for improvement.

   It is useful to see that I have made good progress in my grief. I can consider a holiday abroad. (ID 4)

6. Difficulties and uncertainties: a few participants (4) faced challenges in completing exercises or understanding the objectives.

   I am not sure I am in the requested target. (ID 2)

Identity and autobiographical memory disturbances are common in psychological disorders, particularly in prolonged grief [83], and can hinder recovery [82]. The online module described above offers an innovative approach to address these disruptions. The findings indicate that the identity-focused module was generally beneficial for participants coping with the loss of a closed one. However, addressing the difficulties and uncertainties some participants experienced is crucial to enhance the overall effectiveness and accessibility of the module. Future research should continue to explore the effectiveness of this type of intervention focusing on autobiographical memory and mental projection into the future in treating psychological disorders.

3. Conclusions

IBIs have a tremendous potential to improve mental health access and outcomes. However, the challenge of high dropout rates remains a significant obstacle [88, 89]. To address this issue, researchers and practitioners must work to develop effective strategies for enhancing engagement and reducing attrition. The mHealth psychological intervention LIVIA 2.0 incorporated five key innovations aimed at improving engagement and outcomes compared to its predecessor, LIVIA-FR. These innovations included guidance on demand, automated reminders, tailored recommendations and exercise selection, the assessment of personal resources, and a module focused on identity and autobiographical memory.

The guidance on demand feature showed limited success as only few participants requested help to move forward in the program. Future research could explore the reasons people did not contact us. However, the limited evidence we gathered regarding the application of a MOTR approach shows promise as the response of the participants was clearly positive and it helped them pursue the program with motivation. In light of the current evidence, we would recommend using a weekly guidance and applying MOTR in IBIs targeting grief symptoms.

Automated reminders have gained attention as a promising strategy to enhance participant adherence to IBIs [56–58]. However, to ensure their effectiveness and minimize potential drawbacks, it is crucial to strike a balance in reminder frequency. We recommend considering the individual needs and preferences of participants when determining the timing and frequency of reminders. Finding the right balance is crucial to encourage adherence without becoming burdensome. Moreover, to gain a deeper understanding of the impact of reminders on participant adherence and experiences, further research is needed. Studies with different formats, timing, and wording to identify the most impactful design elements. Quantitative data on completion rates should be complemented with qualitative data to explore the effects of reminders beyond mere completion. Investigating participant perspectives, motivations, and barriers will inform the development of more effective reminder strategies.

Finally, clearly communicate the purpose and benefits of reminders, emphasizing how they support participants' engagement and treatment outcomes. Provide participants with options to manage or modify their reminder preferences, empowering them to have control over their experience. Finally, to assess the impact of reminders, it is important to include comprehensive measures in research protocols. Beyond completion rates, gather data on participant experiences, satisfaction, and perceived helpfulness of reminders. A systematic evaluation will provide insights into the overall effects of reminders on adherence and engagement, enabling researchers to refine their strategies accordingly.

The innovation of providing tailored recommendations and exercise selection showed limited success, as only half of the participants followed the recommended order to complete the modules in LIVIA 2.0, while the remaining participants chose their own path. This indicates that giving the choice to participants to select the order of completion that best suits them appears as a good solution. Additionally, the participants tended to select only the first exercise proposed out of the three options presented in each session. When designing mHealth psychological interventions, it is crucial to consider the diversity of participant needs and incorporate tailored content accordingly. However, our results suggest also that offering multiple exercise options may not be necessary as it is time-consuming to implement compared to the limited use that our participants made of it.

The integration of the AERES tool [75] into a mHealth psychological intervention is a promising innovation, aiming to provide a positive resource-focused approach to therapy. However, participant engagement with this tool in LIVIA 2.0 was quite low, indicating a need for further refinement. Future research should focus on ways to improve user interaction with this tool, potentially through more personalized and interactive methods. This could involve reintegrating components included in the semi-structured interview from the original AERES, such as the selection of resources that the person wishes to develop, discover, or breaking down the resource identification process into more manageable, focused sections in link with the currently proposed content of the intervention. While this innovation signifies a step toward a more resource-oriented therapeutic approach, its effective implementation within mHealth psychological intervention remains a challenge to be addressed.

The module focusing on identity and autobiographical memory disturbances has shown some promise in addressing key issues in prolonged grief, as evidenced by positive participants' feedback on its usefulness. Identity and autobiographical memory disruptions are common features across various psychological disorders and can significantly hinder the recovery process [82]. Therefore, the positive reception of an identity-focused module in LIVIA 2.0 from the participants suggests that it could be a valuable addition to mHealth psychological interventions. The novelty of such an approach underscores the necessity for further rigorous investigation to demonstrate its effectiveness across a broader population. Moreover, it is important to continue improving the content and delivery of this type of interventions with special attention to overcoming potential difficulties and uncertainties of the participants. This endeavor is integral to the advancement of treatment methods in the field of grief therapy and beyond. **Table 3** provides a summary of each innovation implemented in LIVIA 2.0 along with their respective results and recommendations.

Currently, LIVIA 2.0 has not been translated into other languages beyond French. Expanding LIVIA to include more languages could enhance accessibility. Future translations and adaptations should consider cultural nuances to ensure the intervention's effectiveness across diverse settings [90]. This approach underscores the

Innovation	Result	Recommendation
Guidance on demand	This type of contact was not as successful as anticipated. Only a very low proportion of participants contacted us, and mainly for technical reasons.	We recommend using a default weekly guidance.
Automated reminders	Aside from one participant who explicitly shared their experience with email, we do not know what impact the reminders had on other participants.	We recommend the use of reminders since there were no detrimental consequences for not having them.
Tailored recommendations and exercise selection	Half of the participants followed the recommended order to complete the modules in LIVIA 2.0, while the remaining participants chose their own path.	We recommend limiting users to one exercise per session instead of giving them the freedom to choose multiple exercises.
Assessment and promotion of personal resources	e-AERES implementation remained unsatisfactory in view of the low number of times that participants explicitly and purposefully called upon their personal resources.	We recommend splitting up e-AERES to better focus attention on a particular aspect of resources. This way a person will have more opportunity to reflect on the presence and mobilization of their strengths.
A module focused on identity and autobiographical memory	The identity-focused module was generally appreciated and beneficial for participants coping with the loss of a close one.	We recommend using an identity-focused module for IBIs targeting grief because of its successful implementation and positive participant reception.

Table 3.
Summary of each innovation implemented in LIVIA 2.0, along with their respective results and recommendations.

necessity of adapting both the content and delivery of LIVIA 2.0 to resonate with different cultural backgrounds, thereby addressing the global mental health treatment gap more effectively.

By learning from the successes and limitations of innovations such as those in LIVIA 2.0, researchers can further refine and develop effective mHealth psychological interventions to address a wide range of mental health issues. MHealth psychological interventions can transcend traditional barriers of time place or stigma, making mental health support more accessible and personalized. However, the road to fully realizing this potential is challenging. As we navigate this path, continuous collaboration between researchers, mental health professionals, and the people for whom these tools are designed (for example by using co-designs) [91] will remain a vital ingredient.

Acknowledgements

The present study is funded by the Swiss National Science Foundation, Grant 100014_182840 (AD, VP). It is supported by the center LIVES (Swiss Center of Expertise in Life Course Research), which is financed by the Swiss National Science Foundation (grant number: 51NF40-185901). The University of Lausanne, CARLA laboratory (Cognitive and Affective Regulation Laboratory) provides the infrastructure and salaries of a part of the team (AD, RW, LE, VP). This funding source had no role in the design of this study and will not have any role during its execution, analyses, interpretation of the data, or decision to submit.

Conflict of interest

The authors declare no conflict of interest.

Author details

Liliane Efinger*†, Maya Kheyar†, Valentino Pomini, Laurent Berthoud, Robin Wicki and Anik Debrot
Institute of Psychology, University of Lausanne, Lausanne, Switzerland

*Address all correspondence to: efinger.liliane@gmail.com

† The first two authors contributed equally to this work and are listed alphabetically by last name.

References

[1] WHO. World mental health report: Transforming mental health for all. 2022. Available from: https://www.who.int/publications/i/item/9789240049338

[2] Andersson G, Titov N. Advantages and limitations of Internet-based interventions for common mental disorders. World Psychiatry. 2014;**13**: 4-11. DOI: 10.1002/wps.20083

[3] Andersson G. Internet-delivered psychological treatments. Annual Review of Clinical Psychology. 2016;**12**:157-179. DOI: 10.1146/annurev-clinpsy-021815-093006

[4] Richards D, Enrique A, Palacios J, Duffy D, Richards D, Enrique A, et al. Internet-delivered cognitive behaviour therapy. In: Cognitive Behaviour Therapy – Clinical Applications. IntechOpen; 2017. DOI: 10.5772/intechopen.71412

[5] Rochlen AB, Zack JS, Speyer C. Online therapy: Review of relevant definitions, debates, and current empirical support. Journal of Clinical Psychology. 2004;**60**:269-283. DOI: 10.1002/jclp.10263

[6] Cuijpers P, van Straten A, Andersson G. Internet-administered cognitive behavior therapy for health problems: A systematic review. Journal of Behavioral Medicine. 2008;**31**:169-177. DOI: 10.1007/s10865-007-9144-1

[7] Donker T, Blankers M, Hedman E, Ljotsson B, Petrie K, Christensen H. Economic evaluations of Internet interventions for mental health: A systematic review. Psychological Medicine. 2015;**45**:3357-3376. DOI: 10.1017/S0033291715001427

[8] Kazdin AE, Blase SL. Rebooting psychotherapy research and practice to reduce the burden of mental illness. Perspectives on Psychological Science. 2011;**6**:21-37. DOI: 10.1177/1745691610393527

[9] Price M, Yuen EK, Goetter EM, Herbert JD, Forman EM, Acierno R, et al. mHealth: A mechanism to deliver more accessible, more effective mental health care. Clinical Psychology & Psychotherapy. 2014;**21**:427-436. DOI: 10.1002/cpp.1855

[10] Wallin EE, Mattsson S, Olsson EM. The preference for Internet-based psychological interventions by individuals without past or current use of mental health treatment Delivered online: A survey study with mixed-methods analysis. JMIR Mental Health. 2016;**3**:e25. DOI: 10.2196/mental.5324

[11] Summers-Gabr NM. Rural-urban mental health disparities in the United States during COVID-19. Psychological Trauma. 2020;**12**:S222-S224. DOI: 10.1037/tra0000871

[12] Ebert DD, Berking M, Thiart H, Riper H, Laferton JAC, Cuijpers P, et al. Restoring depleted resources: Efficacy and mechanisms of change of an internet-based unguided recovery training for better sleep and psychological detachment from work. Health Psychology. 2015;**34S**:1240-1251. DOI: 10.1037/hea0000277

[13] Erbe D, Eichert HC, Riper H, Ebert DD. Blending face-to-face and Internet-based interventions for the treatment of mental disorders in adults: Systematic review. Journal of Medical Internet Research. 2017;**19**:e306. DOI: 10.2196/jmir.6588

[14] Palmqvist B, Carlbring P, Andersson G. Internet-delivered

treatments with or without therapist input: Does the therapist factor have implications for efficacy and cost? Expert Review of Pharmacoeconomics & Outcomes Research. 2007;7:291-297. DOI: 10.1586/14737167.7.3.291

[15] Kooistra LC, Wiersma JE, Ruwaard J, van Oppen P, Smit F, Lokkerbol J, et al. Blended vs. face-to-face cognitive behavioural treatment for major depression in specialized mental health care: Study protocol of a randomized controlled cost-effectiveness trial. BMC Psychiatry. 2014;**14**:290. DOI: 10.1186/s12888-014-0290-z

[16] Wentzel J, van der Vaart R, Bohlmeijer ET, van Gemert-Pijnen JE. Mixing online and face-to-face therapy: How to benefit from blended care in mental health care. JMIR Mental Health. 2016;**3**:e9. DOI: 10.2196/mental.4534

[17] Berger T, Hammerli K, Gubser N, Andersson G, Caspar F. Internet-based treatment of depression: A randomized controlled trial comparing guided with unguided self-help. Cognitive Behaviour Therapy. 2011;**40**:251-266. DOI: 10.1080/16506073.2011.616531

[18] Klein JP, Berger T, Schroder J, Spath C, Meyer B, Caspar F, et al. Effects of a psychological Internet intervention in the treatment of mild to moderate depressive symptoms: Results of the EVIDENT study, a randomized controlled trial. Psychotherapy and Psychosomatics. 2016;**85**:218-228. DOI: 10.1159/000445355

[19] Carlbring P, Andersson G, Cuijpers P, Riper H, Hedman-Lagerlof E. Internet-based vs. face-to-face cognitive behavior therapy for psychiatric and somatic disorders: An updated systematic review and meta-analysis. Cognitive Behavioral Therapy. 2018;**47**:1-18. DOI: 10.1080/16506073.2017.1401115

[20] Etzelmueller A, Vis C, Karyotaki E, Baumeister H, Titov N, Berking M, et al. Effects of Internet-based cognitive behavioral therapy in routine care for adults in treatment for depression and anxiety: Systematic review and meta-analysis. Journal of Medical Internet Research. 2020;**22**:e18100. DOI: 10.2196/18100

[21] Karyotaki E, Efthimiou O, Miguel C, Bermpohl FMG, Furukawa TA, Cuijpers P, et al. Internet-based cognitive behavioral therapy for depression: A systematic review and individual patient data network meta-analysis. JAMA Psychiatry. 2021;**78**:361-371. DOI: 10.1001/jamapsychiatry.2020.4364

[22] Baumeister H, Reichler L, Munzinger M, Lin J. The impact of guidance on Internet-based mental health interventions: A systematic review. Internet Interventions. 2014;**1**:205-215. DOI: 10.1016/j.invent.2014.08.003

[23] Krieger T, Bur OT, Weber L, Wolf M, Berger T, Watzke B, et al. Human contact in internet-based interventions for depression: A pre-registered replication and meta-analysis of randomized trials. Internet Interventions. 2023;**32**:100617. DOI: 10.1016/j.invent.2023.100617

[24] Koelen JA, Vonk A, Klein A, de Koning L, Vonk P, de Vet S, et al. Man vs. machine: A meta-analysis on the added value of human support in text-based internet treatments ("e-therapy") for mental disorders. Clinical Psychology Review. 2022;**96**:102179. DOI: 10.1016/j.cpr.2022.102179

[25] Moshe I, Terhorst Y, Philippi P, Domhardt M, Cuijpers P, Cristea I, et al. Digital interventions for the treatment of depression: A meta-analytic review. Psychological Bulletin. 2021;**147**:749-786. DOI: 10.1037/bul0000334

[26] Karyotaki E, Kleiboer A, Smit F, Turner DT, Pastor AM, Andersson G, et al. Predictors of treatment dropout in self-guided web-based interventions for depression: An 'individual patient data' meta-analysis. Psychological Medicine. 2015;**45**:2717-2726. DOI: 10.1017/S0033291715000665

[27] Richards D, Richardson T. Computer-based psychological treatments for depression: A systematic review and meta-analysis. Clinical Psychology Review. 2012;**32**:329-342. DOI: 10.1016/j.cpr.2012.02.004

[28] Oakley-Girvan I, Docherty JP. A new approach to enhancing engagement in eHealth Apps. Interactive Journal of Medical Research. 2022;**11**:e38886. DOI: 10.2196/38886

[29] O'Kearney R, Gibson M, Christensen H, Griffiths KM. Effects of a cognitive-behavioural Internet program on depression, vulnerability to depression and stigma in adolescent males: A school-based controlled trial. Cognitive Behaviour Therapy. 2006;**35**:43-54. DOI: 10.1080/16506070500303456

[30] Schneider F, de Vries H, Candel M, van de Kar A, van Osch L. Periodic email prompts to re-use an internet-delivered computer-tailored lifestyle program: Influence of prompt content and timing. Journal of Medical Internet Research. 2013;**15**:e2151. DOI: 10.2196/jmir.2151

[31] Eysenbach G. The law of attrition. Journal of Medical Internet Research. 2005;7:e11. DOI: 10.2196/jmir.7.1.e11

[32] Christensen H, Griffiths KM, Farrer L. Adherence in internet interventions for anxiety and depression. Journal of Medical Internet Research. 2009;**11**:e13. DOI: 10.2196/jmir.1194

[33] Druce KL, Dixon WG, McBeth J. Maximizing engagement in mobile health studies: Lessons learned and future directions. Rheumatic Diseases Clinics of North America. 2019;**45**:159-172. DOI: 10.1016/j.rdc.2019.01.004

[34] Nijland N, van Gemert-Pijnen JE, Kelders SM, Brandenburg BJ, Seydel ER. Factors influencing the use of a web-based application for supporting the self-care of patients with type 2 diabetes: A longitudinal study. Journal of Medical Internet Research. 2011;**13**:e71. DOI: 10.2196/jmir.1603

[35] Titov N, Dear BF, Johnston L, McEvoy PM, Wootton B, Terides MD, et al. Improving adherence and clinical outcomes in self-guided internet treatment for anxiety and depression: A 12-month follow-up of a randomised controlled trial. PLoS One. 2014;**9**:1-8. DOI: 10.1371/journal.pone.0089591

[36] Geraghty AWA, Torres LD, Leykin Y, Pérez-Stable EJ, Muñoz RF. Understanding attrition from international Internet health interventions: A step towards global eHealth. Health Promotion International. 2013;**28**:442-452. DOI: 10.1093/heapro/das029

[37] Barak A, Klein B, Proudfoot JG. Defining Internet-supported therapeutic interventions. Annals of Behavioral Medicine. 2009;**38**:4-17. DOI: 10.1007/s12160-009-9130-7

[38] Musiat P, Johnson C, Atkinson M, Wilksch S, Wade T. Impact of guidance on intervention adherence in computerised interventions for mental health problems: A meta-analysis. Psychological Medicine. 2022;**52**:229-240. DOI: 10.1017/S0033291721004621

[39] Hermes ED, Lyon AR, Schueller SM, Glass JE. Measuring the implementation

of behavioral intervention technologies: Recharacterization of established outcomes. Journal of Medical Internet Research. 2019;**21**:e11752. DOI: 10.2196/11752

[40] Brodbeck J, Berger T, Biesold N, Rockstroh F, Znoj HJ. Evaluation of a guided internet-based self-help intervention for older adults after spousal bereavement or separation/divorce: A randomised controlled trial. Journal of Affective Disorders. 2019;**252**:440-449. DOI: 10.1016/j.jad.2019.04.008

[41] Berthoud L, Efinger L, Kheyar M, Pomini V, Debrot A. Hope may come from Internet in times of COVID-19: Building an online programme for grief (LIVIA). Frontiers in Psychiatry. 2021;**12**:626831. DOI: 10.3389/fpsyt.2021.626831

[42] Efinger L, Debrot A, Pomini V. LIVIA-FR : Implémentation et évaluation d'une intervention par Internet pour des personnes francophones peinant à surmonter la perte de leur partenaire. Annales Médico-Psychologiques, Revue Psychiatrique. 2022;**180**:1000-1007. DOI: 10.1016/j.amp.2021.05.004

[43] Stroebe M, Schut H. The dual process model of coping with bereavement: Rationale and description. Death Studies. 1999;**23**:197-224. DOI: 10.1080/074811899201046

[44] Stroebe M, Schut H. The dual process model of coping with bereavement: A decade on. Omega Westport. 2010;**61**:273-289. DOI: 10.2190/OM.61.4.b

[45] Debrot A, Kheyar M, Efinger L, Berthoud L, Pomini V. Supporting people who have lost a close person by bereavement or separation: Protocol of a randomized controlled trial comparing two French-language Internet-based interventions. JMIR Research Protocols. 2022;**11**:e39026. DOI: 10.2196/39026

[46] Debrot A, Efinger L, Kheyar M, Pomini V, Berthoud L. Effects of a French-language Internet-based intervention targeting grief symptoms after bereavement and separation: A randomized controlled trial. Journal of Medical Internet Research. Forthcoming 2024

[47] Hadjistavropoulos HD, Schneider LH, Edmonds M, Karin E, Nugent MN, Dirkse D, et al. Randomized controlled trial of internet-delivered cognitive behaviour therapy comparing standard weekly versus optional weekly therapist support. Journal of Anxiety Disorders. 2017;**52**:15-24. DOI: 10.1016/j.janxdis.2017.09.006

[48] Hadjistavropoulos HD, Schneider LH, Mehta S, Karin E, Dear BF, Titov N. Preference trial of internet-delivered cognitive behaviour therapy comparing standard weekly versus optional weekly therapist support. Journal of Anxiety Disorders. 2019;**63**:51-60. DOI: 10.1016/j.janxdis.2019.02.002

[49] Caspar F. Optimizing psychotherapy with plan analysis. In: Handbook of Psychotherapy Case Formulation. New York: The Guilford Press; 2022. pp. 209-251

[50] Debrot A, Berthoud L, Caspar F, Berger T, Pomini V. Tailoring guidance in Internet-based interventions with motive-oriented therapeutic relationship. Frontiers in Digital Health. 2022;**4**:842487. DOI: 10.3389/fdgth.2022.842487

[51] Caspar F. Chapter 14 – Plan analysis and the motive-oriented therapeutic relationship. In: Kramer U, editor. Salesforce Case

Formula: A Complete Guide. Amsterdam, NL: Elsevier Academic Press; 2019. pp. 265-290. DOI: 10.1016/B978-0-12-813521-1.00014-X

[52] Breen LJ, O'Connor M. Family and social networks after bereavement: Experiences of support, change and isolation. Journal of Family Therapy. 2011;**33**:98-120. DOI: 10.1111/j.1467-6427.2010.00495.x

[53] Vedder A, Boerner K, Stokes JE, Schut HAW, Boelen PA, Stroebe MS. A systematic review of loneliness in bereavement: Current research and future directions. Current Opinion in Psychology. 2022;**43**:48-64. DOI: 10.1016/j.copsyc.2021.06.003

[54] Terhell EL, Broese van Groenou MI, van Tilburg T. Network dynamics in the long-term period after divorce. Journal of Social and Personal Relationships. 2004;**21**:719-738. DOI: 10.1177/0265407504047833

[55] Pai N, Vella S-L. The physical and mental health consequences of social isolation and loneliness in the context of COVID-19. Current Opinion in Psychiatry. 2022;**35**:305-310. DOI: 10.1097/YCO.0000000000000806

[56] Ritterband LM, Borowitz S, Cox DJ, Kovatchev B, Walker LS, Lucas V, et al. Using the Internet to provide information prescriptions. Pediatrics. 2005;**116**: e643-e647. DOI: 10.1542/peds.2005-0404

[57] Hutchesson MJ, Tan CY, Morgan P, Callister R, Collins C. Enhancement of self-monitoring in a web-based weight loss program by extra individualized feedback and reminders: Randomized trial. Journal of Medical Internet Research. 2016;**18**: 50-60. DOI: 10.2196/jmir.4100

[58] Titov N, Dear BF, Johnston L, Lorian C, Zou J, Wootton B, et al. Improving adherence and clinical outcomes in self-guided Internet treatment for anxiety and depression: Randomised controlled trial. PLoS One. 2013;**8**:e62873. DOI: 10.1371/journal.pone.0062873

[59] Clarke G, Eubanks D, Reid E, Kelleher C, O'Connor E, DeBar LL, et al. Overcoming depression on the Internet (ODIN) (2): A randomized trial of a self-help depression skills program with reminders. Journal of Medical Internet Research. 2005;**7**:e16. DOI: 10.2196/jmir.7.2.e16

[60] Christensen H, Batterham P, Mackinnon A, Griffiths KM, Kalia Hehir K, Kenardy J, et al. Prevention of generalized anxiety disorder using a web intervention, iChill: Randomized controlled trial. Journal of Medical Internet Research. 2014;**16**:e199. DOI: 10.2196/jmir.3507

[61] Fry JP, Neff RA. Periodic prompts and reminders in health promotion and health behavior interventions: Systematic review. Journal of Medical Internet Research. 2009;**11**:e16. DOI: 10.2196/jmir.1138

[62] Schneider F, van Osch L, Schulz DN, Kremers SP, de Vries H. The influence of user characteristics and a periodic email prompt on exposure to an internet-delivered computer-tailored lifestyle program. Journal of Medical Internet Research. 2012;**14**:e40. DOI: 10.2196/jmir.1939

[63] Rimer BK, Kreuter MW. Advancing tailored health communication: A persuasion and message effects perspective. The Journal of Communication. 2006;**56**:S184-S201. DOI: 10.1111/j.1460-2466.2006.00289.x

[64] Lustria MLA, Cortese J, Noar SM, Glueckauf RL. Computer-tailored health

interventions delivered over the web: Review and analysis of key components. Patient Education and Counseling. 2009;**74**:156-173. DOI: 10.1016/j.pec.2008.08.023

[65] Brug J, Oenema A, Campbell M. Past, present, and future of computer-tailored nutrition education. The American Journal of Clinical Nutrition. 2003;**77**:1028S-1034S. DOI: 10.1093/ajcn/77.4.1028S

[66] Frank RI, Davidson J. The Transdiagnostic Road Map to Case Formulation and Treatment Planning: Practical Guidance for Clinical Decision Making. Oakland, CA: New Harbinger Publications; 2014

[67] Hayes SC, Hofmann SG. Process-Based CBT: The Science and Core Clinical Competencies of Cognitive-Behavioral Therapy. New Harbinger Publications; 2018

[68] Boyd-Franklin N, Cleek EN, Wofsy M, Mundy B. Therapy in the Real World: Effective Treatments for Challenging Problems. New York, NY: Guilford Press; 2013

[69] Nezu AM, Maguth NC. Problem-solving–based therapies: Empirical support and transdiagnostic capabilities. In: Emotion-Centered Problem-Solving Therapy: Treatment Guidelines. Springer Publishing Company; 2019. pp. 51-76

[70] Warner RE. Solution-Focused Interviewing: Applying Positive Psychology, A Manual for Practitioners. Toronto, ON: University of Toronto Press; 2013

[71] Rashid T. Positive psychotherapy: A strength-based approach. The Journal of Positive Psychology. 2015;**10**:25-40. DOI: 10.1080/17439760.2014.920411

[72] Bendig E, Erb B, Schulze-Thuesing L, Baumeister H. The next generation: Chatbots in clinical psychology and psychotherapy to Foster mental health – A scoping review. Verhaltenstherapie. 2019:64-76. DOI: 10.1159/000501812

[73] Park N. Classifying and measuring strengths of character. In: Lopez SJ, Snyder CR, editors. Handbook of Positive Psychology. Oxford University Press; 2021. pp. 33-58

[74] Shankland R. Échelles validées en psychologie positive. In: Positive Psychology. 3rd ed. Dunod; 2019. pp. 157-174

[75] Bellier-Teichmann T, Pomini V. Evolving from clinical to positive psychology: Understanding and measuring patients' strengths: A pilot study. Journal of Contemporary Psychotherapy. 2015;**45**:99-108. DOI: 10.1007/s10879-014-9287-7

[76] Bellier-Teichmann T, Golay P, Pomini V. Which are your resources and how do they contribute to your recovery? European Review of Applied Psychology. 2018;**68**:215-226. DOI: 10.1016/j.erap.2018.10.004

[77] Beike DR, Brandon NR, Cole HE. Is sharing specific autobiographical memories a distinct form of self-disclosure? Journal of Experimental Psychology. General. 2016;**145**:434-450. DOI: 10.1037/xge0000143

[78] Schacter DL, Benoit RG, Szpunar KK. Episodic future thinking: Mechanisms and functions. Current Opinion in Behavioral Sciences. 2017;**17**:41-50. DOI: 10.1016/j.cobeha.2017.06.002

[79] Wolf T, Demiray B. The mood-enhancement function of autobiographical memories: Comparisons

with other functions in terms of emotional valence. Consciousness and Cognition. 2019;**70**:88-100. DOI: 10.1016/j.concog.2019.03.002

[80] Bluck S, Alea N, Habermas T, Rubin DC. A TALE of three functions: The self-reported uses of autobiographical memory. Social Cognition. 2005;**23**: 91-117. DOI: 10.1521/soco.23.1.91.59198

[81] Conway MA, Pleydell-Pearce CW. The construction of autobiographical memories in the self-memory system. Psychological Review. 2000;**107**:261-288. DOI: 10.1037/0033-295x.107.2.261

[82] Dalgleish T, Hitchcock C. Transdiagnostic distortions in autobiographical memory recollection. Nature Reviews Psychology. 2023;**2**:166-182. DOI: 10.1038/s44159-023-00148-1

[83] Maccallum F, Bryant RA. A cognitive attachment model of prolonged grief: Integrating attachments, memory, and identity. Clinical Psychology Review. 2013;**33**:713-727. DOI: 10.1016/j.cpr.2013.05.001

[84] Golden AM, Dalgleish T, Mackintosh B. Levels of specificity of autobiographical memories and of biographical memories of the deceased in bereaved individuals with and without complicated grief. Journal of Abnormal Psychology. 2007;**116**:786-795. DOI: 10.1037/0021-843X.116.4.786

[85] Robinaugh DJ, McNally RJ. Remembering the past and envisioning the future in bereaved adults with and without complicated grief. Clinical Psychological Science: A Journal of the Association for Psychological Science. 2013;**1**:290-300. DOI: 10.1177/2167702613476027

[86] Mancini AD, Griffin P, Bonanno GA. Recent trends in the treatment of prolonged grief. Current Opinion in Psychiatry. 2012;**25**:46-51. DOI: 10.1097/YCO.0b013e32834de48a

[87] Braun V, Clarke V. Using thematic analysis in psychology. Qualitative Research in Psychology. 2006;**3**:77-101. DOI: 10.1191/1478088706qp063oa

[88] Donkin L, Christensen H, Naismith SL, Neal B, Hickie IB, Glozier N. A systematic review of the impact of adherence on the effectiveness of e-therapies. Journal of Medical Internet Research. 2011;**13**:e1772. DOI: 10.2196/jmir.1772

[89] Fuhr K, Schröder J, Berger T, Moritz S, Meyer B, Lutz W, et al. The association between adherence and outcome in an Internet intervention for depression. Journal of Affective Disorders. 2018;**229**:443-449. DOI: 10.1016/j.jad.2017.12.028

[90] Heim E, Kohrt BA. Cultural adaptation of scalable psychological interventions. Clinical Psychology in Europe. 2019;**1**(4):1-22. DOI: 10.32872/cpe.v1i4.37679

[91] Eyles H, Jull A, Dobson R, Firestone R, Whittaker R, Te Morenga L, et al. Co-design of mHealth delivered interventions: A systematic review to assess key methods and processes. Current Nutrition Reports. 2016;**5**:160-167. DOI: 10.1007/s13668-016-0165-7

Chapter 15

Perspective Chapter: Integrating Large Language Models and Blockchain in Telemedicine

Thomas F. Heston

Abstract

This perspective paper examines how combining artificial intelligence in the form of large language models (LLMs) with blockchain technology can potentially solve ongoing issues in telemedicine, such as personalized care, system integration, and secure patient data sharing. The strategic integration of LLMs for swift medical data analysis and decentralized blockchain ledgers for secure data exchange across organizations could establish a vital learning loop essential for advanced telemedicine. Although the value of combining LLMs with blockchain technology has been demonstrated in non-healthcare fields, wider adoption in medicine requires careful attention to reliability, safety measures, and prioritizing access to ensure ethical use for enhancing patient outcomes. The perspective article posits that a thoughtful convergence could facilitate comprehensive improvements in telemedicine, including automated triage, improved subspecialist access to records, coordinated interventions, readily available diagnostic test results, and secure remote patient monitoring. This article looks at the latest uses of LLMs and blockchain in telemedicine, explores potential synergies, discusses risks and how to manage them, and suggests ways to use these technologies responsibly to improve care quality.

Keywords: telemedicine, artificial intelligence, large language models, blockchain, interoperability, data privacy, technology convergence

1. Introduction

The practice of telemedicine has accelerated rapidly, with virtual visits growing 38-fold since the start of the COVID-19 pandemic [1]. This massive expansion increased access and convenience for patients consulting remotely with physicians and other healthcare providers [2]. However, fundamental challenges remain in delivering personalized, integrated care. Practitioners face constrained time, administrative support, and technological skills [3]. Patients struggle to coordinate across disconnected providers, lacking holistic records [4]. Despite profound progress, telemedicine still remains more promise than fulfillment.

Emerging technologies like artificial intelligence (AI) and blockchain present important solutions. Natural language processing AI in the form of large language

Feature	Description	Capabilities	Examples
LLMs	Large neural networks are trained on massive amounts of text data to understand and generate human-like text.	Assisting in diagnostic processes, generating patient information, and automating administrative tasks.	ChatGPT, Anthropic, diagnostic tools, and chatbots for patient engagement
Blockchain	A decentralized digital ledger that records transactions across many computers so that the record cannot be altered retroactively.	Interoperability across healthcare systems, secure encryption of patient records, and data immutability. Patients own and control their own medical data.	Bitcoin, Ethereum, Cardano, Hyperledger Fabric
Overlap	Combines LLMs knowledge processing with blockchain's secure, decentralized data management.	Improved patient management while allowing patients to securely control and share their own medical data.	LLM integration into the Cardano blockchain

Table 1.
Synergy of LLMs with blockchain in medicine.

models (LLMs) can supply physicians with contextualized recommendations from an ever-expanding range of journals and cases [5]. Blockchain facilitates decentralized knowledge-sharing across distance and medical specialties [6]. While neither of these newer technologies is a silver bullet, converged together LLMs and blockchain enable improved overall medical care across scattered systems.

This perspective article explores intersecting applications of technology, specifically LLMs and blockchain, propelling the next generation of telemedicine. While drawing upon existing literature to provide context, the main focus is on proposing a novel perspective on how the integration of these technologies can transform telemedicine. The article argues that the synergistic combination of LLMs and blockchain has the potential to address key challenges in telemedicine, such as care personalization, system integration, and patient data privacy/sharing. Opportunities to augment physicians' abilities to diagnose, monitor, and engage patients remotely are reviewed (**Table 1**). Meaningful successes from early adoption are evaluated in light of enduring risks requiring mitigation before mainstream adoption.

Leading medical innovations will combine patient-centered care with advanced technologies. Blockchain technologies can help achieve that by securely transmitting diagnostics and increasing interoperability between electronic health records [7]. LLM-based AI assistants can intelligently adjust guidance based on holistic health records and patient communication [8]. Telemedicine empowered by LLMs and blockchain will potentially expand access to care, decrease costs, and improve community health. While significant challenges exist, this perspective article argues that the next frontier of telemedicine lies in the convergence of these technologies.

2. Literature review

No articles that addressed the specific issue of combining LLMs with blockchain technology in telemedicine could be identified. Therefore, a literature review was performed to provide a foundational logic for the proposal of combining LLMs with blockchain technology in telemedicine. By examining relevant literature on the individual components of LLMs and blockchain technology and their pairwise relationships, this focused review aims to demonstrate the potential for integrating these technologies to enhance telemedicine. A targeted literature search using PubMed and Google Scholar was performed to inform this perspective on integrating LLMs and blockchain in telemedicine.

Recent studies have explored the applications of LLMs in healthcare, highlighting their potential to assist with tasks such as clinical decision support, patient triage, and documentation [9]. They suggest that LLMs can help streamline processes and improve efficiency in healthcare settings. However, data privacy, bias, and reliability challenges have also been noted, underscoring the need for careful implementation and monitoring [10].

Blockchain technology has been investigated for its potential to enhance healthcare security, privacy, and interoperability [11]. Blockchain-based systems have been proposed to manage electronic health records, enable secure data sharing, and facilitate patient consent management [12]. While these applications show promise, scalability, regulatory compliance, and user adoption challenges remain significant [7].

Although the literature on the specific combination of LLMs and blockchain in healthcare is scarce, there is recognition that combining LLMs with blockchain technology can improve data privacy in other fields [13]. Also, Sam Altman, the CEO of OpenAI, and the Cardano blockchain recently have engaged in talks looking into putting an LLM on its distributed network. Since current LLMs are centralized and controlled by a single entity, there are concerns regarding data privacy, bias, and censorship. A decentralized blockchain-based LLM would increase the transparency of LLMs, potentially improving diversity and decreasing costs to the end-user [14].

Telemedicine has been widely studied, with numerous articles discussing its benefits, challenges, and future directions. Key challenges identified in the literature include data security, privacy, licensure, and integration with existing healthcare systems [15]. As telemedicine continues to evolve, researchers have emphasized the need for innovative solutions to address these challenges and improve patient outcomes [16].

A recent literature review provides a complementary overview of key aspects of eHealth systems, including architectures, mHealth advances, and security challenges, that aligns with and reinforces many of the topics discussed in this manuscript [17]. The authors delve into the technical implementation of blockchain, IoT, and cloud-based architectures, detailing, for example, a three-layer IoT architecture consisting of device, network, and application layers. Their discussion of mHealth advances covers wireless sensors, mobile devices, and short-range, satellite, and cellular communication technologies, including the evolution from 3G to 5G networks. Common security threats outlined, such as eavesdropping, data modification, and denial of service attacks, echo the security challenges highlighted in this work. The research challenges identified, spanning areas like standardization, communication speed, blockchain limitations, and mHealth literacy, intersect with and could further inform the key research gaps and future directions presented herein. Collectively, the survey offers some additional context and examples that enrich the core concepts while pointing to the same overarching opportunities and need for continued research and development to realize the full potential of eHealth systems.

By synthesizing insights from these separate bodies of literature, a foundation for this perspective is given on the potential benefits and challenges of integrating LLMs and blockchain in telemedicine. While the specific combination of these technologies in telemedicine has not been extensively studied, the existing literature on their individual applications and pairwise relationships suggests that their integration could offer novel solutions to enhance security, privacy, and decision support in telemedicine. By exploring possible synergies, this perspective article aims to contribute to the ongoing discussion on the future of telemedicine and the role of emerging technologies in transforming healthcare delivery.

3. Large language models in telemedicine

Large language models (LLMs) are a class of AI systems that can analyze, comprehend, and generate content after training on massive amounts of data [18]. Current LLMs are estimated to have over 175 billion parameters training on over 1 trillion words across textbooks, Wikipedia articles, and other digital content [19]. These LLMs utilize neural networks structured in "transformer" architectures, which continue learning through weights and transformations on input [20]. These interconnected nodes enable the rapid interpretation of patterns across extremely large datasets that are not approachable manually. LLMs can recognize relationships and generate natural language responses by absorbing tremendous volumes of information. These LLMs are continually updated by curating training data and integrating feedback from human users to create safety guardrails.

For telemedicine applications, customized LLMs trained on clinical sources can quickly analyze guidelines that synthesize connections in patient charts. The continued maturation of LLMs could potentially enable immediate access to current guidelines at the point of care, revolutionizing telemedicine practice by increasing the speed of informed decision-making. LLMs can also highlight a patient's important and relevant medical background [21]. For instance, an LLM may review patient history and symptoms pre-visit. It would then supply background on aligned conditions ahead of the telemedicine visit with the clinician. Then, during a live consultation, the LLM could cross-check emerging details against a highly curated medical training database. This would prompt physicians with validated recommendations specific to that patient in real-time dialog. LLMs have demonstrated abilities to assist with rapid chart reviews. This capacity to quickly perform a record review and present relevant information and perhaps previously unknown connections or patterns to the clinician presents a major advance in computer technology.

Currently, startups worldwide are actively working to tailor and validate AI usage for telemedicine screening, diagnosis, and care support. Applications are broad, from radiology image evaluation [22] to patient chart reviews [23]. AI, using LLMs, could be integrated into all aspects of the televisit, even including a real-time evaluation of the conversation [24].

However, concerns exist about the use of LLMs in medicine, including their tendency to generate unreliable responses [25]. This can be partly due to randomness parameters, crucial for creating varied and fluent language, but can also introduce uncertainty when analyzing critical medical data. The result is that the analysis of clinical data may not be routinely uniform but will contain inconsistent and unreliable responses inappropriate for clinical practice [26]. While randomness offers benefits like adaptability for generating possible diagnoses, it's essential to consider other factors, such as biases in training data and poorly constructed prompts.

While LLMs incorporate a large amount of knowledge by training on a huge amount of data, this unsupervised learning model can also result in harmful gender and racial biases [27]. These biases can be demographic, reflecting societal inequalities present in the training data, or algorithmic, stemming from how the training algorithms process information. For example, an LLM might underdiagnose certain demographics due to historical data underrepresentation or suggest biased treatment options influenced by algorithmic limitations. Recognizing and mitigating these biases through strategies like diversifying training data, employing fairness-aware algorithms, and ongoing human review is essential for responsible integration into telemedicine.

Another concern about the introduction of AI into telemedicine is medical malpractice. If an AI makes a mistake, will the AI or the human clinician be responsible? Alternatively, if the clinician made a mistake but had consulted an AI at the time of the patient visit, would that decrease their liability [28]? The legal landscape is complex and rapidly evolving. Currently, the recommendation is for clinicians to use LLMs only as assistive or confirmatory tools [29].

Finally, in addition to the concerns about accuracy, reliability, and malpractice, there is great concern regarding the ability of LLMs to maintain patient privacy [30]. Although utilizing locally deployed LLMs instead of a centralized LLM may help maintain privacy [31], anonymization and data encryption remain crucial. There remains concern that online tools are highly insecure and that these LLMs can leak secrets [32, 33].

While material risks exist surrounding validation and responsibility, when applied judiciously, LLMs may meaningfully assist physicians practicing telemedicine. The continued maturation of LLMs could enable immediate access to current guidelines at the point of care. Realizing that potential depends on a disciplined assessment of outcomes from initial implementations rather than speculation. Further refinement must shape their evolving role in supporting compassionate, safe, and high-quality virtual care delivery.

4. Improving security with blockchain technology

Blockchains are distributed ledgers that enable secure, transparent record-keeping without a central authority that can tamper with or modify the data. These distributed ledgers are databases shared across multiple computers. Blockchains can be public and globally distributed, as is the case for cryptocurrencies such as Bitcoin and smart contract platforms such as Ethereum. Private, permissioned blockchains are also common. These blockchains, such as the Hyperledger Fabric framework, only allow approved members to join [34]. Multiple decentralized nodes operate blockchain, while cryptographic techniques secure and verify information.

4.1 Understanding blockchains and distributed ledgers

Blockchains store records across computer networks. A public shared ledger synchronizes data instead of having the data siloed in a proprietary system owned by a healthcare network. Blockchain cryptography secures the distributed database. This high level of security is obvious when noting that the Bitcoin blockchain, with a market capitalization of over $800B available to hackers, has not suffered a breach since its creation in 2009. Although individual wallets and exchanges are vulnerable, the blockchain network itself has remained intact [35].

When users approve transactions like adding records through pre-agreed consensus protocols, blockchains permanently and immutably log those exchanges across a large decentralized network using digital signatures. The consensus protocols ensure all nodes validate new data additions prior to appending the shared database. This establishes a verifiable audit trail, building trust without the vulnerability of intermediaries introducing corruption.

4.2 Healthcare blockchain adoption

In telemedicine, blockchain shows early promise in improving:

- *Security*—permissioned blockchains in healthcare often use private keys like digital passports for secure data encryption and access control. This is an improvement to siloed systems where records are isolated, and securing sharing across institutions is extremely challenging. Only authorized healthcare professionals who have been granted these keys can enter the network and access/update patient records. Without the correct keys, unauthorized parties cannot decrypt data or tamper with information, preventing breaches. Patients, not healthcare providers, insurance companies, or hospitals, control their own keys and, therefore, fully control their personal data.

- *Interoperability*—by consolidating records, shared ledgers can integrate diagnostics across otherwise siloed health systems during care coordination. For example, hospitals today struggle to share lab tests and imaging across different provider networks or medical record platforms. This causes delays, repeat testing, and disconnected care. Blockchain-based ledgers could allow seamless, cross-affiliate sharing of full patient diagnostic history, enabling streamlined specialist consultations, transfers, and treatment continuity.

- *Privacy*—zero-knowledge proofs applied to patient records could allow patients to share specific medical information without revealing their full identity. For example, a patient could prove they have a certain gene variation for research purposes without disclosing their name or other personal details. This privacy goes well beyond research. Blockchain also empowers patients to keep their data private through decentralized storage, pseudonymization, and fine-grained access control, allowing secure sharing with auditability.

Blockchain systems could secure telemedicine data by leveraging decentralized identity standards that provide authentication for individuals, organizations, and connected devices. Digital keys enacted through secure multi-party computation and zero-knowledge proof schemes serve as dynamically verifiable credentials with finely tuned permissions. This allows identity owners to selectively disclose claims required to authorize health data exchange. For instance, a patient could authorize the transmission of diagnostic results to a new specialist by presenting a temporary access credential registered on-chain without revealing unrelated sensitive details. Health networks interfacing with these blockchain frameworks ensure accountability as data requests and permissions are immutably recorded in auditable distributed ledgers. Such identity data marketplaces can balance utility with privacy, allowing patients sovereignty over sharing levels.

4.3 Ongoing opportunities and risk management

As blockchain sees rising adoption in healthcare contexts, maintaining rigorous security, privacy, and interoperability standards is required for responsible scaling of these technologies. Innovations like hardening smart contract code, strengthening consensus protocols to prevent manipulation risks, and advancing encryption techniques resistant to quantum computers will help distributed ledger solutions secure telemedicine care models in the future. While talent shortages in software engineering and the difficulty of integrating legacy systems will need to be overcome, continued progress in blockchain-specific healthcare infrastructure points towards a coming coalescence capable of safely streamlining telemedicine data sharing worldwide. And society has already made tremendous strides. For example, the successful use of blockchain technology in securing medical records dates back to at least 2016, when Estonia began securing its health records [36]. Estonia's successful use of blockchain technology in securing medical records demonstrates the potential for this technology to transform data security in telemedicine. Supporting this promising beginning, analysts project the adoption of blockchain in healthcare is expected to grow significantly by 2030, with a compound annual growth rate of around 40% [37].

5. Opportunities and risks of AI and blockchain in telemedicine

When applied judiciously, integrating AI in the form of LLMs with blockchain technology into telemedicine infrastructure presents noteworthy opportunities to improve care outcomes as well as inherent risks requiring mitigation.

5.1 Opportunities

Integrating blockchain with LLMs poses meaningful opportunities to improve the speed and accuracy of evaluating patient records and improving management. Several key opportunities are associated with thoughtfully incorporating these technologies:

- *Visit efficiency*: LLMs could enhance virtual visit efficiency by rapidly summarizing the pertinent medical history and flagging relevant past conditions ahead of teleconsultations. LLMs excel at rapidly summarizing large volumes of data.

- *Quality control*: LLMs could help improve patient visit consistency by monitoring dialog in real-time and summarizing validated recommendations.

- *Improved triage*: LLM-based chatbots could allow increased throughput of common complaints via automated triaging. Increased speed of appropriate referrals would expand access to care.

- *Better security*: LLMs have an unproven track record in ensuring patient privacy, but combining LLMs with blockchain technology could mitigate these concerns. A blockchain-LLM system could improve security and patient privacy compared to existing systems. Record archiving would be more secure, more private, and immutable.

- *Interoperability*: blockchain technology cuts across geopolitical boundaries, allowing improved data sharing globally.

5.2 Risks

Prudent adoption necessitates actively addressing salient risks of new and advanced technologies, including:

- *Bias*: LLMs are known to be vulnerable to bias and have demonstrated inequitable performance across patient demographics.

- *Unclear responsibility*: malpractice issues remain murky when technology breaks down or provides inaccurate information.

- *Privacy violations*: the inappropriate use of LLMs or programming errors could potentially result in privacy breaches.

- *Integration*: overcoming legacy infrastructure fragmentation will be challenging. Knowledge gaps in the technology development workforce remain significant. A coordinated global effort at establishing interoperability standards could help improve development.

Integrating blockchain with LLMs poses meaningful opportunities to improve the speed and accuracy of evaluating patient records and improving management. When combined with blockchain's security features and interoperability, LLMs have great potential to advance quality, increase patient privacy, decrease costs, and increase access to care.

However, significant challenges exist. Fragmentation, legacy systems, and talent gaps hinder progress [38]. Privacy concerns pose another significant risk when integrating blockchain and LLMs into telemedicine systems. While blockchain provides initial data privacy through encryption and pseudonymity, it remains vulnerable to privacy leakage if sufficient patient information is linked. Privacy-preserving mechanisms can be deployed in conjunction with blockchain technology to address these issues. These include advanced encryption schemes like attribute-based encryption, which ensures fine-grained access control by associating attributes with private keys, and proxy re-encryption, which enables secure data sharing without revealing private keys. Additionally, techniques such as zero-knowledge proofs and homomorphic encryption can further enhance privacy by allowing computation on encrypted data without revealing the underlying information. Smart contracts can also be leveraged to enforce data access control policies and maintain an immutable audit trail. Careful integration of these privacy mechanisms is crucial to realize the full potential of blockchain in enabling secure, privacy-preserving telemedicine systems while mitigating the associated risks [39]. By complementing the contextual analysis capabilities of LLMs with the secure data management afforded by privacy-enhanced blockchain solutions, telemedicine platforms can deliver more personalized and privacy-centric care.

Ethical accountability must be ingrained at every stage of convergence. Safeguarding patient interests must remain the top priority. This demands moving forward with advanced technologies but with a balance of caution, ensuring safe implementation. LLMs and blockchain technologies provide this balance of innovation with safety.

5.3 Regional differences in challenges and barriers

Integrating LLMs and blockchain in telemedicine faces challenges and barriers across different regions. In Europe and the US, data privacy regulations such as the General Data Protection Regulation (GDPR) and the Health Insurance Portability and Accountability Act (HIPAA) pose strict yet slightly different requirements for handling sensitive patient data [40]. Ensuring compliance with these regulations while implementing new technologies can be complex and time-consuming [41].

In Asia, the digital divide between urban and rural areas presents a significant challenge to the widespread adoption of telemedicine [42]. Financial costs and limited access to reliable internet connectivity and digital devices in some regions may hinder the implementation of AI and blockchain solutions. Additionally, cultural differences in healthcare decision-making and patient-provider relationships may influence the acceptance of these technologies [43].

The Middle East faces its own set of challenges, including a lack of standardized electronic health record systems and limited interoperability between healthcare providers [44]. This fragmentation and lack of infrastructure can make it difficult to integrate new technologies seamlessly [45].

Despite these regional differences, there are also common barriers that transcend geographical boundaries. These include concerns about data security and privacy, the need for robust regulatory frameworks, and the requirement for healthcare professionals to adapt to new technologies and workflows. Addressing these shared challenges will be crucial for the successful integration of LLMs and blockchain in telemedicine across all regions.

6. Research applications

For research, the true transformative power of this synergy lies in combining advanced LLMs' ability to rapidly evaluate large amounts of data with blockchain's ability to securely share medical information [13]. Furthermore, this convergence of technologies creates the ability to implement a continuous learning loop with potential major, tangible benefits such as:

- Patient data (wearables, tests, records) is shared via blockchain's distributed ledgers, allowing patients to control their private information while enabling anonymous sharing with researchers.

- Shared data then trains advanced LLMs to provide personalized guidance, augment diagnostics, coordinate interventions, and update patient records.

Early adopters have already demonstrated this powerful synergy between LLMs and blockchain technology. For example, Cardano, a public blockchain platform, is working to develop a decentralized LLM integrated into their blockchain. This pioneering initiative addresses pressing data privacy, fairness, and bias issues [46]. The integration of AI with blockchain technology in cardiovascular medicine has been pursued due to the combination of AI's analytic capabilities with blockchain's secure management of data [47]. The resulting data marketplace could empower patients with more control over their personal medical information, from wearables to lab tests, health records, and medical images. Patients could then voluntarily share anonymized data to help researchers access vast, diverse datasets, leading to improved diagnostic and treatment recommendations. This helps mitigate risks of bias inherent in limited institutional data silos.

7. Discussion

The perspective presented in this article has important implications for the future of telemedicine. By integrating LLMs and blockchain technology, key challenges related to care personalization, system integration, and patient data privacy/sharing can be addressed. The synergistic combination of these technologies has the potential to transform telemedicine by improving diagnostics, coordinating interventions, and creating more personalized medical care.

Real-world pilots combining LLMs and blockchain in telemedicine are currently in the theoretical stage only. However, they will require deliberative caution while evaluating their impact and building physician trust. While the potential exists, priority areas remain around integrating systems, enabling secure data sharing, and providing versatile clinical tools. A global effort at setting standards could greatly assist the development of these technologies.

Global interest in digital health has recently declined after reaching an all-time high investment funding of $59.7B in 2021. In 2022, global digital health funding fell to $25.9B; in 2023, it fell to $13.2B [48, 49]. Momentum continues around narrow, siloed point solutions rather than deeply integrated platforms that can address global issues such as improved access and healthcare equity.

Advancing interoperability frameworks is vital to lower proprietary barriers impeding unified data integration across closed vendor systems. Decentralized data sharing securely at scale requires collaboration to simplify integration burdens through co-designing open APIs and standards. This smoothes connections so physicians can access seamlessly combinable tools, not isolated platforms needing custom interfaces.

Additionally, emerging complementary technologies like extended reality and quantum computing could accelerate personalized interventions combined with AI and blockchain. For example, distributed mentor networks leveraging VR case reviews informed by LLM guidance tracked on blockchain ledgers may enhance clinical learning that can scale globally. Quantum machine learning pattern recognition applied to multi-layer de-identified datasets could also unlock optimal treatment insights. Rather than converging into narrow siloes, transformative progress builds upward through expanding technology synergies centered on patient outcomes globally.

Ultimately, advancement depends on ethical governance, demonstrating consistent improvements to earn trust. Mathematical assurances around algorithmic behaviors must take priority over superficial marketing gestures. Transparency measures on alignment with clinical values, explanatory modes, bias elimination, and advisory monitoring will help anchor possibilities in accountability along with deliberate, patient-focused progress [50].

Moreover, the implementation of these technologies will require collaboration across disciplines and stakeholders, including healthcare providers, technology developers, policymakers, and patient advocates. Establishing clear guidelines and standards for the responsible development and deployment of these technologies will be critical to ensuring their safe and effective use in telemedicine.

The path ahead holds no shortage of collaborative milestones if rooted in expanding access for all people - not merely increasing market share. Realizing the convergence where AI and blockchain enhance telemedicine depends on enlisting diverse expertise to scrutinize limitations courageously while accelerating discoveries proven to uplift universal care quality. This conscious effort could launch platforms enabling augmented diagnostics, orchestrated interventions, and democratized personalized guidance. These ingredients supporting modern telemedicine's next evolution exist through the ethical application of technology.

8. Conclusions

The convergence of LLMs, blockchain technology, and telemedicine holds vast potential; however, its responsible realization hinges significantly on adopting a patient-centric approach. Customized AI tools, such as LLMs, offer the capability to assist and potentially enhance human decision-making by enabling a swifter and more comprehensive analysis of patient records than manual review permits. Blockchains and distributed ledgers enable permission-based data fluidity, ensuring the utmost privacy and security of medical records, accessible globally only to individuals authorized by the patient. Telemedicine extends virtual access and provides uninterrupted healthcare services, regardless of geographical constraints.

By insisting on the highest standards to ensure global development, this synergy between LLMs and blockchain technologies has the potential to facilitate comprehensive advancements, including secure remote patient monitoring, decentralized storage and access to diagnostics, and real-time personalized guidance tailored to individual needs. These capabilities can lead to a reduction in errors, an expansion of human medical expertise, and the confident triaging of cases. However, without governance that prioritizes consistency, explainability, and transparency to establish trust, this promising synergy of technologies will fail to live up to its potential.

In conclusion, the perspective presented here argues that the convergence of LLMs, blockchain technology, and telemedicine holds vast potential for transforming telemedicine. The essential ingredients for this important convergence are within reach. Ultimately, the success of this convergence will depend on our willingness to embrace new advances while simultaneously advancing safety guardrails and prioritizing patient interests. By doing so, we can unlock the full potential of LLMs and blockchain in telemedicine and create a more equitable, accessible, and effective global healthcare system.

Author details

Thomas F. Heston[1,2]

1 University of Washington, Seattle, USA

2 Washington State University, Spokane, USA

*Address all correspondence to: theston@uw.edu

References

[1] Bestsennyy O, Gilbert G, Harris A, Rost J. Telehealth: A post-COVID-19 reality? [Internet]. McKinsey. 2021. Available from: https://www.mckinsey.com/industries/healthcare/our-insights/telehealth-a-quarter-trillion-dollar-post-covid-19-reality

[2] Gajarawala SN, Pelkowski JN. Telehealth benefits and barriers. The Journal for Nurse Practitioners. 2021;**17**(2):218-221. DOI: 10.1016/j.nurpra.2020.09.013

[3] Nene S, Rauch M, Belanger D, Bennett R, Berry G, Saad N, et al. Personalized telehealth: Redesigning complex care delivery for the 65+ during the COVID pandemic: A survey of patients, caregivers, and health-care providers. Canadian Geriatrics Journal. 2023;**26**(1):150-175. DOI: 10.5770/cgj.26.641

[4] Lai YF, Lum AYW, Ho ETL, Lim YW. Patient-provider disconnect: A qualitative exploration of understanding and perceptions to care integration. PLoS One. 2017;**12**(10):e0187372. DOI: 10.1371/journal.pone.0187372

[5] Yang X, Chen A, PourNejatian N, Shin HC, Smith KE, Parisien C, et al. A large language model for electronic health records. npj Digital Med. 2022;**5**(1):194. DOI: 10.1038/s41746-022-00742-2

[6] Elangovan D, Long CS, Bakrin FS, Tan CS, Goh KW, Yeoh SF, et al. The use of blockchain technology in the health care sector: Systematic review. JMIR Medical Informatics. 2022;**10**(1):e17278. DOI: 10.2196/17278

[7] Schmeelk S, Kanabar M, Peterson K, Pathak J. Electronic health records and blockchain interoperability requirements: A scoping review. JAMIA Open. 2022;**5**(3):ooac068. DOI: 10.1093/jamiaopen/ooac068

[8] Nawab K, Ramsey G, Schreiber R. Natural language processing to extract meaningful information from patient experience feedback. Applied Clinical Informatics. 2020;**11**(2):242-252. DOI: 10.1055/s-0040-1708049

[9] Karabacak M, Margetis K. Embracing large language models for medical applications: Opportunities and challenges. Cureus. 2023;**15**(5):e39305. DOI: 10.7759/cureus.39305

[10] Jeyaraman M, Balaji S, Jeyaraman N, Yadav S. Unraveling the ethical enigma: Artificial intelligence in healthcare. Cureus. 2023;**15**(8):e43262. DOI: 10.7759/cureus.43262

[11] Taherdoost H. Privacy and security of blockchain in healthcare: Applications, challenges, and future perspectives. Sci. 2023;**5**(4):41. DOI: 10.3390/sci5040041

[12] Kiania K, Jameii SM, Rahmani AM. Blockchain-based privacy and security preserving in electronic health: A systematic review. Multimedia Tools and Applications. 2023;**82**(18):28493-28519. DOI: 10.1007/s11042-023-14488-w

[13] Rizvi S. Blockchain-based LLMs: A game changer for data privacy protection [Internet]. Dataversity. 2023. Available from: https://www.dataversity.net/blockchain-based-llms-a-game-changer-for-data-privacy-protection/

[14] Decentralized Large Language Model: Cardano and Altman Join Forces [Internet]. HyScaler. 2023. Available from: https://hyscaler.com/insights/large-language-model-cardano-altman/

[15] Linkous J. Challenges in telehealth. In: Board on Health Care Services, Institute of Medicine, editors. The Role of Telehealth in an Evolving Health Care Environment: Workshop Summary. Washington (DC): National Academies Press (US); 2012. pp. 17-19. DOI: 10.17226/13466

[16] Haleem A, Javaid M, Singh RP, Suman R. Telemedicine for healthcare: Capabilities, features, barriers, and applications. Sensors International. 2021;**2**:100117. DOI: 10.1016/j.sintl.2021.100117

[17] Alenoghena CO, Onumanyi AJ, Ohize HO, Adejo AO, Oligbi M, Ali SI, et al. eHealth: A survey of architectures, developments in mHealth, security concerns and solutions. International Journal of Environmental Research and Public Health. 2022;**19**(20):13071. DOI: 10.3390/ijerph192013071

[18] Birhane A, Kasirzadeh A, Leslie D, Wachter S. Science in the age of large language models. Nature Reviews Physics. 2023;**5**(5):277-280. DOI: 10.1038/s42254-023-00581-4

[19] Brown TB, Mann B, Ryder N, et al. Language models are few-shot learners. arXiv. 2020;**2005**:14165v4. DOI: 10.48550/arxiv.2005.14165

[20] Toews R. Transformers Revolutionized AI. What Will Replace Them? [Internet]. Forbes. 2023. Available from: https://www.forbes.com/sites/robtoews/2023/09/03/transformers-revolutionized-ai-what-will-replace-them/?sh=7280a52b9c1f

[21] Meskó B. The impact of multimodal large language models on health care's future. Journal of Medical Internet Research. 2023;**25**:e52865. DOI: 10.2196/52865

[22] Winkel DJ, Heye T, Weikert TJ, Boll DT, Stieltjes B. Evaluation of an AI-based detection software for acute findings in abdominal computed tomography scans: Toward an automated work list prioritization of routine CT examinations. Investigative Radiology. 2019;**54**(1):55-59. DOI: 10.1097/RLI.0000000000000509

[23] Ge J, Li M, Delk MB, Lai JC. A comparison of a large language model vs manual chart review for the extraction of data elements from the electronic health record. Gastroenterology. 2024;**166**(4):707-709.e3. DOI:10.1053/j.gastro.2023.12.019

[24] Zoom. Zoom Debuts New AI Companion Capability for Whiteboard, Expands Availability to Industries [Internet]. 2023. Available from https://news.zoom.us/ai-companion-zoomtopia/ [Accessed: January 30, 2024]

[25] Currie GM. Academic integrity and artificial intelligence: Is ChatGPT hype, hero or heresy? Seminars in Nuclear Medicine. 2023;**53**(5):719-730. DOI: 10.1053/j.semnuclmed.2023.04.008

[26] Heston TF, Lewis LM. ChatGPT provides inconsistent risk-stratification of patients with atraumatic chest pain. medRxiv. 2023;**11**(29):23299214. DOI: 10.1101/2023.11.29.23299214

[27] Zack T, Lehman E, Suzgun M, Rodriguez JA, Celi LA, Gichoya J, et al. Assessing the potential of GPT-4 to perpetuate racial and gender biases in health care: A model evaluation study. Lancet Digital Health. 2024;**6**(1):e12-e22. DOI: 10.1016/S2589-7500(23)00225-X

[28] Schweikart SJ. Who will be liable for medical malpractice in the future? How the use of artificial intelligence in medicine will shape medical tort law. Minnesota

Journal of Law, Science & Technology. 2021;**22**:1

[29] Banja JD, Hollstein RD, Bruno MA. When artificial intelligence models surpass physician performance: Medical malpractice liability in an era of advanced artificial intelligence. Journal of the American College of Radiology. 2022;**19**(7):816-820. DOI: 10.1016/j.jacr.2021.11.014

[30] Blease C. Open AI meets open notes: Surveillance capitalism, patient privacy and online record access. Journal of Medical Ethics. 2024;**50**(2):84-89. DOI: 10.1136/jme-2023-109574

[31] Cai W. Feasibility and prospect of privacy-preserving large language models in radiology. Radiology. 2023;**309**(1):e232335. DOI: 10.1148/radiol.232335

[32] Yu J, Wu Y, Shu D, Jin M, Xing X. Assessing prompt injection risks in 200+ custom GPTs. arXiv. 2023;2311.11538v1. DOI: 10.48550/arXiv.2311.11538

[33] Burgess M. OpenAI's custom chatbots are leaking their secrets [Internet]. Wired. 2023. Available from: https://www.wired.com/story/openai-custom-chatbots-gpts-prompt-injection-attacks/

[34] Androulaki E, Manevich Y, Muralidharan S, Murthy C, Nguyen B, Sethi M, et al. Hyperledger fabric: A distributed operating system for permissioned blockchains. In: Proceedings of the Thirteenth EuroSys Conference on - EuroSys '18. New York, New York, USA: ACM Press; 2018. pp. 1-15. DOI: 10.1145/3190508.3190538

[35] Sterling A. Can bitcoin network Be hacked? The safety of cryptocurrency [Internet]. Doubloin. 2023. Available from: https://www.doubloin.com/learn/can-bitcoin-network-be-hacked

[36] Heston TF. A case study in blockchain health care innovation. International Journal of Current Research. 2017;**9**(11):60587-60588

[37] Blockchain technology in healthcare market projected to reach USD 14.1 billion by 2030 [Internet]. Global Newswire. 2023. Available from: https://www.globenewswire.com/en/news-release/2023/11/30/2788314/0/en/Blockchain-Technology-in-Healthcare-Market-projected-to-reach-USD-14-1-Billion-by-2030-growing-at-a-CAGR-of-37-5-during-the-forecast-period-of-2023-2030-pronounced-by-MarketDigits-.html

[38] AbdelSalam FM. Blockchain revolutionizing healthcare industry: A systematic review of blockchain technology benefits and threats. Perspectives in Health Information Management. 2023;**20**(3):1b

[39] Hiwale M, Walambe R, Potdar V, Kotecha K. A systematic review of privacy-preserving methods deployed with blockchain and federated learning for the telemedicine. Healthcare Analytics (New York, N.Y.). 2023;**3**:100192. DOI: 10.1016/j.health.2023.100192

[40] HIPAA vs. GDPR compliance: What's the difference? [internet]. OneTrust. 2022. Available from: https://www.onetrust.com/blog/hipaa-vs-gdpr-compliance/

[41] Polsinelli PC. GDPR Implementation and HIPAA Compliance: An Analysis of the GDPR and HIPAA for U.S. Health & Life Sciences Organizations [Microsoft White paper]. 2018

[42] Wang X, Shi J, Lee KM. The digital divide and seeking health information on smartphones in Asia: Survey study of ten countries. Journal of Medical

Internet Research. 2022;**24**(1):e24086. DOI: 10.2196/24086

[43] Saha S, Beach MC, Cooper LA. Patient centeredness, cultural competence and healthcare quality. Journal of the National Medical Association. 2008;**100**(11):1275-1285. DOI: 10.1016/S0027-9684(15)31505-4

[44] Al-Samarraie H, Ghazal S, Alzahrani AI, Moody L. Telemedicine in middle eastern countries: Progress, barriers, and policy recommendations. International Journal of Medical Informatics. 2020;**141**:104232. DOI: 10.1016/j.ijmedinf.2020.104232

[45] Parkes P, Pillay TD, Bdaiwi Y, Simpson R, Almoshmosh N, Murad L, et al. Telemedicine interventions in six conflict-affected countries in the WHO eastern Mediterranean region: A systematic review. Conflict and Health. 2022;**16**(1):64. DOI: 10.1186/s13031-022-00493-7

[46] LLM integration unleashes AI advancements: 5 remarkable breakthroughs [Internet]. Hyscaler. 2023. Available from: https://hyscaler.com/insights/llm-integration-advancing-ai/

[47] Krittanawong C, Aydar M, Hassan Virk HU, Kumar A, Kaplin S, Guimaraes L, et al. Artificial intelligence-powered blockchains for cardiovascular medicine. The Canadian Journal of Cardiology. 2022;**38**(2):185-195. DOI: 10.1016/j.cjca.2021.11.011

[48] Diaz N. Digital health funding hits a wall [Internet]. Becker's Hospital Review. 2024. Available from: https://www.beckershospitalreview.com/digital-health/digital-health-funding-hits-a-wall.html

[49] State of digital health 2022 report [Internet]. CB Insights. 2023. Available from: https://www.cbinsights.com/research/report/digital-health-trends-2022/

[50] Sharma S, Rawal R, Shah D. Addressing the challenges of AI-based telemedicine: Best practices and lessons learned. Journal of Education Health Promotion. 2023;**12**:338. DOI: 10.4103/jehp.jehp_402_23

Chapter 16

Digital Frontiers in Healthcare: Integrating mHealth, AI, and Radiology for Future Medical Diagnostics

Reabal Najjar

Abstract

In an era where technology and healthcare increasingly intertwine, we stand on the precipice of a seismic shift in the future of healthcare and medicine. This chapter unravels the confluence of mHealth, artificial intelligence (AI), and radiology as it navigates the labyrinth of these advancements, dissecting their unique qualities, historical evolution, and projected trajectories. From the democratising potential of mHealth to AI's analytical might, and the transformative journey of medical imaging from film to digital—the chapter offers a deep dive into current realities and future horizons. Further, the intersection of these domains is explored, illuminating AI's revolutionary role in enhancing mHealth capabilities through advances in medical imaging. An exhaustive review of cutting-edge applications and the ethico-regulatory conundrums they pose, forms a substantial part of the discourse, followed by a foresight into anticipated technological breakthroughs, their potential impacts, and the critical role of policymakers and health leaders in this odyssey. The chapter culminates in a holistic synthesis, tying together the strands of the preceding sections to underscore the transformative potential of this technological triumvirate. The text is designed as a captivating exploration, a reflective critique, and a roadmap for the future as we collectively navigate towards a technologically empowered healthcare era.

Keywords: mHealth, artificial intelligence, machine learning, healthcare, medical imaging, radiology

1. Introduction

In the rapidly evolving landscape of healthcare, the merging of mobile health (mHealth), artificial intelligence (AI), and medical imaging signifies a critical transformation, offering a multidimensional, patient-centred, data-driven model optimised for enhanced diagnostic and therapeutic outcomes.

mHealth, a subset of eHealth, capitalises on the pervasive nature of mobile technologies to augment the reach and efficacy of healthcare services [1]. The omnipresence of smartphones has spawned an era of ubiquitous health monitoring and services. No longer tethered by geographical constraints, we are now able to furnish real-time health data, diminishing healthcare disparities and enabling timely interventions [2].

AI, the broad umbrella under which machine learning (ML), deep learning (DL), and neural networks reside, has woven itself into the fabric of healthcare. It plays an integral role in predicting, diagnosing, and managing diseases [3–5]. The sheer power of AI to unravel intricate health datasets is ushering in a new era of personalised care that's nothing short of extraordinary [5].

This transformative potential of AI is particularly evident in the realm of medical imaging, an indispensable pillar of modern medicine. While traditional imaging techniques hold undeniable value, they are contingent on the clinician's expertise and are not impervious to human error. Enter AI algorithms, particularly those rooted in machine learning. These tools swiftly dissect complex imaging data with extraordinary precision, minimising human error [4]. Equipped with vast image databases, these algorithms discern nuanced patterns beyond the reach of human cognition and lay the groundwork for predictive analytics in medicine [4–6].

When we interweave mHealth, AI, and medical imaging, we unlock the potential to revolutionise healthcare delivery. AI uncovers the diagnostic treasures hidden in medical images, while mHealth ensures their accessibility, thereby accelerating diagnoses, optimising treatment plans, and improving patient outcomes [7].

mHealth, AI, and medical imaging, in isolation, boast formidable capabilities. However, their combined potential is the spark that may ignite a full-scale transformation in healthcare. As we navigate the industry's shift towards a preventative, personalised, and precision-focused model, the integration of these three domains becomes all the more critical. This chapter delves deep into the advantages, challenges, and future implications of this promising coalescence for the future of healthcare.

2. Understanding mHealth

2.1 Definition and key features of mHealth

mHealth, a derivative of eHealth, represents the utilisation of mobile and wireless technologies to support the attainment of health objectives [8]. Defined by the Global Observatory for eHealth as "medical and public health practice supported by mobile devices, such as mobile phones, patient monitoring devices, personal digital assistants (PDAs), and other wireless devices", mHealth has opened new avenues for the delivery of healthcare services [9].

Key features of mHealth include the facilitation of data collection in real-time, provision of access to healthcare services irrespective of geographic location, ensuring timely healthcare interventions, and improving patient adherence to medical advice and prescriptions [10, 11]. The ability to incorporate a variety of applications, ranging from telemedicine, electronic health records (EHRs), and healthcare analytics, to wearable technology and health-related IoT applications, underscores the flexibility of mHealth [2].

mHealth promotes an individualised and patient-centric approach to healthcare, affording a comprehensive health perspective of each patient through a combination of real-time and longitudinal data [12]. Furthermore, by enabling remote patient monitoring and diagnostics, mHealth minimises unnecessary hospital visits, thereby reducing the strain on healthcare systems [11]. With the integration of artificial intelligence and machine learning algorithms, mHealth has the potential to revolutionise healthcare by providing personalised, predictive, and preventive care. Despite its transformative capacity, mHealth implementation must negotiate challenges related to privacy, security, interoperability, and regulatory considerations.

2.2 Tracing the path: historical progression and evolution

The inception of mHealth in the early 2000s, coinciding with the mobile telecommunications boom, signified the harnessing of mobile and wireless technologies for health objectives [8]. Initially, mHealth primarily facilitated health information dissemination and communication among healthcare providers, reaching even remote areas [1].

The debut of the first iPhone in 2007 significantly broadened the mHealth landscape. These 'smartphones,' essentially handheld computers with advanced processing capacities and sophisticated software, evolved beyond mere communication tools to potent health platforms [13].

The subsequent introduction of app stores ushered in a wave of health-related applications, drastically expanding mHealth's scope [13]. These apps ranged from fitness trackers promoting healthy habits to telemedicine interfaces enabling virtual consultations, thus empowering individuals to actively manage their health.

The late 2000s saw the emergence of wearable technologies and the Internet of Things (IoT) [14]. Wearables, equipped with biometric sensors, facilitated real-time health monitoring, promoting proactive and preventative care. Concurrently, the IoT interconnected these devices, creating a synchronised health data ecosystem [14].

The transition from 3G to 4G and 5G further propelled mHealth. Enhanced data transfer rates and reduced latencies of these mobile networks enabled real-time transmission of large, complex data, such as medical imaging, improving care quality and speed [2].

Over the past decade, mHealth has evolved from a technological novelty to a crucial component of global healthcare delivery systems. This swift integration of mHealth has been propelled by shifting societal habits, relentless technological advancements, and dynamic healthcare demands [15]. The COVID-19 pandemic underscored the necessity for remote healthcare delivery and patient monitoring, further elevating mHealth's relevance and urgency.

2.3 mHealth today and beyond: current status and future implications

At the confluence of the technological era and healthcare, mHealth emerges as a dynamic catalyst. The current state is characterised by broad utilisation across diverse applications: chronic disease management, patient monitoring, health education, and telehealth consultations, among others [11]. mHealth technologies facilitate improved patient outcomes by fostering proactive health management and personalised healthcare.

Pervasive use of smartphones and wearable devices, combined with growing health consciousness, has driven mHealth integration into routine healthcare. Telehealth services, catalysed by the COVID-19 pandemic, remain an exemplary adaptation of mHealth, bridging patient-provider geographical disparities [16].

mHealth's future appears laden with potential. An anticipated trajectory involves the marriage of mHealth and AI, facilitating predictive analytics and personalised medicine. The wealth of data procured by mHealth devices could be harnessed to predict health outcomes and prompt preventative interventions, amplifying the healthcare paradigm shift towards prevention over cure.

Furthermore, incorporating genomics and precision medicine within the mHealth spectrum could revolutionise patient management, transitioning from symptom-based to molecular-based treatment [10, 15].

Yet, the path forward also raises concerns: ethical, privacy, and cybersecurity issues must be scrupulously addressed. As mHealth continues its journey towards seamless integration into healthcare, continuous innovation, stringent regulation, and user acceptance remain vital elements influencing its future prospects. Thereby, mHealth stands on the precipice of defining the next healthcare epoch, embodying a blend of ubiquitous computing, personalised medicine, and predictive analytics.

3. Harnessing artificial intelligence and machine learning in healthcare

3.1 Decoding AI and ML

Artificial Intelligence, in its simplest form, refers to the capability of machines to emulate human cognitive functions such as understanding, learning, problem-solving, and decision-making [17]. This complex field of computer science was designed with the intention of creating intelligent machines that can behave, react, and work like human beings. They can execute a wide array of tasks with precision and efficiency, ranging from performing simple tasks to solving intricate problems.

There are two main types of AI—Narrow AI, which is designed to perform a narrow task such as voice recognition, and General AI, which is a type of machine intelligence that has the potential to perform any intellectual task that a human being can do [3]. The present era predominantly features Narrow AI, where AI technologies specialise in particular domains such as customer service through chatbots, voice recognition in virtual assistants, or image interpretation in medical imaging.

Machine learning, on the other hand, is an application of AI that grants systems the ability to automatically learn and improve from experience without explicit programming [17]. ML operates under the fundamental principle that machines should access data and learn autonomously.

ML is typically categorised into three types: *supervised learning*, where algorithms are trained on labelled data; *unsupervised learning*, where algorithms learn from unlabelled data to discover hidden patterns or intrinsic structures; and *reinforcement learning*, where an agent learns to make decisions by interacting with its environment, receiving rewards for positive actions and penalties for negative actions [3].

A further extension of ML is deep learning, which is an algorithm-based model that aims to mimic the human brain. DL algorithms utilise artificial neural networks with multiple layers—sometimes consisting of hundreds—that process the data, each layer providing a distinct interpretation [18]. This layered interpretation allows DL models to handle complex data and draw accurate conclusions or make predictions effectively. **Figure 1** provides a brief overview of AI and its various subsets.

3.2 AI and ML in contemporary medicine

AI and ML are revolutionising healthcare, impacting a spectrum of areas from diagnosis to administration. A fundamental application of these technologies lies in managing copious amounts of patient data, encompassing laboratory results, imaging studies, genetic profiles and comprehensive electronic health records, thereby facilitating the extraction of invaluable insights [6].

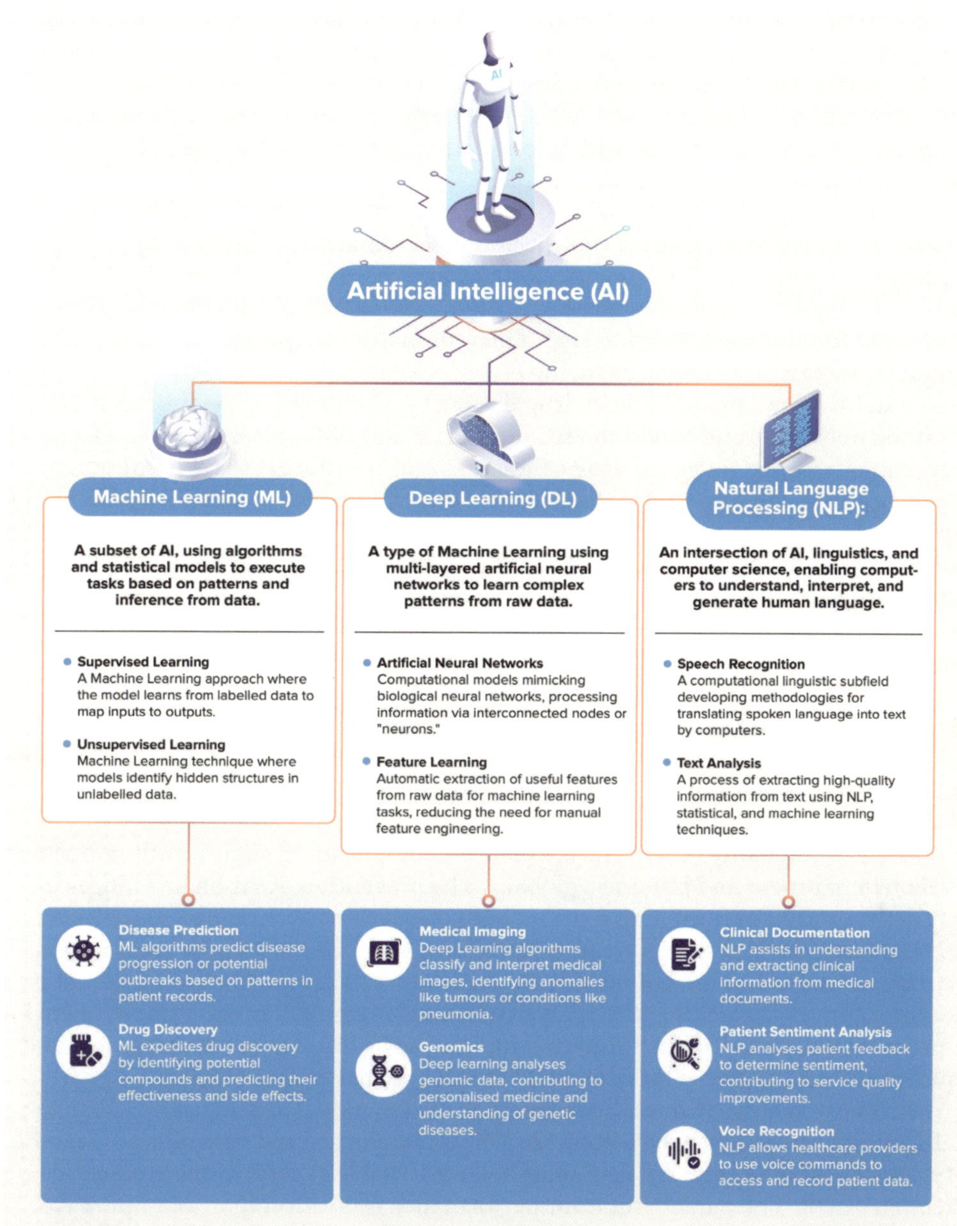

Figure 1.
An overview of artificial intelligence, machine learning, deep learning, and natural language processing.

In the sphere of personalised medicine, ML underpins the derivation of significant patterns from patient data [19]. This empowers the provision of bespoke therapeutic approaches, tailored to individual genetic, environmental, and lifestyle factors, heralding a departure from traditional methodologies. ML models, when applied to large-scale biomedical datasets, can illuminate associations between genetic variations and disease susceptibility, thereby enriching our comprehension of disease pathogenesis and progression [20].

Integral to contemporary healthcare are AI-driven clinical decision support systems. These sophisticated systems decode complex patient data, providing clinicians with essential insights that inform diagnostic and treatment decisions. Furthermore, predictive analytics, underpinned by AI, represent a potent tool for early disease detection, identifying patterns within longitudinal patient data to predict disease risks, thus optimising patient outcomes [19].

In the domain of medical imaging, AI introduces transformative enhancements. Notably, computer vision, an AI sub-discipline, automates the interpretation of a myriad of imaging modalities, such as radiographs, computed tomography (CT) scans, and magnetic resonance imaging (MRI), often equalling or surpassing the accuracy of human interpretation [21]. This automation supports radiologists by mitigating their workload and reducing error incidence.

AI and ML play a pivotal role in drug discovery, streamlining the process and curtailing both costs and timeframes. Through utilising ML, researchers can forecast interactions between potential drug candidates and specific diseases, predicated upon extensive, multi-dimensional biological datasets, thus expediting the drug discovery trajectory [4, 5].

AI-powered robotics have ushered in unprecedented precision and consistency within surgical practice. Robotic surgical systems, guided by AI algorithms, can execute complex surgical tasks with minimal invasiveness, resulting in reduced postoperative discomfort and accelerated recovery [22].

3.3 Case studies: practical applications of ML in mHealth

3.3.1 Diabetic retinopathy

Diabetic retinopathy (DR), a severe diabetes complication, significantly contributes to vision impairment and blindness globally. The prevention of vision loss hinges on early detection and prompt intervention, both of which require regular retinal screening. However, such screenings are often unachievable or unavailable in many regions, particularly those with limited resources. This is where ML and AI technologies present a robust solution, automating the analysis of retinal images for precise and efficient DR detection [23]. One such transformative application of ML is in the development and deployment of a DL model for detecting DR from retinal images (**Figure 2**).

A striking example of this advancement is the DL model developed by Gulshan et al. [24]. By employing a dataset of 128,175 retinal images and convolutional neural networks (CNNs), this model demonstrated remarkable success in the automatic detection of DR. The model's superior performance was reflected in an impressive area under the receiver operating characteristic curve (AUC-ROC) of 0.991 for DR detection, a clear improvement over previous methodologies and a testament to the potential of AI and ML in DR screening [24].

The application of AI and ML in mHealth, as epitomised by this case study, offers several advantages over traditional DR screening methods. The primary benefit is a significant reduction in healthcare professionals' workload, enabling concentration on complex cases and direct patient care [25]. AI-driven systems also deliver swift, accurate retinal image analysis, facilitating timely diagnosis and intervention to prevent vision loss [23]. Furthermore, the automation of DR screening using AI and ML can enhance healthcare access in underserviced areas, where the availability of specialist ophthalmologists is often scarce [26].

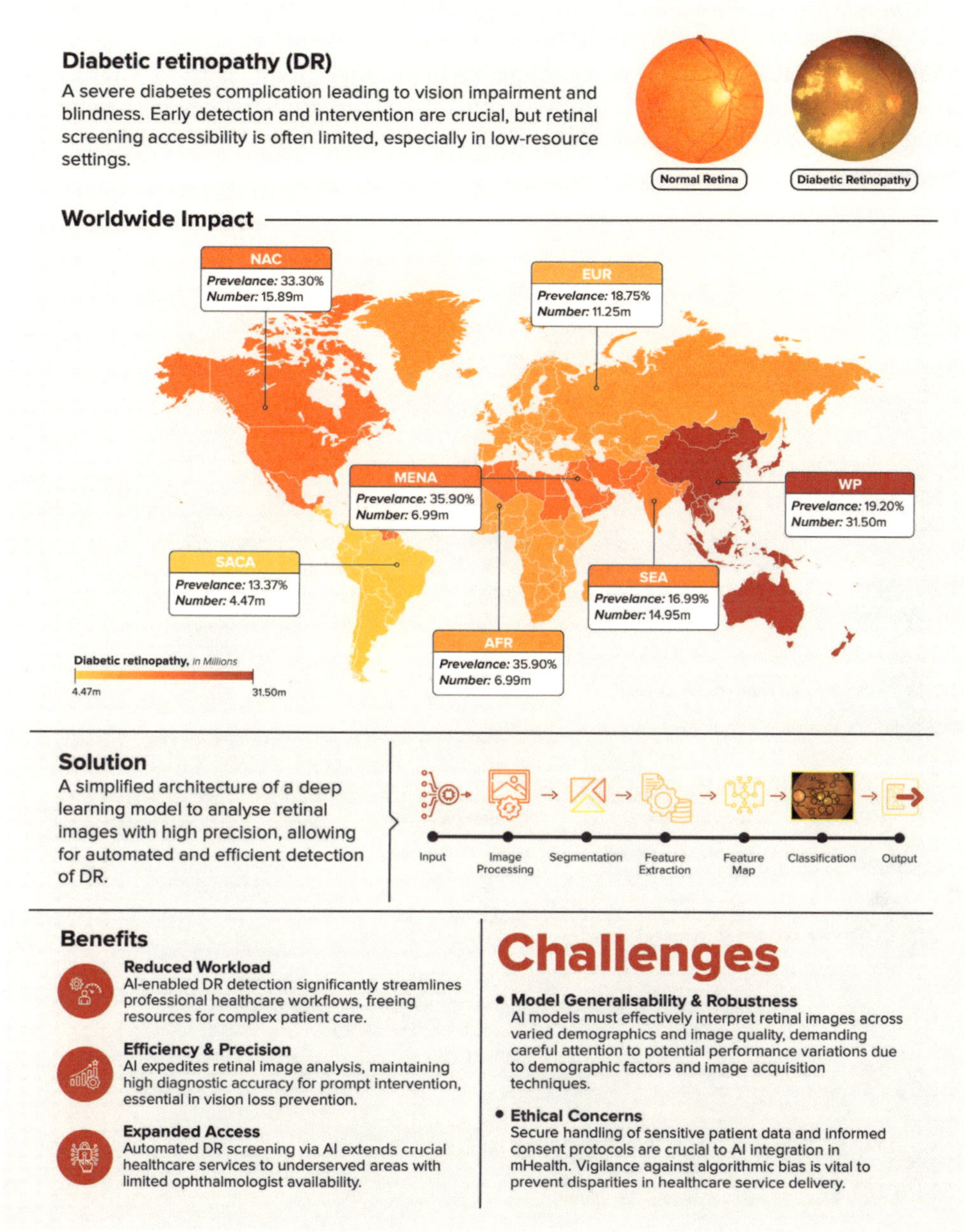

Figure 2.
Machine learning applications in diabetic retinopathy.

Nonetheless, it's important to recognise the challenges accompanying the implementation of AI and ML for DR detection in mHealth. The success of AI models hinges on their generalisability and robustness across diverse populations and varied retinal image quality [27]. Additionally, addressing ethical considerations surrounding data privacy, informed consent, and algorithmic bias is essential for the responsible use of AI in mHealth applications [28].

3.3.2 Chronic obstructive pulmonary disease (COPD)

This case study examines a practical use of ML models in mHealth for COPD management and monitoring. It provides crucial insights and challenges encountered during this process, offering valuable guidance for future AI and ML healthcare integration efforts [29].

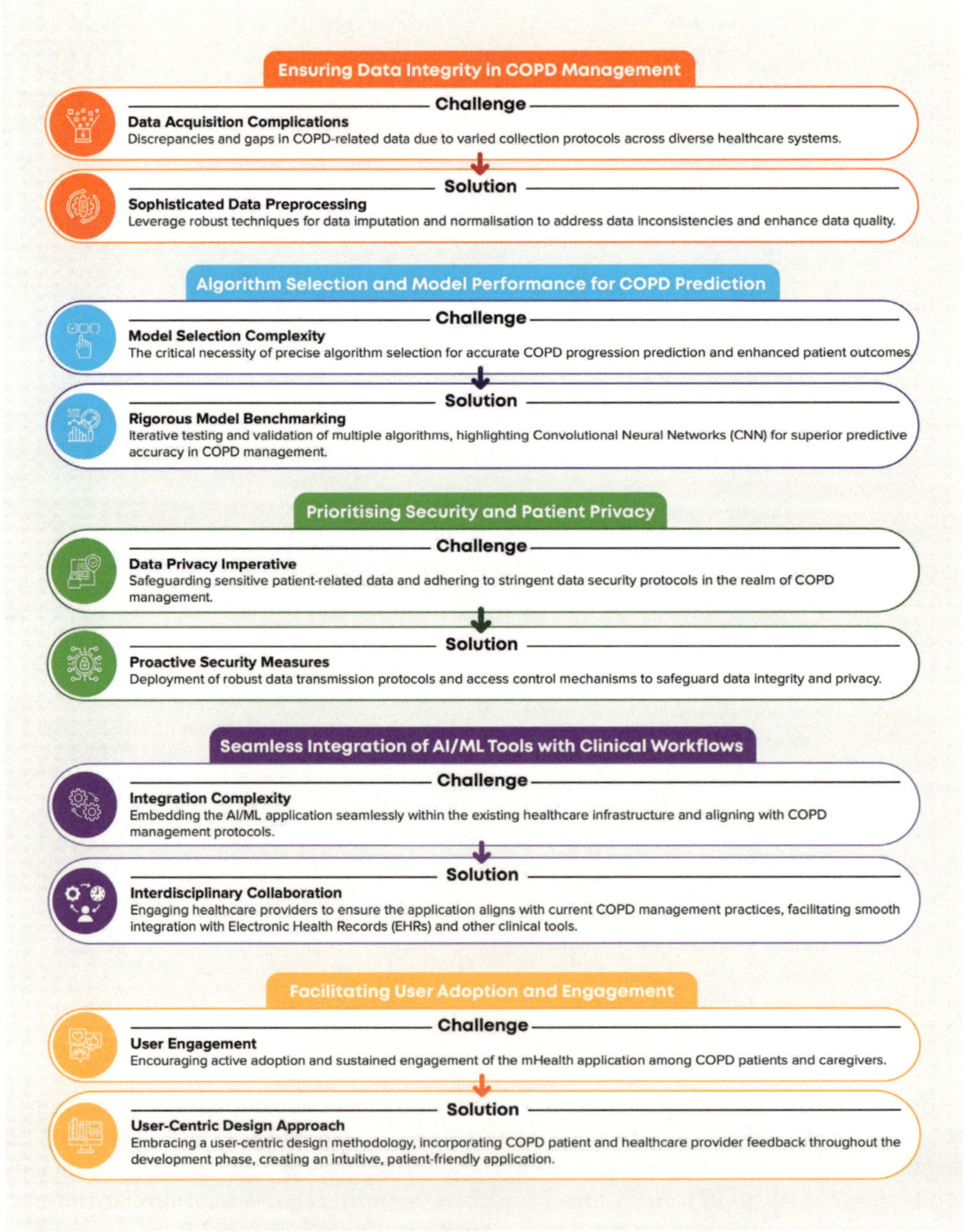

Figure 3.
Machine learning applications in COPD.

COPD is a persistent respiratory disorder characterised by continuous symptoms and airflow limitation due to airway and/or alveolar anomalies [30]. mHealth applications could revolutionise COPD care by enabling remote patient monitoring and delivering real-time, personalised health feedback [31].

The development of the COPD mHealth application encountered various obstacles (**Figure 3**).

1. *Data collection and quality*: the collection of high-quality data is essential for the effective deployment of AI and ML in mHealth [29]. Data collection challenges included incomplete data and quality discrepancies due to variations in data collection protocols across healthcare providers. Data preprocessing techniques, such as imputation and normalisation, were used to overcome these issues.

2. *Algorithm selection and model performance*: choosing the right AI and ML algorithms is critical for precise prediction and improved patient outcomes [32]. Various algorithms, including support vector machines (SVM), random forest (RF), and DL models, were assessed, with convolutional neural networks (CNNs) proving most effective for predicting patient outcomes and providing personalised feedback [29].

3. *Security and privacy*: preserving patient confidentiality and protecting sensitive health data was a priority [33]. Robust security measures, such as secure data transmission protocols and access control systems, were implemented to address these concerns.

4. *Integration with clinical workflows*: the incorporation of the mHealth application into existing healthcare systems and clinical workflows required strategic partnerships with healthcare providers to tailor the application for smooth integration with electronic health records (EHRs) and other clinical tools [34].

5. *User adoption and engagement*: encouraging user adoption and engagement with the mHealth application was critical [35]. A user-centric design approach and the inclusion of feedback from COPD patients and healthcare providers during the design and development stages resulted in an intuitive application with high user adoption rates.

3.4 A glimpse into the future: potential applications

AI and ML are progressively transforming the healthcare ecosystem with a myriad of applications that span diagnostics, therapeutics, patient care management, and health system optimisation, presenting a vision of future healthcare marked by individualised and efficient care [5].

- *Predictive analytics and disease modelling*: AI/ML algorithms, meticulously trained on expansive datasets, possess the capability to discern patterns that elude human cognitive processes. For instance, sophisticated DL models can prognosticate the progression of chronic ailments such as diabetes or chronic kidney disease, thereby allowing for proactive interventions to mitigate disease progression [10].

  Unintrusive wearable IoT devices persistently collate and transmit integral patient health data, including heart rate variability, blood glucose metrics, and sleep patterns, into a designated ML model. This dynamic model, continually learning and evolving, has the potential to recognise early indications of disease progression, substantially reducing the burden of chronic diseases by facilitating proactive health management [36].

- *Radiomics and imaging diagnostics*: AI/ML has made significant strides in radiomics, an area dedicated to extracting large volumes of features from radiographic images via data characterisation algorithms. ML models, specifically CNNs, have demonstrated superior diagnostic accuracy in identifying conditions such as lung cancer from CT scans and breast cancer from mammograms [37]. As these models evolve, their predictive accuracy is likely to improve, leading to a decrease in both false positives and negatives, curtailing the need for invasive diagnostic procedures, and consequently enhancing patient outcomes. Additionally, the incorporation of federated learning—an approach allowing ML across multiple datasets at their original location—could augment model generalisability without jeopardising patient data privacy [38].

- *Personalised medicine and therapeutics*: AI/ML algorithms, through the comprehensive analysis of both genotypic and phenotypic patient data, have the capability to discern the most effective therapeutic intervention for an individual, thereby reducing the dependency on the often-inherent trial-and-error methodology in treatment strategies [39].

Through the use of a single blood examination and genomic sequencing, an AI algorithm can propose the most suitable pharmacological regimen for a patient with complex comorbidities. The AI model integrates factors such as drug interactions, individual metabolic responses, and potential adverse effects into its decision-making process. This degree of precision in therapeutics has the potential to significantly improve patient outcomes and elevate the standard of patient care [39].

- *Health systems improvement*: AI/ML holds the capability to enhance health systems, streamlining administrative tasks, optimising patient flow, and improving resource allocation. Future application of natural language processing (NLP) algorithms could sift through electronic health records, automate billing, facilitate appointment scheduling, and augment workflow efficiency, thus allowing healthcare professionals to devote more time to patient care [40].

4. Medical imaging: a journey from radiography to superintelligence

4.1 Overview of traditional medical imaging techniques

The genesis of modern medical imaging can be traced back to the discovery of X-rays by Wilhelm Conrad Roentgen in 1895 (**Figure 4**). The initial technique, radiography, leveraged the differential absorption of X-ray radiation among tissues, with denser structures, such as bones, appearing white due to increased absorption [41]. Further sophistication was introduced through the utilisation of contrast agents, enhancing the perceptibility of specific structures in procedures such as angiography or barium swallow examinations [41].

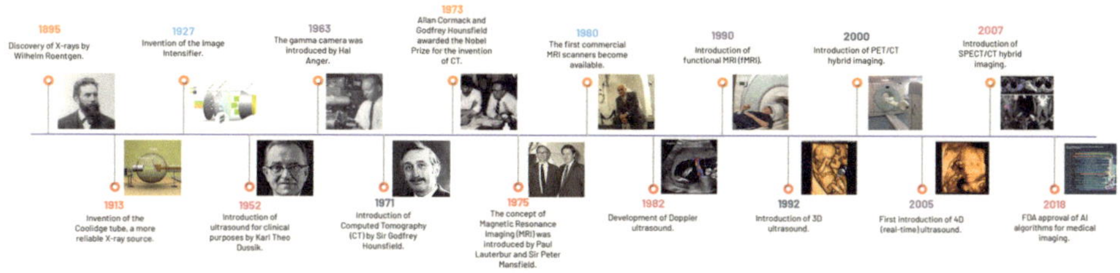

Figure 4.
A historical timeline of the key discoveries in medical imaging.

Fluoroscopy, conceived in the early twentieth century as a dynamic extension of radiography, facilitated real-time visualisation of internal body structures. This capability has proved invaluable for executing minimally invasive procedures like catheter placement and joint injections, solidifying its irreplaceable role in the clinical scenario [42]. Thereafter, the 1940s heralded the introduction of ultrasound imaging, a modality leveraging high-frequency sound waves to generate real-time images of internal organs (Edler). Embodying safety, portability, and cost-effectiveness, ultrasound has emerged as a cornerstone in diverse fields such as obstetrics, cardiology, and emergency medicine (Bushberg).

The 1970s witnessed another breakthrough with the introduction of CT scanning by Sir Godfrey Hounsfield. CT employs multiple X-ray measurements taken from distinct angles, yielding cross-sectional images or 'slices' of the body [43]. The three-dimensional vistas offered by CT scans supersede conventional X-rays in visualising intricate structures such as the brain, lungs, and abdominal organs.

Medical imaging took another significant leap forward in the early 1980s with the clinical adoption of MRI. Devoid of ionising radiation, MRI creates high-resolution images by harnessing the principles of nuclear magnetic resonance [44, 45]. Particularly efficacious for imaging soft tissues and organs, MRI is an unrivalled tool for studying structures such as the brain, spinal cord, and musculoskeletal system [44, 45].

Nuclear medicine techniques of the contemporary era, such as Positron Emission Tomography (PET) and Single-Photon Emission Computed Tomography (SPECT), afford functional imaging by tracking radiation from an introduced radioactive tracer [46, 47]. These techniques impart critical insights into the physiological function and metabolic processes of organs, facilitating diagnostic and therapeutic applications in fields as diverse as cardiology, neurology, and oncology [46, 47].

Nevertheless, the remarkable benefits accrued from traditional medical imaging are somewhat offset by inherent limitations. These include exposure to ionising radiation (pertinent to X-rays and CT scans), variable image resolution, dependence on operator skill (in ultrasound imaging), significant economic implications, and protracted scanning times (particularly in MRI). The transition to digital imaging, bolstered by the integration of AI, promises to counter many of these challenges, a perspective explored in subsequent sections.

4.2 The digital revolution in imaging

The digital era has heralded pivotal developments in medical science, presenting an array of advantages whilst concurrently introducing novel complexities. Digital medical imaging, essentially a transformation of images into numerical data for computational interpretation, has facilitated a period of enhanced diagnostic precision, efficient data archiving, and accelerated transmission of medical imagery, encapsulating X-rays, CT scans, MRI, and ultrasounds [48].

The transition to digital has primarily eclipsed analogue imaging methodologies, underscoring its potential to revolutionise diagnostic efficacy and accuracy. The intricacy afforded by digital images, attributable to superior resolution and contrast, has been instrumental in augmenting the sensitivity and specificity of disease detection [49]. This aspect is indispensable across numerous clinical scenarios, including the discernment of diminutive tumours or the delineation of nuanced stroke lesions. Additionally, digital images facilitate manipulations for optimal visualisation without compromising the image integrity, offering adjustable contrast, brightness, and magnification parameters tailored to individual patient contexts and specific clinical requisites.

Another salient advantage of digital imaging is its capacity for streamlined storage and retrieval. The physical archiving of analogue images poses significant challenges, occupying substantial space and risking degradation over time. Conversely, digital images can be effectively preserved within electronic databases such as Picture Archiving and Communication Systems (PACS), thus ensuring sustained image integrity [50]. The integration of digital imaging with EHRs further optimises retrieval and bolsters the continuity of patient care.

The capability for instantaneous and remote transmission of digital images represents a key benefit, particularly relevant in the burgeoning field of telemedicine. Physicians can access diagnostic images virtually anywhere, encouraging global collaboration irrespective of geographical barriers [51]. Nevertheless, the digitisation of medical imaging is not devoid of challenges. Foremost, the substantial costs associated with the acquisition and maintenance of digital imaging equipment and software can impose a significant financial encumbrance on numerous healthcare providers.

While digital imaging expedites storage, the vast increase in data consequent of this transition presents a formidable challenge. This voluminous data surge necessitates robust data management strategies to ensure data integrity, security, and accessibility. Confidentiality and security concerns also underscore the hurdles inherent to digital imaging. As medical images become an integral component of an interconnected digital health ecosystem, potential breaches of confidentiality and unauthorised access emerge, thereby necessitating rigorous cybersecurity protocols. Lastly, the assimilation of digital imaging into established healthcare workflows may necessitate substantial change management efforts, encompassing training healthcare professionals to operate innovative technologies, interpret digital images, and adapt to evolving workflow dynamics [52].

4.3 The impact of AI on the transformation of radiology

Within the ambit of medical imaging, AI has substantially expedited the evolution from traditional to digital techniques, reinventing diagnostics and prognostics by providing more accurate, rapid, and efficient tools that redefine clinical decision-making.

The transformative capacity of AI in medical imaging is primarily grounded in its sophisticated pattern recognition ability [53]. As such, a gamut of AI algorithms, particularly those harnessing DL approaches, are making substantial strides in medical imaging interpretation. For instance, CNNs, a type of DL model inspired by the visual cortex, has been especially impactful in the realm of radiology, demonstrating exceptional competence in identifying complex patterns in voluminous image data sets.

CNNs can process both 2D and 3D images, discerning nuanced details that may elude the human eye, thereby extending the capacity of radiologists. By learning from vast data sets and continuously improving its accuracy with each data interaction, ML can potentially uncover novel imaging biomarkers, facilitating earlier detection, better prognostication, and personalised treatment.

AI is also instrumental in expediting the image acquisition and reconstruction processes in imaging modalities like CT and MRI [54]. For instance, AI has proven adept at producing high-quality images from undersampled data, mitigating the traditionally extended MRI scan times and enhancing patient comfort. Additionally, it aids in reducing exposure to ionising radiation in CT imaging by enabling superior image quality from lower dose acquisitions.

The significant progress in AI-powered medical imaging extends beyond diagnostics. The predictive potential of AI, paired with imaging, holds promise in enhancing patient management by forecasting disease progression and therapeutic response [55]. This predictive capacity is particularly relevant in chronic conditions, such as cardiovascular diseases and cancer, where timely and accurate assessment can significantly influence therapeutic outcomes. Moreover, AI's integration in interventional imaging promotes the development of image-guided therapies, thus further optimising patient care.

Furthermore, AI can be a potent tool in managing the substantial data generated in medical imaging [56]. With digital imaging systems producing a tremendous amount of data daily, traditional methods of data handling prove increasingly inadequate. AI, with its capacity to analyse and extract meaningful insights from large-scale imaging data, offers an effective solution to this challenge. This data-driven approach can potentially foster a move towards precision medicine, tailoring therapies based on individual patient profiles.

However, while AI's potential in medical imaging is substantial, it should be viewed as a tool to augment, not replace, clinicians. Ideally, AI serves as a secondary reader, assisting clinicians in improving efficiency and reducing diagnostic errors, whilst maintaining human oversight to validate the final clinical decision.

5. Intersection of mHealth and AI in medical imaging

5.1 Real-world applications: mHealth meets AI

The capability of mHealth platforms to collect and share healthcare data provides an unprecedented avenue for AI to influence patient care. These applications broadly fall under two categories: *diagnosis assistance* and *image analysis*. Both these functionalities, powered by AI and delivered through mHealth, can significantly contribute to streamlined and efficient medical imaging processes [57].

Firstly, AI has been applied in numerous diagnostic imaging applications, where its machine learning algorithms can enhance the accuracy of interpreting images by leveraging CNNs adept at processing image data. A notable example is Google's *DeepMind*, which demonstrated its potential in diagnosing age-related macular degeneration and diabetic retinopathy from retinal scans, performing at par or better than human experts [58]. Its deployment via mHealth platforms could provide timely and accurate diagnosis, thereby improving patient outcomes, particularly in remote or resource-poor settings.

Another breakthrough has been the use of AI algorithms in analysing mammograms to detect breast cancer. For instance, ScreenPoint Medical's *Transpara*™

employs AI to interpret mammograms and tomosynthesis exams, helping radiologists identify potential anomalies with improved accuracy [59]. This mHealth-accessible tool allows healthcare professionals to utilise advanced AI-assisted diagnosis, even on their handheld devices.

Furthermore, the intersection of mHealth and AI is revolutionising ultra-sound imaging. Butterfly Network's *Butterfly iQ*, for instance, uses a handheld, pocket-sized ultrasound device that connects to a smartphone and uses AI to capture and interpret images [60]. This democratises the use of ultrasound technology, particularly in rural or low-resource settings where conventional ultrasound machines are not readily available.

Shifting our focus to AI-assisted image analysis, AI algorithms are now capable of providing real-time insights, making them vital tools during surgical procedures. A case in point is the AI software developed by Aidoc, designed to flag acute conditions like strokes, pulmonary embolisms, and cervical spine fractures in CT scans [61]. By integrating such AI software into mHealth platforms, the potential for immediate, round-the-clock analysis could transform acute care.

It is noteworthy to highlight the advent of smart wearable devices and biosensors that collate and interpret an abundance of physiological data. Companies such as Apple and Fitbit are spearheading this trend with AI-powered interpretation of ECG data to detect irregular cardiac rhythms, an established risk factor for cerebrovascular conditions [62]. Similarly, Google's *Project Nightingale* strives to anticipate patient deterioration and optimise corresponding treatment plans through real-time data analytics [63].

5.2 The synergy of mHealth and AI in radiology: key benefits

The synthesis of mobile health with AI within the context of medical imaging proffers a cornucopia of benefits, engendering a fundamental shift in the paradigm of healthcare delivery. In order to comprehend these advantages, it is critical to understand the unique attributes each technology contributes to this potent amalgamation.

The integration of mHealth and AI within the realm of medical imaging offers an array of benefits, facilitating a substantive shift in the landscape of healthcare delivery. To fully appreciate these merits, it is crucial to understand the unique characteristics that each technology contributes to this powerful fusion.

- *Accessibility and expediency*: a primary and compelling merit of mHealth is its capacity to democratise healthcare through enhanced accessibility. This is critically vital in remote and underserved regions where the scarcity of medical resources and expertise exacerbates health inequities [4, 64]. By integrating mHealth with AI in medical imaging, we enable remote diagnostics and patient monitoring, thereby negating the requirement for physical proximity to advanced medical facilities. Additionally, AI-driven algorithm within mHealth applications can significantly hasten the diagnostic process and turnaround time of imaging interpretation. In emergency scenarios, this swift response may constitute the difference between life and death, underscoring the immense potential of this symbiosis.

- *Precision and consistency*: AI algorithms demonstrate remarkable proficiency in extracting salient features from medical images, outperforming humans in some instances [4]. When harnessed in mHealth applications, these AI tools offer the dual advantage of precision and consistency. They can effectively eliminate human errors arising from fatigue or oversight, which are not uncommon in traditional, human-dependent diagnostic processes. AI's prowess in detecting minute aberrations in medical images that may be overlooked by the human eye could potentially enhance early disease detection, improving prognostic outcomes.

- *Patient empowerment and engagement*: mHealth solutions are inherently patient-centred, promoting active patient involvement in managing their health [64]. The incorporation of AI in mHealth for medical imaging further empowers patients by providing them with actionable insights. Patients can monitor health trends, understand potential health risks, and participate more effectively in shared decision-making processes. This paradigm shift from a reactive to a proactive healthcare model cultivates a more engaged, informed patient populace.

- *Efficient resource utilisation*: The healthcare sector, particularly in developing regions, is often beleaguered by resource constraints. The combination of mHealth and AI in medical imaging can engender more efficient utilisation of resources [4]. AI-powered tools, with their automated image analysis capabilities, can alleviate the workload of overburdened healthcare professionals, enabling them to focus on more critical tasks. In the context of growing patient numbers and a limited healthcare workforce, such efficiency gains are indispensable.

- *Data-driven decision making*: AI's capability to process and learn from vast datasets can imbue mHealth with powerful predictive and prescriptive analytics [64]. These data-driven insights can inform both population health strategies and individual patient care plans. By identifying patterns and trends in medical imaging data, AI can help predict disease progression or response to treatment, enabling healthcare providers to tailor therapeutic interventions for optimal outcomes.

5.3 Pioneering advances of AI-driven radiology

AI/ML have revolutionised medical imaging, facilitating a swift shift from traditional reactive medical practices to more proactive and predictive healthcare. Its integration into medical imaging has yielded a panoply of innovative applications that have enhanced both the accuracy and speed of diagnostics.

One of the most groundbreaking applications of AI in medical imaging pertains to *computer-aided detection and diagnosis* (*CAD*) [65]. AI algorithms, through DL techniques, are capable of detecting subtle changes in imaging scans that may elude the human eye. For instance, CNNs have been utilised to identify anomalous patterns in images, successfully aiding in the diagnosis of conditions ranging from cancerous tumours to cardiovascular diseases. Research shows that CNNs have demonstrated exemplary performance in detecting lung nodules in CT scans, enhancing early-stage lung cancer detection and ultimately improving patient prognoses [65, 66] (**Figure 5**). Additionally, CNNs demonstrate profound capabilities in detecting intracranial infarcts or haemorrhages and in the identification of large vessel occlusion. Their incorporation into these sectors has markedly revolutionised the paradigm of stroke treatment, as showcased in **Figure 6**.

Another notable application is the use of AI in *image segmentation*. Traditionally, the demarcation of regions of interest (ROIs) in medical images was performed

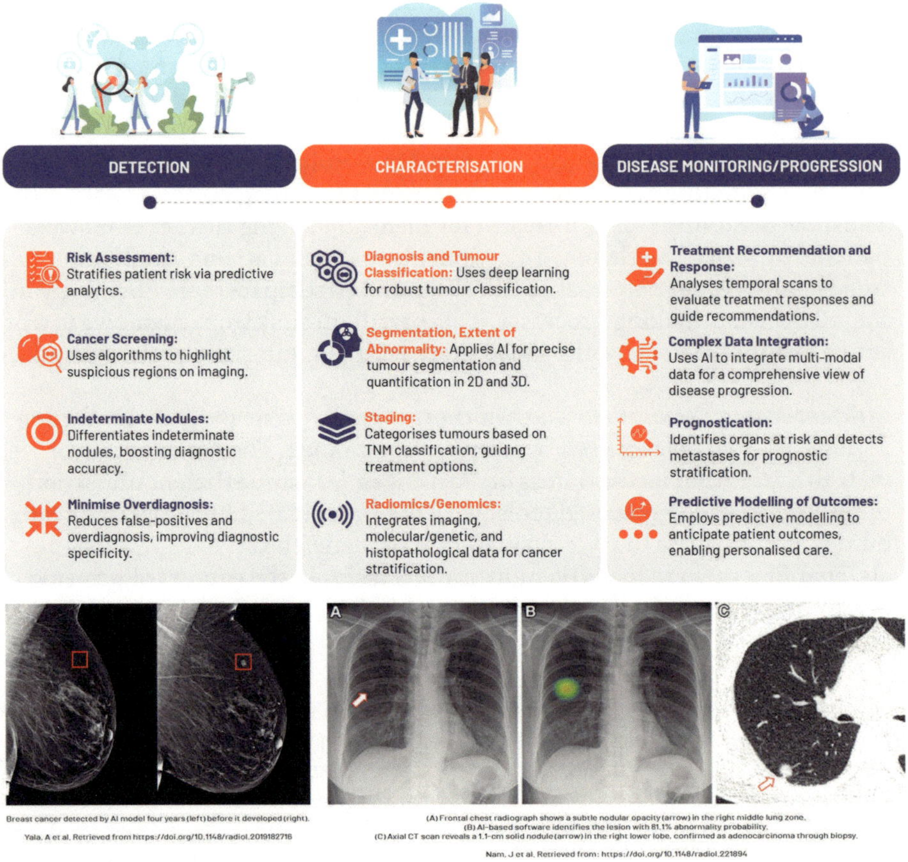

Figure 5.
Machine learning applications in oncological imaging.

manually, a laborious process often fraught with variability and inconsistencies. The emergence of AI has streamlined this process, ensuring higher precision and reproducibility [67]. For instance, in radiation oncology, the accurate segmentation of tumour regions and adjacent healthy tissues in CT or MRI scans is crucial for treatment planning [68]. AI algorithms can automate this process, minimising human error and enabling more accurate and targeted treatments.

AI has also proven instrumental in *predictive modelling* in medical imaging [56]. By leveraging machine learning algorithms, it's possible to predict patient outcomes based on imaging data. For example, the progression of neurodegenerative diseases such as Alzheimer's can be predicted by analysing structural changes in brain MRI scans over time using AI algorithms. Similarly, the risk of cardiovascular events can be predicted by analysing coronary artery calcium scoring in CT scans.

AI is also being deployed in *automated quality control* in medical imaging. In an environment where the acquisition of high-quality images is paramount for accurate diagnosis and treatment, AI can play a pivotal role in identifying sub-optimal images and suggesting adjustments to improve quality [21]. This application of AI not only enhances the accuracy of diagnoses but also improves the efficiency of the imaging workflow.

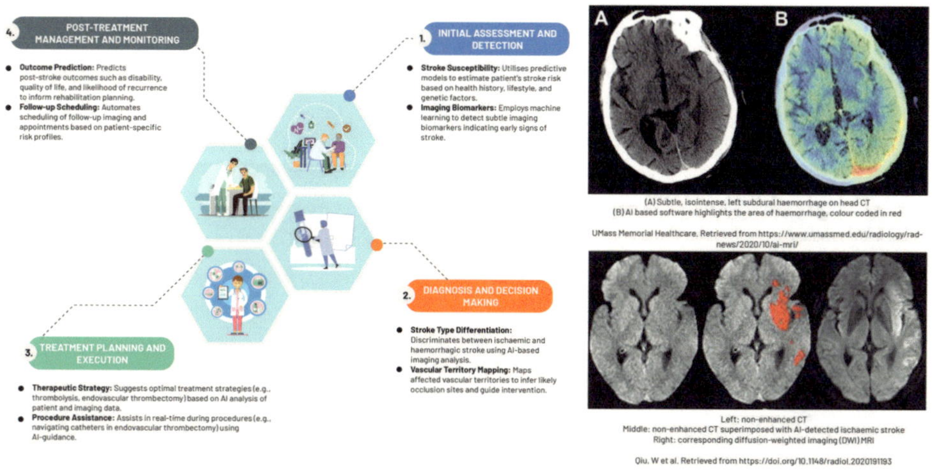

Figure 6.
Machine learning applications in neuroradiology.

In the realm of *real-time imaging*, AI is increasingly being used to facilitate immediate analysis and interpretation of images during procedures such as ultrasounds, potentially expediting diagnoses and enabling more immediate therapeutic interventions [40]. The application of AI in real-time imaging could reduce the need for specialist involvement during image acquisition, thereby streamlining workflows and improving access to healthcare services.

Furthermore, *AI-aided radiogenomics* represents another cutting-edge application [65]. This field aims to correlate imaging features with genomic data, thus providing a non-invasive means of determining the genetic profile of tumours. This method can potentially guide more personalised therapeutic strategies, enhancing treatment efficacy and patient outcomes.

6. Forecasting the future: mHealth, AI, and medical imaging

6.1 The technological horizon: projected advancements

The impending healthcare revolution is forecasted to be driven by major advancements in mHealth, AI/ML, and medical imaging technologies, all enabled by the rapid progress in AI algorithms, computation, sensor technology, and network connectivity (**Figure 7**).

ML models and AI algorithms are set to undergo significant refinement, with increasingly prevalent application of DL networks for complex tasks like medical image-based disease diagnosis. These models are expected to evolve, taking on multifaceted tasks such as comprehensive treatment plan formulation and patient outcome prediction with heightened precision. AI-empowered predictive analytics will facilitate accurate forecasting of disease trajectories, potentially even before symptom manifestation [69].

Medical imaging technologies are also on a trajectory of considerable improvement. Development is underway for imaging modalities capable of elucidating biological processes at cellular or molecular level. Hybrid imaging technologies like

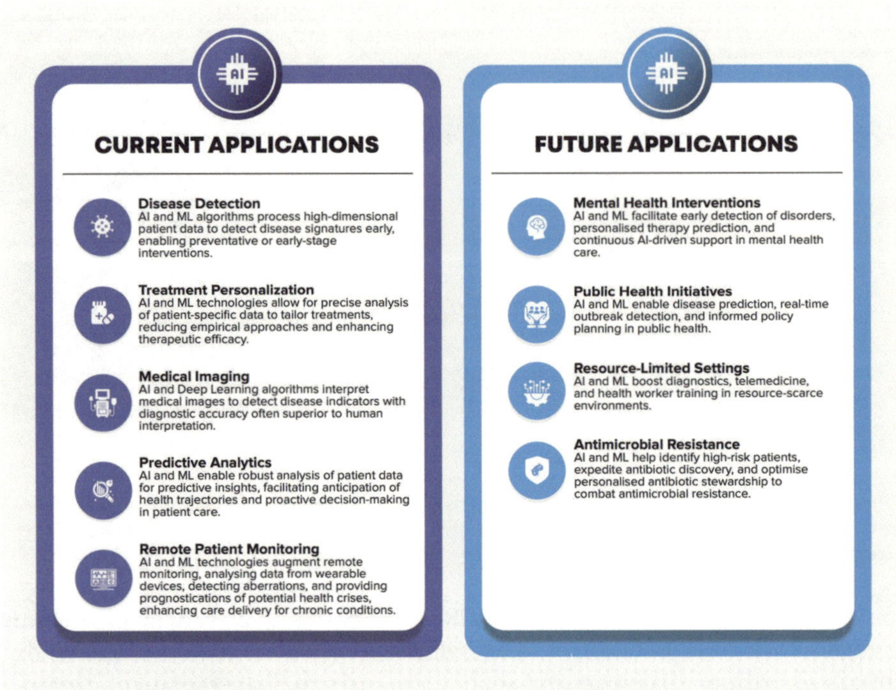

Figure 7.
Current and future applications of artificial intelligence and machine learning in healthcare.

PET/MRI and PET/CT are expected to gain wider acceptance due to their combined strengths [67]. Simultaneously, advancements in imaging resolution will provide hitherto unattainable anatomical and physiological details. The symbiosis of AI and medical imaging is projected to strengthen, with machine learning models proficiently interpreting imaging data, identifying patterns, and making accurate predictions (Rajpurkar; Salameh). Through exposure to real-world data, these algorithms will progressively improve diagnostic precision, reducing misdiagnosis and enhancing patient outcomes [70].

mHealth technologies are set for remarkable advancement, with the next generation of wearable and implantable devices likely to offer broader real-time health monitoring [71]. The immense data generated by these devices will be harnessed by sophisticated AI systems for personalised health guidance [72]. Additionally, the roll-out of 5G and anticipated 6G networks will significantly enhance the capacity of mHealth applications for data management and real-time stakeholder synchronisation [73]. This will support superior remote patient monitoring and telemedicine services, improving healthcare accessibility and efficiency [74].

The integration of AI and blockchain technologies offers promising solutions for data security and patient privacy in mHealth, with blockchain's decentralised and tamper-proof structure providing secure platforms for storing and sharing sensitive health data. Moreover, virtual and augmented reality are poised to revolutionise medical training, surgical planning, rehabilitation, and patient education, further facilitating remote patient care and contributing to healthcare democratisation [75].

While these advancements promise transformative impacts, they also raise challenges related to data privacy, ethics, and regulatory frameworks. The subsequent sections will delve into the implications of these advancements on healthcare delivery and patient outcomes, along with the role of policymakers and healthcare leaders in shaping this future.

6.2 Impact on healthcare delivery and patient outcomes

The impending era of digital healthcare is anticipated to profoundly reshape patient care, healthcare delivery, and clinical outcomes. It is essential to comprehensively explore the potential implications of this transformation.

One key impact will be increased healthcare accessibility. The integration of AI and mHealth liberates medical imaging from the restrictive, stationary hospital equipment, enabling portable imaging devices enhanced by AI algorithms for immediate interpretations [76]. This shift could decentralise diagnostic services, particularly benefiting remote or underserved regions and potentially reducing healthcare disparities [77].

Simultaneously, the precision and speed of diagnostics are set to improve substantially. AI algorithms excel in extracting meaningful information from complex imaging data, often outperforming human capacity for pattern recognition [78]. This advanced capacity could promote early disease identification and personalised care, refining treatment plans and enhancing patient outcomes. Furthermore, AI's machine learning models promise standardisation in image interpretation, mitigating interobserver variability and human error [79].

In addition, patient monitoring is poised for significant advancement. AI-embedded wearable technology provides continuous, real-time health monitoring, transforming chronic disease management and early detection of complications [80]. This ongoing surveillance could streamline interventions, optimise outcomes, and reduce hospital admissions.

Telemedicine is also expected to evolve, driven by AI, mHealth, and medical imaging. This transition from hospital-focused to home-based care may enhance patient safety and satisfaction, supporting a more patient-centred model [81]. AI's predictive capacity could guide remote patient management and preempt potential health issues, reducing emergency hospitalisations.

Advanced language models like ChatGPT are emerging as vital tools in this changing healthcare landscape [82]. Acting as an interface between complex AI algorithms and users, these models can synthesise large volumes of medical data into actionable insights, and provide immediate responses to patient queries, education, and psychological support [83]. They also aid research by scanning vast literature to identify novel findings and research trends [83].

At a broader scale, AI-enhanced medical imaging can offer population-level insights into disease trends, informing public health strategies and resource allocation [84]. The aggregation of health data from mHealth apps creates a rich repository for AI to uncover new medical knowledge, accelerating research and clinical innovation [85].

The synergy between AI, mHealth, and medical imaging stands to deliver substantial economical advantages through increased diagnostic precision, timely interventions, and enhanced preventive measures [83]. However, this necessitates the development of regulatory and ethical frameworks to safeguard patient confidentiality and autonomy, ensuring these technologies are oriented towards maximising patient benefit [86]. The fundamental role of healthcare leaders in directing this course underlines the importance of preserving human empathy within the healthcare system.

6.3 Policymakers and health leaders: their role in shaping the future

Policymakers and health leaders hold the reins in guiding this anticipated seismic shift in healthcare, their strategies and directives having the potential to significantly determine the future trajectory and impact of these emerging technologies.

The junction of AI and mHealth brings an array of opportunities for medical imaging, encompassing enhanced diagnostic accuracy, optimisation of workflow processes, and the personalisation of healthcare delivery. Conversely, this technological advancement introduces intricacies related to privacy, equity, regulation, and professional roles. Policymakers and health leaders are tasked with steering this complex landscape, delicately balancing between fostering innovation and ensuring regulation, privacy, and safety [87–89].

Understanding that innovation does not transpire in isolation is crucial in appreciating the role of these leaders. The intricacies of AI-driven mHealth applications must be contextualised and regulated within societal, legal, and ethical frameworks. The ability to comprehend the potential and perils of these technologies is paramount in formulating balanced and forward-thinking regulations that protect interests without inhibiting innovation [88, 89].

One potential regulatory hurdle pertains to data privacy. AI and mHealth technologies function on the collection, storage, and processing of extensive patient data, creating potential privacy and security risks. Policymakers are tasked with modernising privacy laws and regulations, demanding rigorous data security measures while empowering patients with the autonomy over their health data [90].

The question of algorithmic transparency and accountability also arises. Given the often 'black-box' nature of AI algorithms, unintended, discriminatory, or harmful outcomes may occur. Ensuring transparency and explicability of AI systems in healthcare is critical, allowing for accountability during adverse events [91].

From an equity standpoint, these technologies pose a risk of widening the healthcare divide. High-tech solutions frequently necessitate considerable resources, potentially exacerbating disparities between affluent and impoverished, urban and rural. Health leaders are obligated to strive for equitable distribution of these technologies, ensuring their benefits permeate all demographics [92].

In terms of professional roles, AI-driven mHealth applications may catalyse significant shifts in the healthcare workforce. Policymakers and health leaders are required to predict and navigate these changes, aiding healthcare professionals in developing the requisite skills to collaborate with AI, and ensuring that these technologies augment, rather than substitute, the human element in healthcare [93].

Health leaders are further mandated to cultivate a culture of change and innovation within healthcare institutions. Their role includes advocating for AI-driven mHealth applications, propelling adoption, and managing resistance to change among healthcare providers.

7. Challenges and strategies in AI integration

7.1 Technical obstacles in implementation

The marriage of AI/ML and mHealth inaugurates an unprecedented aeon in healthcare, offering personalised, accessible, and streamlined care [94]. Despite this, the deployment of these advanced technologies presents a multitude of complex issues. The obstacles encountered in this integration demand careful contemplation and tactical planning to ensure success (**Figure 8**).

The primary hurdle is *data compatibility and interoperability*. AI algorithms require extensive and high-quality annotated data for efficient training and accurate results [95]. mHealth applications, conversely, yield diverse data types such as electronic health records, real-time sensor data, images, and text, often in varying formats and standards. This heterogeneity can result in compatibility issues, hampering effective data utilisation by AI algorithms. Consequently, harmonising these disparate data forms for AI applications represents a significant technical challenge.

Simultaneously, *scalability and integration* present their unique challenges. The exponential number of mHealth users concomitantly generates a growing volume and variety of data. AI systems must possess scalability to accommodate this growth, necessitating substantial computational resources and robust algorithms that can manage increasing complexity [77]. Integrating AI systems into established healthcare information systems, known for their complexity and structured workflows, demands careful strategising to avert disruption and ensure seamless and efficient AI tool integration.

The inherent *complexity of AI algorithms* further complicates the process. Particularly, DL models comprise intricate networks with potentially millions of parameters. Training these models requires a data abundance, significant computational power, and technical expertise [96]. Coupled with their 'black box' characteristic, making the prediction process opaque, these complexities can impede the broader adoption of AI in mHealth, as healthcare professionals might hesitate to utilise tools that are not transparent.

The *reliability and validity* of AI-powered mHealth applications present another major hurdle. Given their crucial role in assisting health decisions, consistent accuracy and reliability of outputs are paramount [85]. This necessitates rigorous testing and validation methods, ensuring performance across diverse scenarios and patient

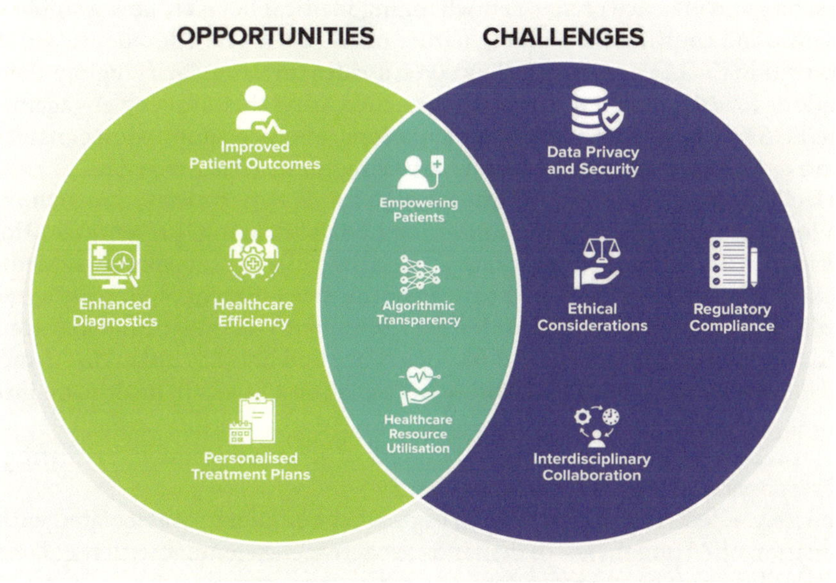

Figure 8.
Opportunities and challenges of AI integration into clinical practice.

demographics. Additionally, these algorithms must be resilient to changes and anomalies in the input data, safeguarding against erroneous outputs when confronted with unfamiliar data.

To surmount these technical obstacles, it is proposed that potential solutions include the development of standardized data protocols and comprehensive testing methodologies [97]. Enhanced collaboration among AI developers, mHealth creators, healthcare professionals, and policymakers could expedite the creation of efficient integration strategies and scalability solutions. Ongoing training and education in AI for healthcare professionals could help demystify the 'black box', fostering trust in AI-driven mHealth applications [98]. These challenges can only be overcome through collective effort, enabling the full potential of AI and mHealth integration in healthcare.

7.2 Regulatory challenges and how to navigate them

The advent and adoption of artificial intelligence and mHealth in medical imaging introduces multifaceted regulatory considerations, shaped by the converging factors of data privacy, algorithmic accountability, clinical responsibility, and policy enforcement [99]. Successfully manoeuvring this regulatory landscape calls for a considered and rigorous strategy.

Data protection stands out as a key challenge, as AI and mHealth involve handling significant volumes of personal health information. Safeguarding this data in accordance with health information privacy regulations, including Australia's Privacy Act 1988, is an imposing undertaking [100]. Effective navigation of this terrain may be achieved through implementing robust data governance protocols, stringent encryption techniques, anonymisation processes, and rigorous controls on data access and sharing. This will not only ensure regulatory compliance but will also fortify user trust and confidence, thereby enhancing adoption and endorsement [99].

The interpretation of regulations concerning software as a medical device introduces another challenge. Regulatory authorities, traditionally accustomed to assessing the safety and efficacy of static, unchanging medical devices, now grapple with the dynamic and continually evolving nature of AI [101]. The Therapeutic Goods Administration (TGA) in Australia has taken strides towards clarifying regulatory expectations for AI-imbued medical devices, indicating that ongoing engagement with the TGA, awareness of emerging regulations, and pre-submission consultations may serve as valuable strategies to traverse this regulatory challenge [102].

The lack of global regulatory harmonisation for AI applications, due to the expansive potential of mHealth solutions and AI in medical imaging, presents additional difficulties. Participation in international initiatives like the International Medical Device Regulators Forum (IMDRF) can aid in the development of globally agreed standards, easing the regulatory burden associated with AI integration in mHealth [103]. Lastly, clarification of clinical responsibility and liability linked to AI-mediated medical decisions is crucial. The growing influence of AI tools in healthcare introduces ambiguity concerning accountability [95]. Addressing this necessitates fostering a comprehensive understanding of the roles of AI systems and demarcating clinical responsibilities in healthcare delivery.

Ultimately, effectively navigating the regulatory complexities associated with the amalgamation of AI and mHealth demands proactive engagement with regulatory bodies, the establishment of stringent data governance and cybersecurity infrastructures, prioritisation of transparency and accountability in AI algorithms, active involvement in international standardisation efforts, and clarification of clinical responsibilities.

The ultimate goal extends beyond mere compliance with regulations, striving instead to champion responsible innovation that genuinely enhances patient care.

7.3 Transversing the ethical landscape: confidentiality and patient privacy

The integration of AI/ML with mHealth platforms holds promise for improved healthcare delivery and patient outcomes. However, these advancements also trigger significant ethical dilemmas, primarily concerning patient privacy and data protection [104]. The mHealth applications, combined with AI's advanced data processing capabilities, continually accumulate and analyse personal health data, necessitating an immediate focus on these issues.

A major ethical issue arises from the vast quantity of health-related data generated and disseminated by mHealth applications. This collected information is not only extensive but highly personal, covering a wide range of biometric, physiological, and lifestyle data. Without robust data security measures, the pervasiveness of mHealth applications might expose sensitive data to misuse [105]. AI algorithms' data needs for training and validation further amplify privacy concerns. The limitations of data anonymisation as a privacy preservation strategy have been underscored by advancements in re-identification techniques [106].

The 'black box' nature of certain AI algorithms clouds the decision-making process, posing issues of transparency and accountability [107]. This opacity has implications for informed patient consent and intensifies the risk of algorithmic bias, which could lead to potentially harmful healthcare decisions [108].

Current regulatory structures struggle to adapt to these rapidly evolving technologies, with global data flows and multinational tech companies compounding the challenge. Emerging solutions, proposed via interdisciplinary efforts, include implementing robust data governance frameworks with secure data transmission protocols, data minimisation strategies, and dynamic consent models [109]. Innovative cryptography-based methods, such as homomorphic encryption and differential privacy, offer promising pathways for balancing data utility with patient confidentiality [110].

Creating interpretable and explainable AI models can help address transparency and accountability issues. The push for 'explainable AI' aims to make AI decision-making processes more understandable and reliable [111]. Addressing algorithmic bias requires the mindful collection of diverse and representative datasets and the inclusion of fairness-centric evaluation metrics within AI systems [68].

The advancement of AI in mHealth necessitates a strong ethical framework, prioritising human dignity, autonomy, and privacy. While these challenges are substantial, they are not insurmountable. Through collective efforts from technologists, healthcare professionals, ethicists, regulators, and patients, the successful integration of AI with mHealth can be achieved. Thus, ethical responsibility, privacy respect, and a steadfast commitment to improving patient outcomes should guide us in navigating this transformative healthcare landscape.

8. Concluding remarks

8.1 Recap and reflections

The interplay between mHealth, AI, and medical imaging delineates a transformative trajectory in healthcare, which this review has sought to explore comprehensively.

The merger of mHealth with AI holds the promise of personalisation and efficiency in healthcare service delivery.

AI, specifically machine learning, has exhibited extensive capacities in enhancing clinical decision-making processes, encompassing a spectrum from disease diagnosis to prognosis. This review has analysed the current significance of AI in healthcare and proposed potential future trends.

The evolution of medical imaging from conventional to digital modalities has been a linchpin in clinical diagnosis. The introduction of AI in this field has catalysed transformative changes in image acquisition, interpretation, and management. The synthesis of AI and mHealth in this realm is incrementally improving healthcare quality, with the review providing a detailed overview of innovative applications and case studies in diagnostic imaging, radiology, and pathology imaging. Despite the myriad benefits, these technologies also introduce a set of challenges that demand attention from a technical and regulatory standpoint, underlining the necessity for equilibrium between innovation, patient safety, and privacy.

Looking towards the future, this review highlights the potential ramifications of these advancements on healthcare delivery and patient outcomes. It emphasises the crucial role policymakers and health leaders must assume in steering this transformation while preserving the ethos of patient-centred care.

8.2 Highlighting the transformative impetus

To underscore the transformative potential of AI, mHealth, and medical imaging is to herald a new era in healthcare. The integration of these technologies paves the way for ubiquitous, personalised, and proactive healthcare that transcends theoretical speculation and edges towards actualisation.

AI, primarily through machine learning, bolsters the healthcare ecosystem via its proficiency in real-time, high-throughput data analytics, diagnostic precision, and prognostic accuracy. Concurrently, medical imaging is being reshaped, with AI algorithms fuelling advancements in image acquisition, interpretation, and analysis.

The efficacy of mHealth is underlined by its inherent accessibility, with an ever-increasing prevalence of mobile devices surmounting geographical barriers and enabling patient autonomy. The confluence of AI with mHealth technologies in the sphere of medical imaging enables sophisticated diagnostics at one's fingertips, marking a significant stride towards equitable healthcare.

Collectively, these advancements herald an era of proactive, predictive, personalised, and participative medicine. As we navigate policy, regulatory, and ethical hurdles, we stand to gain a healthcare system that epitomises patient-centred, data-driven, and equitable care. The potential for these technologies in healthcare is vast and tantalisingly within our grasp.

Author details

Reabal Najjar
Canberra Health Services, Canberra, Australia

*Address all correspondence to: reabal.najjar@act.gov.au

References

[1] Kumar S, Nilsen WJ, Abernethy A, Atienza A, Patrick K, Pavel M, et al. Mobile health technology evaluation: The mhealth evidence workshop. American Journal of Preventive Medicine. 2013;**45**(2):228-236

[2] Ratanawong JP, Naslund JA, Mikal JP, Grande SW. Achieving the potential of mhealth in medicine requires challenging the ethos of care delivery. Primary Health Care Research & Development. 2022;**23**:e18

[3] Russell SJ, Norvig P. Artificial Intelligence: A Modern Approach. Malaysia: Pearson Education Limited; 2016

[4] Esteva A, Robicquet A, Ramsundar B, Kuleshov V, DePristo M, Chou K, et al. A guide to deep learning in healthcare. Nature Medicine. 2019;**25**(1):24-29

[5] Topol EJ. High-performance medicine: The convergence of human and artificial intelligence. Nature Medicine. 2019;**25**:44-56

[6] Ching T, Himmelstein DS, Beaulieu-Jones BK, Kalinin AA, Do BT, Way GP, et al. Opportunities and obstacles for deep learning in biology and medicine. Journal of The Royal Society Interface. 2018;**15**(141):20170387

[7] Lundervold AS, Lundervold A. An overview of deep learning in medical imaging focusing on mri. Zeitschrift f ür Medizinische Physik. 2019;**29**(2):102-127

[8] Steinhubl SR, Muse ED, Topol EJ. The emerging field of mobile health. Science Translational Medicine. 2015;**7**(283):283rv3

[9] World Health Organization. Global Diffusion of eHealth - Making Universal Health Coverage Achievable: Report of the Third Global Survey on eHealth. World Health Organization. 2017

[10] Becker S, Miron-Shatz T, Schumacher N, Krocza J, Diamantidis C, Albrecht U-V. mhealth 2.0: Experiences, possibilities, and perspectives. JMIR Mhealth Uhealth. 2014;**2**(2):e24

[11] Rowland SP, Fitzgerald JE, Holme T, Powell J, McGregor A. What is the clinical value of mhealth for patients? npj Digital, Medicine. 2020;**3**(1):4

[12] Fiordelli M, Diviani N, Schulz PJ. Mapping mhealth research: A decade of evolution. Journal of Medical Internet Research. 2013;**15**(5):e95

[13] Kamel Boulos MN, Wheeler S, Tavares C, Jones R. How smartphones are changing the face of mobile and participatory healthcare: An overview, with example from ecaalyx. Biomedical Engineering Online. 2011;**10**(1):1-14

[14] Islam SMR, Kwak D, Kabir MH, Hossain M, Kwak K-s. The internet of things for health care: A comprehensive survey. IEEE Access. 2015;**3**:678-708

[15] Marcolino MS, de Oliveira JAQ, D'Agostino M, Ribeiro ALP, Alkmim MBM, Novillo-Ortiz D. The impact of mhealth interventions: Systematic review of systematic reviews. JMIR mHealth and uHealth. 2018;**6**(1):e8873

[16] Ting DSW, Carin L, Dzau V, Wong TY. Digital technology and covid-19. Nature Medicine. 2020;**26**:459-461

[17] Alpaydin E. Introduction to Machine Learning. 2nd ed. Cambridge, MA, USA: The MIT Press; 2010

[18] Mitchell TM. Machine Learning. 1st ed. USA: McGraw-Hill, Inc.; 1997

[19] Thomas LB, Mastorides SM, Viswanadhan NA, Jakey CE, Borkowski AA. Artificial intelligence: Review of current and future applications in medicine. Federal Practitioner. 2021;**38**(11):527-538

[20] Tagde P, Tagde S, Bhattacharya T, Tagde P, Chopra H, Akter R, et al. Blockchain and artificial intelligence technology in e-health. Environmental Science and Pollution Research. 2021;**28**(38):52810-52831

[21] Tadavarthi Y, Makeeva V, Wagstaff W, Zhan H, Podlasek A, Bhatia N, et al. Overview of noninterpretive artificial intelligence models for safety, quality, workflow, and education applications in radiology practice. Radiology: Artificial Intelligence. 2022;**4**(2):e210114

[22] Bhandari M, Zeffiro T, Reddiboina M. Artificial intelligence and robotic surgery: Current perspective and future directions. Current Opinion in Urology. 2020;**30**(1):48-54

[23] Burlina PM, Joshi N, Pekala M, Pacheco KD, Freund DE, Bressler NM. Automated grading of age-related macular degeneration from color fundus images using deep convolutional neural networks. JAMA Ophthalmology. 2017;**135**(11):1170-1176

[24] Gulshan V, Rajan R, Widner K, Lily Z, Xu L, Zhu B, et al. Performance of a deep-learning algorithm vs manual grading for detecting diabetic retinopathy in India. JAMA Ophthalmology. 2019;**137**(9):987-993

[25] Ting DSW, Cheung CY-L, Lim G, Tan GSW, Quang ND, Gan A, et al. Development and validation of a deep learning system for diabetic retinopathy and related eye diseases using retinal images from multiethnic populations with diabetes. JAMA. 2017;**318**(22):2211-2223

[26] Rajalakshmi R, Subashini R. Ranjit Mohan Anjana, and Viswanathan Mohan, Automated diabetic retinopathy detection in smartphone-based fundus photography using artificial intelligence. Eye. 2018;**32**:1138-1144

[27] Krause J, Gulshan V, Rahimy E, Karth P, Widner K, Corrado GS, et al. Grader variability and the importance of reference standards for evaluating machine learning models for diabetic retinopathy. Ophthalmology. 2018;**125**(8):1264-1272

[28] Devin M. Mann, Jingjing Chen, Rumi Chunara, Paul A Testa, and Oded Nov, Covid-19 transforms health care through telemedicine: Evidence from the field. Journal of the American Medical Informatics Association. 2020;**27**(7):1132-1135

[29] De Ramón Fernández A, Ruiz Fernández D, Gilart Iglesias V, Marcos Jorquera D. Analyzing the use of artificial intelligence for the management of chronic obstructive pulmonary disease (copd). International Journal of Medical Informatics. 2021;**158**:104640. Epub ahead of print

[30] Halpin DMG, Criner GJ, Papi A, Singh D, Anzueto A, Martinez FJ, et al. Global initiative for the diagnosis, management, and prevention of chronic obstructive lung disease. the 2020 gold science committee report on covid-19 and chronic obstructive pulmonary disease. American Journal of Respiratory and Critical Care Medicine;**203**(1):24, 2021-36

[31] Ambrosino N, Vagheggini G, Mazzoleni S, Vitacca M. Telemedicine in

chronic obstructive pulmonary disease. Breathe. 2016;**12**(4):350-356

[32] Miotto R, Wang F, Wang S, Jiang X, Dudley JT. Deep learning for healthcare: Review, opportunities and challenges. Briefings in Bioinformatics. 2018;**19**(6):1236-1246

[33] Klonoff DC. Cybersecurity for connected diabetes devices. Journal of Diabetes Science and Technology. 2015;**9**(5):1143-1147

[34] Bashi N, Karunanithi M, Fatehi F, Ding H, Walters D. Remote monitoring of patients with heart failure: An overview of systematic reviews. Journal of Medical Internet Research. 2017;**19**(1):e18

[35] Wang JB, Cadmus-Bertram LA, Natarajan L, White MM, Madanat H, Nichols JF, et al. Wearable sensor/device (fitbit one) and sms text-messaging prompts to increase physical activity in overweight and obese adults: A randomized controlled trial. Telemedicine Journal and E-Health. 2015;**21**(10):782-792. Epub 2015 Jun 2

[36] Shah P, Kendall F, Khozin S, Goosen R, Hu J, Laramie J, et al. Artificial intelligence and machine learning in clinical development: A translational perspective. npj Digital Medicine. 2019;**2**:69

[37] Ardila D, Kiraly AP, Bharadwaj S, Choi B, Reicher JJ, Peng L, et al. End-to-end lung cancer screening with three-dimensional deep learning on low-dose chest computed tomography. Nature Medicine. 2019;**25**(6):954-961. Erratum in: Nat Med. 2019 Aug;25(8):1319

[38] Sheller MJ, Edwards B, Reina GA, et al. Federated learning in medicine: Facilitating multi-institutional collaborations without sharing patient data. Scientific Reports. 2020;**10**:12598

[39] Zhou Y, Hou Y, Shen J, Huang Y, Martin W, Cheng F. Network-based drug repurposing for novel coronavirus 2019-ncov/sars-cov-2. Cell Discovery. 2020;**6**:14

[40] Martínez-García M, Hernández-Lemus E. Data integration challenges for machine learning in precision medicine. Frontiers in Medicine. 2022;**8**:784455

[41] Tubiana M. Wilhelm Conrad röntgen et la découverte des rayons x [wilhelm conrad röntgen and the discovery of x-rays]. Bulletin de l'Académie Nationale de Médecine. 1996;**180**(1):97-108

[42] Lorenz JM. Management of malignant biliary obstruction. Seminars in Interventional Radiology. 2016;**33**(4):259-267

[43] Hounsfield GN. Computerized transverse axial scanning (tomography). 1. Description of system. British Journal of Radiology. 1973;**46**(552):1016-1022

[44] Lauterbur PC. Image formation by induced local interactions: Examples employing nuclear magnetic resonance. Nature. 1973;**242**:190-191

[45] Mansfield P, Grannell PK. Nmr 'diffraction' in solids? Journal of Physics C: Solid State Physics. 1977;**10**(3):L55-L58

[46] Cherry SR, Jones T, Karp JS, Qi J, Moses WW, Badawi RD. Total-body pet: Maximizing sensitivity to create new opportunities for clinical research and patient care. Journal of Nuclear Medicine. 2018;**59**(1):3-12

[47] Hutton BF, Buvat I, Beekman FJ. Review and current status of spect scatter correction. Physics in Medicine and Biology. 2011;**56**(14):R85-R112

[48] European Society of Radiology (ESR) and European Federation of

Radiographer Societies (EFRS). Patient safety in medical imaging: A joint paper of the european society of radiology (ESR) and the european federation of radiographer societies (EFRS). Insights Imaging. 2019;**10**(1):45

[49] Fedorov A, Clunie D, Ulrich E, Bauer C, Wahle A, Brown B, et al. Dicom for quantitative imaging biomarker development: A standards based approach to sharing clinical data and structured pet/ct analysis results in head and neck cancer research. PeerJ. 2016;**4**:e2057

[50] Huang HK. PACS and Imaging Informatics: Basic Principles and Applications. Hoboken, New Jersey, USA: John Wiley & Sons; 2011

[51] Langlotz CP, Allen B, Erickson BJ, Kalpathy-Cramer J, Bigelow K, Cook TS, et al. A roadmap for foundational research on artificial intelligence in medical imaging: From the 2018 nih/rsna/acr/the academy workshop. Radiology. 2019;**291**(3):781-791

[52] Mun SK, Wong KH, Lo SB, Li Y, Bayarsaikhan S. Artificial intelligence for the future radiology diagnostic service. Frontiers in Molecular Biosciences. 2021;**7**:614258

[53] Lee JG, Jun S, Cho YW, Lee H, Kim GB, Seo JB, et al. Deep learning in medical imaging: General overview. Korean Journal of Radiology. 2017;**18**(4):570-584

[54] Hosny A, Parmar C, Quackenbush J, Schwartz LH, Aerts HJWL. Artificial intelligence in radiology. Nature Reviews. Cancer. 2018;**18**:500-510

[55] Brady AP, Bello JA, Derchi LE, Fuchsjäger M, Goergen SK, Krestin GP, et al. Radiology in the era of value-based healthcare: A multi-society expert statement from the acr, car, esr, is3r, ranzcr, and rsna. Insights into Imaging. 2020;**11**(1):1-15

[56] Pires PB, Santos JD, Pereira IV. Artificial neural networks: History and state of the art. Sixth Edition. Encyclopedia of Information Science and Technology. 2023:1-25

[57] Bashshur R, Doarn CR, Frenk JM, Kvedar JC, Woolliscroft JO. Telemedicine and the covid-19 pandemic, lessons for the future. Telemedicine Journal and E-Health. 2020;**26**(5):571-573

[58] De Fauw J, Ledsam JR, Romera-Paredes B, Nikolov S, Tomasev N, Black-well S, et al. Clinically applicable deep learning for diagnosis and referral in retinal disease. Nature Medicine. 2018;**24**(9):1342-1350

[59] Kooi T, Litjens G, van Ginneken B, Gubern-Mérida A, Sánchez CI, Mann R, et al. Large scale deep learning for computer aided detection of mammographic lesions. Medical Image Analysis. 2017;**35**:303-312

[60] Huang S, Yang J, Fong S, Zhao Q. Artificial intelligence in cancer diagnosis and prognosis: Opportunities and challenges. Cancer Letters. 2020;**471**:61-71

[61] Chilamkurthy S, Ghosh R, Tanamala S, Biviji M, Campeau NG, Venugopal VK, et al. Deep learning algorithms for detection of critical findings in head ct scans: A retrospective study. Lancet. 2018;**392**(10162):2388-2396

[62] Martínez-Sellés M, Marina-Breysse M. Current and future use of artificial intelligence in electrocardiography. Journal of Cardiovascular Development and Disease. 2023;**10**(4):175

[63] Schneble CO, Elger BS, Shaw DM. Google's project nightingale highlights

the necessity of data science ethics review. EMBO Molecular Medicine. 2020;**12**(3):e12053. Epub 2020 Feb 17

[64] Rajkomar A, Dean J, Kohane I. Machine learning in medicine. New England Journal of Medicine. 2019;**380**(14):1347-1358

[65] Habehh H, Gohel S. Machine learning in healthcare. Current Genomics. 2021;**22**(4):291-300

[66] Luchini C, Pea A, Scarpa A. Artificial intelligence in oncology: Current applications and future perspectives. British Journal of Cancer. 2022;**126**:4-9

[67] Qian J, Li H, Wang J, He L. Recent advances in explainable artificial intelligence for magnetic resonance imaging. Diagnostics. 2023;**13**:1571

[68] Wang F, Preininger A. Ai in health: State of the art, challenges, and future directions. Yearbook of Medical Informatics. 2019;**28**(1):16-26. Epub 2019 Aug 16

[69] Rajpurkar P, Chen E, Banerjee O, et al. Ai in health and medicine. Nature Medicine. 2022;**28**:31-38

[70] Rana M, Bhushan M. Machine learning and deep learning approach for medical image analysis: Diagnosis to detection. Multimedia Tools and Applications. 24 Dec 2022:1-39. DOI: 10.1007/s11042-022-14305-w. PMID: 36588765; PMCID: PMC9788870. Epub ahead of print

[71] Al-Antari MA. Artificial intelligence for medical diagnostics-existing and future ai technology! Diagnostics (Basel). 2023;**13**(4):688

[72] Bhattamisra SK, Banerjee P, Gupta P, Mayuren J, Patra S, Candasamy M. Artificial intelligence in pharmaceutical and healthcare research. Big Data and Cognitive Computing. 2023;**7**(1):10

[73] Salameh AI, El Tarhuni M. From 5g to 6g—challenges, technologies, and applications. Future Internet. 2022;**14**(4):117

[74] Devi DH, Duraisamy K, Armghan A, Alsharari M, Aliqab K, Sorathiya V, et al. 5g technology in healthcare and wearable devices: A review. Sensors (Basel). 2023;**23**(5):2519

[75] Yeung AWK, Tosevska A, Klager E, Eibensteiner F, Laxar D, Stoyanov J, et al. Virtual and augmented reality applications in medicine: Analysis of the scientific literature. Journal of Medical Internet Research. 2021;**23**(2):e25499

[76] Kumar K, Kumar P, Deb D, Unguresan ML, Muresan V. Artificial intelligence and machine learning based intervention in medical infrastructure: A review and future trends. Healthcare (Basel). 2023;**11**(2):207

[77] Bhatt P, Liu J, Gong Y, Wang J, Guo Y. Emerging artificial intelligence-empowered mhealth: Scoping review. JMIR Mhealth Uhealth. 2022;**10**(6):e35053

[78] Panayides AS, Amini A, Filipovic ND, Sharma A, Tsaftaris SA, Young A, et al. Ai in medical imaging informatics: Current challenges and future directions. IEEE Journal of Biomedical and Health Informatics. Jul 2020;**24**(7):1837-1857

[79] Iqbal S, Qureshi N, Li J, et al. On the analyses of medical images using traditional machine learning techniques and convolutional neural networks. Archives of Computational Methods in Engineering. 2023;**30**:3173-3233

[80] Shaik T, Tao X, Higgins N, Li L, Gururajan R, Zhou X, et al. Remote

patient monitoring using artificial intelligence: Current state, applications, and challenges. WIREs Data Mining and Knowledge Discovery. 2023;**13**(2):e1485

[81] El-Sherif DM, Abouzid M, Elzarif MT, Ahmed AA, Albakri A, Alshehri MM. Telehealth and artificial intelligence insights into healthcare during the covid-19 pandemic. Healthcare. 2022;**10**(2):385

[82] Radford A, Narasimhan K, Salimans T, Sutskever I. Improving language understanding by generative pre-training. San Francisco: OpenAI; 11 Jun 2018. Available from: https://s3-us-west-2.amazonaws.com/openai-assets/research-covers/language-unsupervised/language_understanding_paper.pdf

[83] Sallam M. Chatgpt utility in healthcare education, research, and practice: Systematic review on the promising perspectives and valid concerns. Healthcare. 2023;**11**(6):887

[84] do Nascimento IJB, Marcolino MS, Abdulazeem HM, Weerasekara I, Azzopardi-Muscat N, Gonçalves MA, et al. Impact of big data analytics on people's health: Overview of systematic reviews and recommendations for future studies. Journal of Medical Internet Research. 2021;**23**(4):e27275

[85] Hogg HDJ, Al-Zubaidy M, Technology Enhanced Macular Services Study Reference Group, Talks J, Denniston AK, Kelly CJ, et al. Stakeholder perspectives of clinical artificial intelligence implementation: Systematic review of qualitative evidence. Journal of Medical Internet Research. 2023;**25**:e39742

[86] Vignali V, Hines PA, Cruz AG, Zietek B, Herold R. Health horizons: Future trends and technologies from the European medicines agency's horizon scanning collaborations. Frontiers in Medicine. 2022;**9**:1064003

[87] Thimbleby H. Technology and the future of healthcare. Journal of Public Health Research. 2013;**2**(3):e28

[88] Kristiansen TB, Kristensen K, Uffelmann J, Brandslund I. Erroneous data: The achilles' heel of ai and personalized medicine. Frontiers in Digital Health. 2022;**4**:862095

[89] Weintraub P, McKee M. Leadership for innovation in healthcare: An exploration. International Journal of Health Policy and Management. 2019;**8**(3):138-144

[90] Kuziemsky CE, Gogia SB, Househ M, Petersen C, Basu A. Balancing health information exchange and privacy governance from a patient-centred connected health and telehealth perspective. Yearbook of Medical Informatics. 2018;**27**(1):48-54. Epub 2018 Apr 22

[91] He J, Baxter SL, Xu J, Xu J, Zhou X, Zhang K. The practical implementation of artificial intelligence technologies in medicine. Nature Medicine. 2019;**25**(1):30-36. Epub 2019 Jan 7

[92] Brewer LC, Fortuna KL, Jones C, Walker R, Hayes SN, Patten CA, et al. Back to the future: Achieving health equity through health informatics and digital health. JMIR Mhealth Uhealth. 2020;**8**(1):e14512

[93] Roski J, Maier EJ, Vigilante K, Kane EA, Matheny ME. Enhancing trust in ai through industry self-governance. Journal of the American Medical Informatics Association. 2021;**28**(7):1582-1590

[94] Bohr A, Memarzadeh K. The rise of artificial intelligence in healthcare applications. In: Artificial Intelligence in

Healthcare. Amsterdam, Netherlands: Elsevier; 2020. pp. 25-60. Epub 2020 Jun 26

[95] Deniz-Garcia A, Fabelo H, Rodriguez-Almeida AJ, Zamora-Zamorano G, Castro-Fernandez M, Ruano MDPA, et al. Quality, usability, and effectiveness of mhealth apps and the role of artificial intelligence: Current scenario and challenges. Journal of Medical Internet Research. 2023;**25**:e44030

[96] Davenport T, Kalakota R. The potential for artificial intelligence in healthcare. Future Healthcare Journal. 2019;**6**(2):94-98

[97] Diaz O, Kushibar K, Osuala R, Linardos A, Garrucho L, Igual L, et al. Data preparation for artificial intelligence in medical imaging: A comprehensive guide to open-access platforms and tools. Physica Medica. 2021;**83**:25-37. Epub 2021 Mar 5

[98] Wadden JJ. Defining the undefinable: The black box problem in healthcare artificial intelligence. Journal of Medical Ethics. 2022;**48**(10):764-768

[99] Cohen IG, Amarasingham R, Shah A, Xie B, Lo B. The legal and ethical concerns that arise from using complex predictive analytics in health care. Health Affairs. 2014;**33**(7):1139-1147

[100] Hassanaly P, Dufour JC. Analysis of the regulatory, legal, and medical conditions for the prescription of mobile health applications in the United States, the European union, and France. Medical devices (Auckland, N.Z.). 2021;**14**:389-409

[101] Gerke S, Minssen T, Cohen G. Ethical and legal challenges of artificial intelligence-driven healthcare. In: Artificial Intelligence in Healthcare. Amsterdam, Netherlands: Elsevier; 2020. pp. 295-336. Epub 2020 Jun 26

[102] Therapeutic Goods Administration. 2022. Available from: https://www.tga.gov.au/

[103] International Medical Device Regulators Forum. 2021. Available from: http://www.imdrf.org/

[104] Floridi L, Taddeo M. What is data ethics? Philosophical Transactions of the Royal Society A: Mathematical, Physical and Engineering Sciences. London: The Royal Society; 2016;**374**:20160360. DOI: 10.1098/rsta.2016.0360

[105] Price WN, Cohen IG. Privacy in the age of medical big data. Nature Medicine. 2019;**25**:37-43

[106] Rocher L, Hendrickx JM, de Montjoye YA. Estimating the success of re-identifications in incomplete datasets using generative models. Nature Communications. 2019;**10**:3069

[107] Castelvecchi D. Can we open the black box of ai? Nature. 2016;**538**(7623):20-23

[108] Gianfrancesco MA, Tamang S, Yazdany J, Schmajuk G. Potential biases in machine learning algorithms using electronic health record data. JAMA Internal Medicine. 2018;**178**(11):1544-1547

[109] Jobin A, Ienca M, Vayena E. The global landscape of ai ethics guidelines. Nature Machine Intelligence. 2019;**1**:389-399

[110] Yu KH, Beam AL, Kohane IS. Artificial intelligence in healthcare. Nature Biomedical Engineering. 2018;**2**:719-731

[111] Adadi A, Berrada M. Peeking inside the black-box: A survey on explainable artificial intelligence (xai). IEEE Access. 2018;**6**:52138-52160